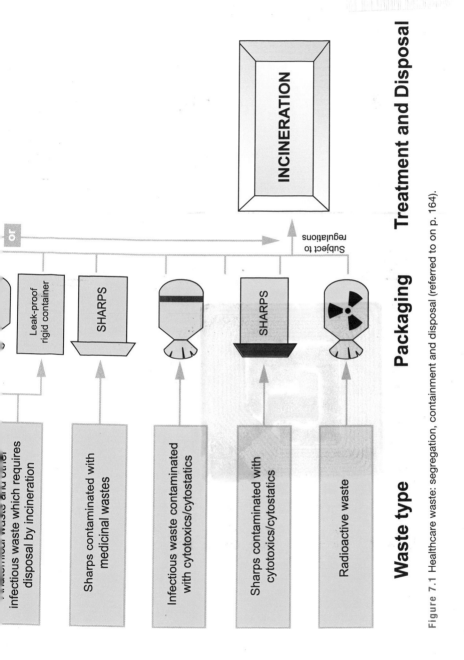

Figure 7.1 Healthcare waste: segregation, containment and disposal (referred to on p. 164).

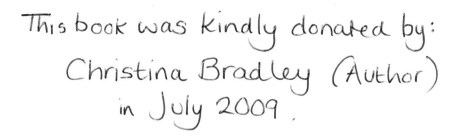

This book was kindly donated by:
Christina Bradley (Author)
in July 2009.

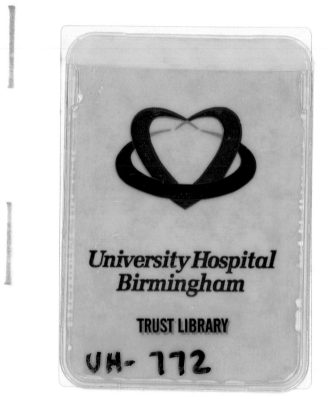

Ayliffe's Control of Healthcare-Associated Infection

Fifth edition

Fifth edition

Ayliffe's Control of Healthcare-Associated Infection

A practical handbook

Edited by:

Adam P Fraise MB BS FRCPath
Consultant Medical Microbiologist and Director,
Hospital Infection Research Laboratory,
University Hospital Birmingham, Birmingham, UK

Christina Bradley MIBMS
Manager, Hospital Infection Research Laboratory,
University Hospital Birmingham, Birmingham, UK

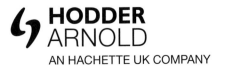

HODDER
ARNOLD

AN HACHETTE UK COMPANY

First published in Great Britain in 1975 by Chapman & Hall
This fifth edition published in 2009 by
Hodder Arnold, an imprint of Hodder Education,
an Hachette UK company, 338 Euston Road, London NW1 3BH

http://www.hoddereducation.com

Hachette UK's policy is to use papers that are natural, renewable and recyclable products and made
from wood grown in sustainable forests. The logging and manufacturing processes are expected to
conform to the environmental regulations of the country of origin.

Whilst the advice and information in this book are believed to be true and accurate at the date of
going to press, neither the author[s] nor the publisher can accept any legal responsibility or liability
for any errors or omissions that may be made. In particular (but without limiting the generality of the
preceding disclaimer) every effort has been made to check drug dosages; however it is still possible
that errors have been missed. Furthermore, dosage schedules are constantly being revised and new
side effects recognized. For these reasons the reader is strongly urged to consult the drug
companies' printed instructions before administering any of the drugs recommended in this book.

British Library Cataloguing in Publication Data
A catalogue record for this book is available from the British Library

Library of Congress Cataloging-in-Publication Data
A catalog record for this book is available from the Library of Congress

ISBN-13 978-0-340-91451-9

1 2 3 4 5 6 7 8 9 10

Commissioning Editor: Philip Shaw
Project Editor: Amy Mulick
Production Controller: Karen Dyer
Cover Designer: Andrew Campling
Indexer: Laurence Errington

Cover image © CDC/Science Photo Library

Typeset in 10.5 on 13pt Berling by Phoenix Photosetting, Chatham, Kent
Printed and bound in Great Britain
Text printed on FSC accredited material

What do you think about this book? Or any other Hodder Arnold title?
Please visit our website: www.hoddereducation.com

CONTENTS

LIST OF CONTRIBUTORS

Tar-Ching Aw Professor and Head, Department of Community Medicine, Faculty of Medicine and Health Sciences, United Arab Emirates University, Al-Ain, United Arab Emirates, and Visiting Professor, Canterbury Christ Church University, Canterbury, UK

Iain Blair Associate Professor, Department of Community Medicine, Faculty of Medicine and Health Sciences, UAE University, Al Ain, United Arab Emirates

Christina Bradley Manager, Hospital Infection Research Laboratory, University Hospital Birmingham, Birmingham, UK

Richard PD Cooke Consultant Microbiologist, Honorary Senior Lecturer, University Hospital Aintree, Liverpool, UK

Mike Cooper Consultant Microbiologist, New Cross Hospital, Wolverhampton, UK

Elizabeth SR Darley Director of Infection Prevention and Control, North Bristol NHS Trust, Bristol, UK

Samir Dervisevic Consultant Virologist and Clinical Lead in Virology, Norfolk and Norwich University Hospitals NHS Foundation Trust, Norwich, UK

Georgia J Duckworth National HCAI and AMR Surveillance Lead and Director, Department of Healthcare Associated Infection and Antimicrobial Resistance, Centre for Infections, Health Protection Agency, London, UK

Rebecca Evans Head of Infection Control Nursing Services, Sandwell and West Birmingham Hospital NHS Trust, Birmingham, UK

Adam P Fraise Consultant Medical Microbiologist and Director, Hospital Infection Research Laboratory, University Hospital Birmingham, Birmingham, UK

Gary L French Professor of Microbiology and Consultant Microbiologist, King's College London and Department of Infection, Guy's and St Thomas' Hospital, London, UK

Savita Gossain Consultant Medical Microbiologist, Health Protection Agency West Midlands Public Health Laboratory, Heart of England NHS Foundation Trust, Birmingham, UK

Kate Gould Consultant Microbiologist, Freeman Hospital, Newcastle upon Tyne, UK

Alison Hames Specialist Registrar Microbiology, Microbiology Department, Freeman Hospital, Newcastle, UK

Peter M Hawkey School of Immunity and Infection, University of Birmingham, and Health Protection Agency West Midlands Public Health Laboratory, Heart of England NHS Foundation Trust, Birmingham, UK

Dawn Hill Nurse Consultant, Welsh Healthcare Associated Infection Programme, National Public Health Service for Wales, UK

Peter Hoffman Consultant Clinical Scientist, Laboratory of Healthcare-associated Infection, Health Protection Agency, London, UK

Peter Hooper Authorizing Engineer (Decontamination), Banbury, Oxfordshire, UK

Julie Hughes Nurse Consultant in Infection Control, University Hospital Aintree, Liverpool, UK

Conor Jamieson Pharmacy Team Leader – Antimicrobial Therapy, Department of Microbiology, City Hospital, Birmingham, UK

Donald J Jeffries Emiritus Professor of Virology, University of London; Chair ACDP TSE Working Group

Alasdair P MacGowan Professor of Clinical Microbiology and Antimicrobial Therapeutics, University of Bristol and Department of Medical Microbiology, North Bristol NHS Trust, Bristol, UK

Susan Millward Infection Prevention Nurse Consultant (working with Nuffield Health Group, UK), and Director, Infection Prevention Ltd, UK

Manjusha Narayanan Consultant Microbiologist, Freeman Hospital, Newcastle upon Tyne, UK

Said Noorazar Quality Control Pharmacist, Pharmacy Department, City Hospital, Birmingham, UK

Jonathan North Consultant Immunologist, Immunology Department, City Hospital, Birmingham, UK

Christine Perry Director, Infection Prevention and Control, University Hospitals Bristol NHS Foundation Trust, Bristol, UK

Deenan Pillay Professor of Virology, University College London Hospitals NHS Foundation Trust and University College London, London, UK

Muhammad Waqar Raza Consultant Microbiologist, Microbiology Department, Freeman Hospital, Hon Sen Lecturer, University of Newcastle, Newcastle, UK

Andrew J Smith Senior Lecturer/Honorary Consultant in Microbiology, Infection Research Group, Glasgow Dental Hospital and School, University of Glasgow, Glasgow, UK

E Grace Smith Consultant Microbiologist and Clinical Service Director, Regional Centre for Mycobacteriology, Heartlands Hospital, Birmingham, UK

Eric W Taylor Consultant Surgeon, Greater Glasgow and Clyde Acute Hospitals NHS Trust, Inverclyde Royal Hospital, Greenock, UK

Avril Weaver Health Protection Nurse, West Midlands West Health Protection Unit, Kidderminster, UK

Michael J Weinbren Consultant Microbiologist, University Hospital of Coventry and Warwickshire NHS Trust, Coventry, UK

Mark H Wilcox Professor of Medical Microbiology, Head of Microbiology, and Clinical Director of Pathology, Leeds Teaching Hospitals and University of Leeds; Lead on *Clostridium difficile* for the Health Protection Agency Regional Microbiology Network, UK

Peter Wilson Consultant Microbiologist, Royal London Hospital, London, UK

FOREWORD

It is a great honour for me to be associated with the fifth edition and to be asked to write the foreword. The book has been in existence for over 30 years and the advice it has provided has always been useful and reliable, not only in the UK but around the world.

Hospital infection, particularly when associated with multiple antibiotic resistance, still remains a major problem. In the early 1960s some *Staphylococcus aureus* strains, resistant to most of the available antibiotics, including methicillin, were spreading in hospitals. Gram-negative bacilli, particularly *Pseudomonas aeruginosa*, were often responsible for severe outbreaks. Aseptic methods were often poor, the use of disinfectants was excessive and inadequately controlled, and defects in sterilization were common. A West Midlands Regional Working Party was set up at this time, chaired by Professor Edward Lowbury, consisting of microbiologists, infection control nurses, clinicians, engineers, administrators and others as necessary to tackle these problems. Meanwhile, the Hospital Infection Research Laboratory was carrying out prevalence surveys of infection and practices in West Midlands hospitals, providing useful data for the Working Party. It was then decided to produce a Regional Code of Practice which was so successful that a hardback book, *Control of Hospital Infection: a practical handbook*, was published and the first editors were EJL Lowbury, GAJ Ayliffe, AM Geddes and JD Williams. Since then, three more editions have been published.

This new edition has been expanded and updated and has a distinguished team of authors. The title has been altered to *Control of Healthcare-Associated Infection* since the increase in day surgery, minor surgery in general practice, and shorter hospital stay has meant that many more infections become manifest in the community.

Most of the recommendations in this book are, as previously, found to be effective in practice. Although methods based on good controlled clinical studies are desirable, these are rarely practical for hospital infection owing to the multiplicity of routes of spread of organisms and the varying number of factors influencing the emergence of infection. As an example, handwashing or disinfection is widely accepted as the most important technique in preventing the spread of infection but it is still uncertain whether an alcohol rub is more effective clinically than washing with soap and water, despite the laboratory evidence in favour of alcohol. The importance of cleaning the environment to control infection is often stressed by patients and politicians, although a risk assessment shows floors to be a minimal risk for transferring infection.

The principles of infection control have changed little over the years, but new problems have continued to emerge, such as multi-resistant tuberculosis and *Clostridium difficile*, which is now one of the major hospital infections in the elderly. Vancomycin-resistant enterococci are causing increasing numbers of infections in some specialized units. Cross-infection with MRSA remains mainly a hospital problem, but highly virulent strains of MRSA are now occurring in the community. Multi-resistant *Escherichia coli* and other Gram-negative infections, although less common than MRSA, can be difficult to control, and outbreaks with gastrointestinal viruses are often reported. The development of molecular techniques has also improved the speed and accuracy of diagnosis. The control of use of antibiotics is a continuing problem and the necessity of good antibiotic stewardship is stressed as well as the possible appointment of antibiotic pharmacists. Improved disinfectants and decontamination equipment are described, particularly for heat-labile items. This book also contains useful advice on hospital design for control of infection, and architects should obtain advice from infection control staff.

Governments, on pressure from patients, are taking a greater interest in healthcare infection and have produced numerous guidelines, legal requirements and other recommendations. National surveillance of infection has been increased and audits and annual targets are increasingly popular. European standards for disinfectant testing have been introduced. All these aspects are well covered in the book but every effort has been made to ensure that the recommendations will have a wide application in other countries. Healthcare establishments in different hospitals, even in the same country may have different problems and the on-site advice of the trained and experienced microbiologist or infection control nurse is still required. Decisions should be based on sound clinical and microbiological expertise rather than adherence to rigid rules. This book will help infection control staff to make such sound decisions.

Despite the plethora of guidelines, regulations and even the internet, infection control staff will still find that this book is a good source of information and advice from experts and will be particularly useful for infection control nurses and microbiologists in training. Finally, I would like to thank Adam Fraise and Tina Bradley for all their hard work in editing such an excellent book.

Graham AJ Ayliffe
Emeritus Professor of Medical Microbiology, University of Birmingham
Former Director of Hospital Infection Research Laboratory, Birmingham
February 2009

PREFACE TO THE FIFTH EDITION

This handbook was first produced as infection control guidance for the West Midlands Region of the UK in the early 1970s. The first edition, published in 1975, was widely used throughout the UK and many other countries. The original contributors were mainly microbiologists, surgeons and physicians from the Midlands, and the original editors, Edward Lowbury, Graham Ayliffe, Alasdair Geddes and David Williams continued to edit and contribute to the recommendations in the second and third editions. For this, the fifth edition, the editors are Adam Fraise and Christina Bradley. It became clear to the current editors that tasks such as this can no longer be based on the opinion of a small group of experts. No matter how knowledgeable the group may be, there is now a requirement for recommendations to be based on sound published evidence or, at the least, the experience of an acknowledged expert in the field concerned. For this reason, a decision was taken to extend the authorship to bring in experts in particular areas of infection prevention and control. All chapters have been revised and some have been significantly overhauled. Others are completely new contributions.

In recent years the focus has changed from infection control to that of prevention. In the UK the introduction of the Code of Practice for the prevention and control of healthcare-associated infection has been paramount in bringing the importance of infection prevention and control to a higher level. In addition, guidelines and standards now identify the roles and responsibilities of individuals when it comes to the management of infection prevention.

The basic techniques and problems of prevention of infection are mainly similar to those described in previous editions, but clinical techniques have progressed and some 'new' and 'old' infections have emerged or re-emerged as major problems.

The increased use of heat-labile equipment, particularly flexible endoscopes, has highlighted the necessity for effective decontamination methods. The importance of cleaning medical and other equipment, particularly with respect to minimizing the risk of transmission of prion-related disease, continues to be stressed, and automated machines have provided improved standards of cleaning and patient and staff safety.

The problems of bloodborne viruses (hepatitis B and C, and HIV) continue to influence hospital practice, and guidance on preventing transmission to and from healthcare workers has been published by government agencies in most countries. One of the major problems world-wide is the increase in antibiotic-resistant strains of bacteria, mainly in hospitals, but also in the community and in animal husbandry. Epidemic strains of methicillin-resistant *Staphylococcus aureus* (MRSA) have spread in hospitals in most countries, and have proved difficult to control without considerable resources and expenditure. The reports of vancomycin-resistant strains are particularly worrying. Highly resistant strains of Gram-negative bacilli also continue to spread in hospitals, and outbreaks of *Clostridium difficile* and norovirus are an unfortunate, but frequent occurrence. Highly resistant strains of *Mycobacterium tuberculosis* are causing therapy problems in many parts of the world, particularly in developing countries, and isolation facilities for patients with resistant organisms are often inadequate.

The possibility of reducing resistance by controlling the use of antibiotics is a logical approach, but so far the implementation of effective policies has proved difficult in most situations. Clinicians are loath to restrict the use of any effective antibiotic in the treatment of individual patients. Infection control techniques can have a greater initial influence on the spread of resistant organisms in hospitals, and are easier to implement. However, a combined approach of antibiotic restriction, effective surveillance and good infection control practices is essential if antibiotic resistance is to be overcome.

The costs of hospital care have increased considerably, and the use of evidence-based guidelines and the elimination of rituals applies as much to infection prevention and control as to other aspects of care. Claims for negligence in many countries are now very high and they redirect urgently needed funds away from patient care. Improvements in quality control, the use of audits and risk assessment are therefore being encouraged by most governments. The effect of these methods on patient outcome (e.g. infection rates) is an obvious criterion for administrators wishing to demonstrate the quality of their services. Surveillance of infection alone can reduce infection but, depending on the method chosen, it can also provide useful information on infection rates. However, the use of rates to compare the incidence of infection in different hospitals is still rarely possible owing to the problem of correcting for risk factors and the early discharge of patients from hospital. Patient care in hospitals and the community is becoming more closely integrated, and the community section in this book has been expanded in order to address administrative structure, outbreaks of infection and the particular problems of infection control in the community.

In recent years, Directives and many international and European standards have been published, as well as guidelines from government agencies and professional organizations. European legislation and standards represent a consensus of opinion from many countries, often with different infection control philosophies, and they may not be appropriate throughout Europe or elsewhere. Many of these regulations and guidelines have been referenced in this book, but these recommendations are not necessarily endorsed where they are considered to be inappropriate.

It is hoped that the book will continue to be of interest and useful to infection control workers in all countries. Infection prevention and control staff should make their own assessments based, where possible, on scientific evidence or on knowledge of the behaviour of micro-organisms in the patient and in the environment. The safety of patients and staff is the main consideration, and all hospitals should have infection control procedures based (where relevant) on national guidelines.

Although this edition is more thoroughly referenced than previous editions, it is still intended as a practical guide. It has been prepared for use by all personnel involved, either directly or indirectly, with infection prevention and control. It is intended for infection control staff, other doctors and nurses, physiotherapists, radiographers and others involved in the treatment and care of patients. It will also be useful in part for administrators, architects, engineers, pharmacists, sterile services staff, domestic and catering managers and others whose work may influence the risk of infection among patients and staff.

Sadly, Professor Lowbury who was co-editor of the first three editions of this book died in 2007 and we would like to acknowledge the contribution that he played in the field of infection control and prevention.

Adam P Fraise
Christina Bradley
February 2009

PART ONE

Basic principles

1 INTRODUCTION

Adam Fraise

Over the past few decades, the discipline of infection control has moved from a relatively quiet subject, which existed in the shadow of clinical specialities to a scientific discipline with a high political profile. It has become clear that healthcare-associated infection contributes significantly to healthcare costs and the public, press and governments are aware of the avoidable morbidity associated with these infections. As a result of the increasing public awareness of healthcare-associated infection, governments have introduced a range of initiatives aimed at both reducing the risk of such infections and increasing public confidence in healthcare systems. These initiatives have included compulsory reporting of infection rates (followed inevitably by the publication of these rates, usually in the form of 'league tables' so that the public can compare institutions with each other), guideline publications (such as those produced by the Centers for Disease Control in the USA and the appointment of individuals (e.g. the Inspector of Microbiology and Infection Control in the UK) charged with reducing healthcare-associated infections in public hospitals. It is open to debate how successful these initiatives have been; however, the increased political and public profile has been viewed as a good thing by many infection control practitioners, as this allows views to be heard by those with influence and may even result in increased resources for this important healthcare function.

Infection control services are provided by a variety of individuals with a range of backgrounds, training and expertise. Hospitals in many countries, such as the USA, employ hospital epidemiologists who run the service utilizing their background in statistics and epidemiology to identify problems and adopt control strategies. European countries frequently have infection control doctors managing the service, which is largely delivered by infection control nurses. Frequently other staff, such as laboratory scientists or other paramedical staff (usually termed infection control practitioners) assist in the delivery of the service. Other staff might be involved, such as statisticians, data collection clerks and administrative support staff. Whatever the local structure, the emphasis has to be on team-working such that strategy and service delivery are integrated. It is helpful to think of a multidisciplinary infection control team, usually consisting of a mixture of staff and invariably including both doctors and nurses.

The aims of the infection control team are to prevent and control healthcare-associated infections. Various techniques are used to achieve this goal, including surveillance, feedback, education, antimicrobial control and outbreak management.

THE IMPORTANCE OF HOSPITAL INFECTION

Prevalence surveys of hospital infection in many countries have shown that about one in ten patients in hospital have acquired an infection (Emmerson *et al.*, 1996) and a similar number of infections are acquired in the community. The main acquired infections are those of the urinary tract, surgical wounds, lower respiratory tract and skin. The frequency and severity vary with the age of the patient, the type of operation in surgical cases, the duration of catheterization (urinary and vascular), immunosuppressive treatment and other factors. It is necessary to take these 'risk' factors into account when comparing the incidence or prevalence of infection in different hospitals, and in the prediction of expected infection in individual patients or wards in hospitals (Emmerson and Ayliffe, 1996).

The *prevalence* rate is the proportion of a defined group that has an infection at any one point in time. The *incidence* rate is the proportion of a defined group that develops an infection within a stated period, and is lower than the prevalence rate. The incidence of hospital-acquired infection is about 5 per cent. This continuous and apparently universal, although variable, incidence is described as *endemic* infection. However, there is sometimes a large increase in the commonly occurring types of infection (e.g. post-operative wound sepsis) or the appearance of infection of a type that is not normally present in the hospital (e.g. salmonella infections in babies, or pseudomonas infections after eye surgery); this is called *epidemic* infection. Typing, usually by serological molecular methods, shows that epidemic infection is usually due to a single type, which can often be traced to a source (e.g. a carrier of a virulent strain of *Staphylococcus aureus*, or a solution contaminated with *Pseudomonas aeruginosa*). If aseptic and hygienic infection control measures in a hospital break down, the frequency of infection caused by multiple types of bacteria (i.e. *endemic* infection as defined above) may be increased to epidemic proportions.

The importance of hospital infection can be considered in terms of both the patient's illness and the prolonged occupancy of hospital beds. Illness owing to hospital infection is now rarely a cause of death, although this may occur in patients with poor resistance (e.g. those with extensive burns or multi-system failure) or from highly pathogenic organisms (e.g. some strains of hepatitis B virus). The cost of a prolonged stay is a convenient measure of the cost of infection, as it equates to a reduction in the number of beds available to fulfil contracts and reduce waiting-lists (Daschner, 1989).

Additional costs may include consumables, such as wound-care dressings and antibiotics. Estimates of the mean number of extra in-patient days in hospital range from 2 to 24, with costs per patient ranging from £250 to £3000 (Coello *et al.*, 1993; Department of Health, 1995). The overall reduction in length of stay means that many patients who would previously have been treated for an infection in hospital will now be treated in the community. This will increase the costs of medical and nursing care in the community. Other more personal 'costs' include the emotional and psychological trauma to the patient and their family, loss of income and the cost of financial support.

DEFINITIONS

It is important to be clear about the meaning of words used in any field and infection control is no exception;

The term *infection* is generally used to refer to the deposition and multiplication of bacteria and other micro-organisms in tissues or on surfaces of the body with an associated tissue reaction. If the response of the host is slight or absent, it is usually termed *colonization*. A carriage site is a normal area of skin or mucous membrane (e.g. nose) in which organisms are multiplying, but without any host response. *Sepsis* is the presence of inflammation, pus formation and other signs of illness in wounds that are colonized by micro-organisms and in tissues to which such infection has spread. Other types of infective illness are described by terms which refer to the site of infection (e.g. tonsillitis, peritonitis, gastroenteritis, pneumonia), or to the specific disease when this is distinctive (e.g. tuberculosis, measles, tetanus). The term *contamination* refers to the soiling of inanimate objects or living material with harmful, potentially infectious or unwanted matter.

Hospital (or '*nosocomial*') *infection* is infection acquired either by patients while they are in hospital, or by members of hospital staff. The term *healthcare-associated infection* (HAI) is becoming widely used to reflect the fact that infections associated with the delivery of healthcare can arise in a variety of settings. *Cross-* (or *exogenous*) *infection* means infection acquired from other people, either patients or staff. *Self-* (or *endogenous*) *infection* refers to infection caused by microbes that the patient carries on normal or septic areas of his or her own body (normal bacterial flora), including organisms that these areas have acquired in hospital (e.g. self-infection supervening on cross-infection or on infection from the environment).

For obvious reasons, all infections of operation wounds are healthcare associated. However, in other sites, it is often impossible to say whether an infection was acquired by the patient in hospital or before he or she came into hospital.

A *source* of hospital infection may be defined as a place where *pathogenic* (i.e. potentially disease-producing) micro-organisms are growing or have grown, and from which they are transmitted to patients (e.g. an infected wound, the nose or faeces of a carrier, contaminated food, contaminated solutions). A *reservoir* is a place where pathogens can survive or sometimes grow outside the body and from which they could be transferred – directly or indirectly – to patients (e.g. static equipment, furniture, floors). Although the term is sometimes used interchangeably with the term *source*, it is usually accepted that the source is the part of the reservoir containing organisms that infect or colonize one or more patients. A *vehicle* is a mobile object that can carry pathogenic organisms to a patient (e.g. dust particles, bedpans, blankets, toys, etc.). The word *vector* is commonly used interchangeably with vehicle, but it is sometimes used in the specialized sense of an insect that carries pathogenic micro-organisms (i.e. an *insect vector*), and should probably be restricted to this usage. These categories overlap. For example, a fluid in which bacteria multiply may be a vehicle as well as a source of infection and will have acquired the organism from some antecedent source (e.g. a patient with *Pseudomonas* infection).

In addition to the need for clear definitions to aid communication, types of infections also need to be defined carefully so that rates can be compared between institutions and even between different countries. The former allows poor practices or inadequacies in training to be identified, whereas the latter may be useful to inform policy-making at a national level. For example, the rates of methicillin-resistant *Staphylococcus aureus* (MRSA) bacteraemia in the UK are much higher than those in countries such as Holland or Denmark. Assuming these differences are real (in other words; as long as the same definitions are used), the difference may be due to variations in the way healthcare is delivered in the respective countries, such as hospital design, bed occupancy and staffing levels. The Centers for Disease Control in Atlanta, Georgia, USA has developed robust and reproducible definitions for the main categories of infections, which are helpful in any prevalence surveys (Garner *et al.*, 1988).

ACTIVITIES OF THE INFECTION CONTROL TEAM

Surveillance

'If you aren't measuring it, you aren't managing it' is a widely used expression in business management circles but is just as valid when applied to infection control. Surveillance is the cornerstone of good infection control practice because it allows one to identify areas where outcomes are below expectations thereby concentrating resources (both time and money) in the areas where they are most needed. Often, underperforming areas are also the areas where the most benefit will result from the same effort; consequently, targeting these areas increases the cost effectiveness of infection control activity.

Surveillance may be centrally (i.e. government) or locally organized, and most professionals in infection control spend time collecting data for both of these purposes. Examples of centrally driven surveillance include MRSA bacteraemia surveillance and national schemes to monitor antimicrobial resistance, and are frequently set up in response to political pressure.

Locally driven surveillance would typically concentrate on surgical-site infection rates or bacteraemia rates associated with intravenous lines.

Feedback

Merely collecting data and filing it away, or publishing it in a report achieves little. It is only when the results are fed back to those who have the power to make change that benefits will accrue. At the local level it has been clearly demonstrated that feeding surgical wound infections back to practising surgeons results in lower infection rates. The precise reasons for this are not clear, but probably relate to the fact that any surgeon identified as having higher rates than average will want to know why and will therefore critically analyse his or her practices and look to see if alternative methods should be adopted. Such high rates may also identify trainees or assistants who need more intensive training to allow them to achieve acceptable standards of care. Of course, the higher rates identified by such surveillance may be purely due to case mix. Some surgeons are recognized as being particularly good and therefore tend to have the higher-risk patients referred to them. It is important, therefore, that any surgical-site surveillance system is corrected for confounding factors such as co-morbidity, intrinsic operative risk and length of procedure. A simple and useful risk index has been developed in the USA (Russo and Spelman, 2002).

Antimicrobial control

It is being increasingly recognized that antimicrobial use is a double-edged sword where healthcare-associated infection is concerned. On one hand the availability of broad-spectrum agents allows immediate empirical therapy to be instituted with a high chance of success, and the increasing use of antimicrobial prophylaxis has a significant impact on the risk of HAI. However, widespread antimicrobial use is now recognized as a risk factor for infections with resistant organisms and is a driver for ongoing endemic MRSA, vancomycin-resistant enterococci (VRE) and *Clostridium difficile* infection.

The concept of antimicrobial stewardship is one that is gaining international support and a programme of education in antimicrobial use combined with closely policed policies to encourage rational antimicrobial prescribing is the norm in many hospitals. To assist in this role, pharmacists with a special interest in antimicrobial prescribing have been appointed by healthcare institutions. They are charged with developing evidence-based policies and developing systems to ensure adherence to such policies. Techniques such as automatic stop orders (where antimicrobials prescribed for a specific condition are discontinued after a predetermined course), automatic switch to oral treatment when indicated, and restriction of some antimicrobials to prescription by senior medical staff or infection specialists all enhance the effectiveness of the antimicrobial pharmacist's role.

Policy development

The development of policies and procedures is a key role for any infection control team. The central document is a collection of procedures (sometimes called an infection control policy or infection control manual), which should outline the accepted way of dealing with a range of issues including:

- isolation of the infected patient;
- handling of linen;
- sharps injuries;
- hand hygiene;
- collection and disposal of waste;
- disinfection and sterilization of instruments;
- decontamination of the environment;
- kitchen practices;
- personal protective equipment;
- specimen collection;
- pest control

as well as measures for the management of specific infections (e.g. MRSA and other resistant organisms, tuberculosis, viral haemorrhagic fevers, etc.).

Outbreak management

Although major outbreaks are, fortunately, a relatively rare event, all infection control teams need an agreed plan for the management of these incidents. A major outbreak plan should form part of the main infection control documentation and should include the key individuals who will be involved as well as how they relate to each other. The roles, responsibilities and membership of the major outbreak committee should be clearly described and the presence of managers (usually the chief executive officer), clinicians, epidemiologists and other interested parties should be explicit within the document. Arrangements for holding meetings of outbreak committees, as well as the reporting mechanisms to key organizational committees should be included in the major outbreak plan.

Decontamination

The days when decontamination took place either in a sterile services department (SSD) or on wards (with little quality control of the latter) are long gone. Decontamination is now a complex subject, which requires training of staff who are involved at all levels. The SSDs still exist, generally run by highly trained and dedicated individuals; however, there is an international trend to consolidate such departments into large centralized facilities serving several hospitals plus a range of community services. As many of these large SSDs are run by commercial companies, this has resulted in a loss of expertise in individual hospitals. Consequently large healthcare organizations have increasingly appointed decontamination managers to oversee the local aspect of decontamination policy.

Issues that need to be addressed include the use of single-use devices and local decontamination policies for items (e.g. endoscopes), which cannot be shipped to a central facility for reprocessing. Single-use items create significant challenges for any organization as their adoption often results in a greater annual expenditure than for reusable items (although, when the cost of reprocessing is included in the calculations, the cost differential is reduced and may even be reversed). Consequently, there is a temptation to reuse single-use items to reduce costs. European legislation makes it quite clear that items marketed for single use must not be reused, and individuals who choose to reuse single-use items may be open to criminal or civil legal proceedings. Similarly, choice of reprocessing methods for endoscopes is a complex issue and a full risk assessment must take place to ensure that health and safety concerns are considered along with any financial issues. It is clear therefore that development of decontamination policy in any healthcare institution is a complex field and needs input from staff with a variety of skills. The input to the process typically comes from microbiologists, infection control practitioners, engineers and managers.

Input into new builds

New builds within the healthcare sector tend to be complex projects involving a variety of different agencies. In the past, healthcare organizations would engage architects and would use in-house staff or sub-contractors to perform the construction phase. This would allow the healthcare institution to oversee the entire project and ensure the end product is fit for purpose. This method of creating new buildings is quite rare now and third-party organizations are used in most cases. Frequently commercial organizations are given a brief to design a facility for a specific purpose, oversee the construction and hand over the final facility to the healthcare organization (so-called 'design and build'). An important variation on this is commonplace in the UK and comes under the heading of 'private finance initiative' (PFI). In a PFI build, a commercial organization is given a brief to design and build a facility, which is then leased to the healthcare organization over a period of several years. This lease will cover maintenance of the building and may include cleaning and portering services as well.

Whatever system is used to create a new build, the involvement of infection control teams from the beginning is paramount. Architects are aware of legislation but will regard guidance as exactly that – optional not imperative. The infection control team should have detailed discussions with the architects from the earliest stages of the build so that guidance for operating theatres, endoscopy suites, intensive care units and isolation rooms are followed. Often guidance from professional societies as well as government departments is not easily obtainable by architects, and the infection control team should make the design and commissioning teams aware of any guidance or legislation that it feels are relevant.

An ongoing dialogue with the architects and commissioners of the build is essential if the end product is to satisfy infection control requirements. Regular meetings should be scheduled and plans formally signed off by a senior member of the infection control team at key stages. Pre-handover visits to the facility are also important; it is often only at this stage that problems such as inaccessible sinks or surfaces that are impossible to clean are identified.

Laundry

Although many hospitals no longer have on-site laundry services, the importance of laundry for infection control cannot be denied. Laundry from infected patients may be heavily contaminated with pathogenic organisms and the infection control team must be assured that all relevant legislation is being followed. The detailed requirements for this service are discussed in detail in Chapter 7.

Kitchens

Foodborne infection is an important risk for any healthcare provider (Department of Health and Social Security, 1986). Catering often takes place on a large scale and the population consuming the food may be frail and have increased susceptibility to gastrointestinal pathogens. Infection control teams should regularly (at least annually) inspect catering facilities that are within the healthcare organization. This will include main kitchens, any cook-chill units, ward kitchens, and staff and visitor facilities. Key points to look for are separation of cooked and raw food, adequate pest control measures, and records of temperatures of food on delivery and after reheating.

Education

Without doubt, the main role of any infection control team is to instil safe practices into the minds and activities of all healthcare workers. While it is tempting for other staff to take a view that infection control should be a job for the infection control team, in reality, effective infection control relies on all staff ensuring that they are adequately trained and that their actions are safe. This is often encapsulated in the adage 'infection control is everyone's responsibility' and requires input from the infection control team to ensure that appropriate training is available. The form of training varies from didactic classroom session to ad hoc one-on-one training following the observation of poor practice in a clinical area. For the latter method to be effective, it is essential that members of the team spend as much time as possible in clinical areas, auditing practice and supporting staff in their desire to protect patients from harm.

Making time available for staff to attend teaching sessions is often difficult in hard-pressed clinical areas and many teams have experimented with workbooks or web-based training material, which can be completed in the healthcare worker's own time.

Mandatory training

Although the training described above is important, some staff will inevitably miss this; either because they do not attend formal sessions or because the infection control team, by pure chance, rarely interacts with them. It is essential, therefore that a safety net is provided so that all staff receive a minimum level of training in infection control. This training must not be optional and mechanism must be in place to identify staff who do not attend these mandatory training sessions. It is normal to arrange mandatory training in fire safety and lifting and handling techniques, and infection control training can be added to this. Alternatively, a workbook approach with a register of completion may be the most effective way of ensuring this training is followed. Whatever system is used, it must be emphasized that the contents of mandatory training is a minimum and conscientious staff will want to add to this. The infection control team should ensure that supplementary training is available for all who desire it.

Effecting change – educational psychology

Arguably, the most important challenge for infection control practitioners is to overcome the reluctance of humans to change their behaviour. Most educated healthcare workers are familiar with the main means by which pathogens can spread from one patient to another, and are fully aware of the importance of hand hygiene and sterile technique. Nevertheless repeated studies have shown that hand-hygiene compliance is poor amongst healthcare workers and, even after intensive education, only improves marginally (Pittet *et al.*, 2000). It is possible that, by using techniques developed by psychologists at motivating behaviour change (utilized in antismoking campaigns as well as drives to increase the wearing of seat-belts in cars), the infection control community can positively influence behaviour and overcome what may be described as the last barrier to effective infection control.

REFERENCES

Coello R, Glenister H, Fereres J *et al.* (1993) The cost of infection in surgical patients: a case-controlled study. *Journal of Hospital Infection* **25**, 239.

Daschner F (1989) Cost-effectiveness in hospital infection control – lessons for the 1990s. *Journal of Hospital Infection* **13**, 325.

Department of Health (1995) *Hospital infection control: guidance on the control of infection in hospitals.* Paper prepared by the DHSS/PHLS Hospital Infection Working Group. London: HMSO.

Department of Health and Social Security (1986) *The report of the Committee of Inquiry into an outbreak of food-poisoning at Stanley Royd Hospital.* London: HMSO.

Emmerson AM and Ayliffe GAJ (eds) (1996) Surveillance of nosocomial infections. In *Bailliére's clinical infectious diseases.* Vol. 3. London: Bailliére Tindall.

Emmerson AM, Enstone JE, Griffin M, Kelsey MC and Smyth ETM (1996) The Second National Prevalence Survey of infection in hospitals – overview of the results. *Journal of Hospital Infection* **32**, 175.

Garner JS, Jarvis WR, Emori TG, Horan TC and Hughes JM (1988) CDC definitions for nosocomial infections, *American Journal of Infection Control* **16**, 28.

Pittet D, Hugonnet S, Harbarth S *et al.* (2000) Effectiveness of a hospital-wide programme to improve compliance with hand hygiene. *Lancet* **356**, 1307.

Russo PL and Spelman DW (2002) A new surgical-site infection risk index using risk factors identified by multivariate analysis for patients undergoing coronary artery bypass graft surgery. *Infection Control and Hospital Epidemiology* **23**, 372.

2 ADMINISTRATION AND RESPONSIBILITY

Adam Fraise

The administrative arrangements for infection control will vary in different countries, but most will include an Infection Control Doctor or Officer (ICD or ICO), an Infection Control Nurse or Practitioner (ICN or ICP) and a Committee (ICC) (Department of Health, 1995). This chapter concentrates on the situation in England, although many of the administrative arrangements described have counterparts in other countries; for example, the commissioning and funding of healthcare in England, as well as the rest of the UK, is within a government infrastructure but similar issues arise when it is the responsibility of health maintenance organizations (HMOs) or private insurers.

The UK has undergone significant changes in the structure of healthcare provision over the last two decades which have affected the administration and responsibility for management of infection control services, and further changes continue to occur with changes in government policy and new Department of Health guidelines.

England is currently divided into Strategic Health Authorities (SHAs) covering populations of varying sizes (Scotland and Wales have similar administrative organizations termed Health Boards and Health Authorities, respectively). The role of the SHAs, as the name implies, is to give strategic guidance to the commissioners of healthcare. The commissioning of healthcare is the responsibility of Primary Care Trusts (PCTs), while provision is the responsibility of acute hospitals, termed acute National Health Service (NHS) Trusts, other healthcare organizations (e.g. ambulance or community Trusts) or family practitioners. Primary Care Trusts are responsible for determining the healthcare requirements for the local population, and will stipulate what monies are available and how these monies will be allocated to hospital or community Trusts via contracts, service agreements and other financial links. Linked to this framework is the Health Protection Agency (HPA), an independent body funded by central government monies (termed a non-departmental public body) charged with protecting public health in England through the provision of support and advice to the NHS and other organizations. The HPA employs Consultants in Communicable Disease Control (CCDCs) who have responsibility for co-ordination of infection control activities, including outbreaks involving hospital Trusts and the community at large.

National Health Service Trusts will usually deliver acute hospital services, community and long-term services, or mental health services, although some may incorporate both hospital and community services. NHS Trusts and private hospitals are monitored by the Healthcare Commission (an independent body, set up to promote and drive improvement in the quality of healthcare and public health) and are expected to follow national guidelines. All acute Trusts are expected to have a Director of Infection Prevention and Control (DIPC) who retains responsibility for hospital infection control, and is directly accountable to the Chief Executive and the Trust Board, and will collaborate with the CCDC. In the event of a major outbreak involving both hospital Trusts and the community, overall responsibility for the coordination of the outbreak rests with the CCDC (see Chapter 16).

All healthcare Trusts are now responsible for the provision of appropriate infection control services, although purchasers can enforce reasonable infection control standards through explicit clauses in contracts. Within this structure in acute Trusts, the Infection Control Team (ICT) will normally be provided by the organization, with the costs of the service recouped by the provider from the prices it charges to the purchasers. The cost of providing an infection control service must be considered an essential part of a Trust. In addition to the annual budget for the ICD and ICNs for routine control purposes, costs of an outbreak may be borne by a contingency fund, although frequently no such fund actually exists. In major outbreaks, additional funding may be provided by the purchaser. Non-acute Trusts (e.g. Mental Health Trusts or Ambulance Trusts) will typically contract infection control services from a nearby acute Trust.

There are also ICNs working within the PCTs, advising them of the measures required for effective infection control and stipulating ways of monitoring the effectiveness via audit of infection control standards.

It is the responsibility of the Chief Executive of the Trust and the board to ensure that adequate arrangements are made to control hospital infection (Department of Health, 2006). These arrangements should include the setting up of an ICC, and the appointment of a DIPC, an ICD and adequate ICN cover in every Trust.

The Trust Board should seek to implement the recommendations of the DIPC, who in turn will seek information and opinions from ICDs and ICNs. Within each Trust, a Directorate structure exists for different services (e.g. surgical or medical services), usually with a Clinical Director, Business Manager and Senior Nurse Manager. Each Directorate has budgetary control and has to work within an agreed business plan of services and care to be provided.

The DIPC and ICC should influence these Directorates via the Chief Executive to ensure that infection control recommendations are communicated to them and implementation is then supported through the planning process. It is particularly important that Directorates' adherence to recommendations and infection control performance are monitored through organizational governance structures. Furthermore, it is the responsibility of all members of staff within the Trust to inform the DIPC, ICD or ICN of potential hazards of infection. Without this cooperation, the ICT cannot be fully effective. In addition to the official responsibilities of the Chief Executive and ICT, the individual clinician in charge of each patient's care and the senior nurse in a unit has a personal responsibility for preventing infection.

INFECTION CONTROL TEAM

The team consists of members of staff with a specialist knowledge and interest in infection control in hospitals. The ICT will include the microbiologist (who will usually be either the DIPC or the ICD), ICNs and (where available) members of the scientific or technical staff with responsibilities in infection control. The ICD and ICN should meet frequently, preferably daily.

More than one ICD and ICN may be appointed in a large Trust, depending on the size and also the type of patient. The Trust Director of Operations or Hospital Manager or a representative may be a member of the team, attending meetings when a major problem arises. If they are not a member of the team, they (or a representative) should always be available to the ICD for discussion of problems.

The role of the ICT is to implement the annual programme and policies and to be responsible for providing advice to the Trust or hospital staff on a 24-hour basis.

The team is responsible for the following:

• surveillance of infections and monitoring methods of control;
• rapid identification and investigation of outbreaks or potentially hazardous procedures;
• providing advice on isolation of infected patients and on hazardous or ineffective procedures;
• giving advice, making day-to-day decisions and liaising with staff in all areas where potential risks of infection exist, especially laboratories, occupational health departments and clinical directorates;
• providing, monitoring and evaluating policies for the prevention of infection and its spread;
• audit of infection control procedures as appropriate;
• a staff education programme in collaboration with the occupational health department, including communication and provision of readily available information to staff on measures of infection control;
• preparing the annual infection control programme and reporting to the ICC.

The particular duties of the ICD and ICN are described below, but there is a considerable overlap in duties and responsibilities between the various members of the team.

Director of Infection Prevention and Control

The individual holding this appointment should be a senior member of the organization with access to the Trust Board and management committees, and should have sufficient authority to command respect from all categories of staff. They are directly responsible to the Chief Executive. They should have a special interest and training in hospital infection, and should be aware of recent developments in the subject. They may be expected to complete the course for the diploma in hospital infection control in the UK or an equivalent qualification in the future, and they should be appointed by the Trust Board. The medical microbiologist is the logical choice, being suitably qualified and in an ideal position to keep the surveillance and record systems under constant scrutiny and review, although the Medical Director, Director of Nursing Services or Director of Operations could fulfil this role. The functions of the DIPC are to develop infection control strategy, formulate an annual infection control plan and to report progress against this plan to the board of the institution.

Infection Control Doctor

The ICD should be a senior member of the medical staff and will have a close working relationship with the DIPC. He or she will share much of the work of the DIPC or, if the DIPC is not a medical microbiologist or ICN, will perform the operational side of the DIPC role under the DIPC's managerial direction. A medical microbiologist is often best suited to this role, being suitably qualified and in an ideal position to keep the surveillance and record systems under constant scrutiny and review. However, some healthcare institutions may not have access to a microbiologist and another clinician with interest in the subject may be suitable. The functions of the ICD in conjunction with other members of the team are to assess risks of infection, to advise on preventative measures and to check their efficacy in all parts of the hospital, including the laundry, sterile services department (SSD), domestic, pharmaceutical and engineering departments, as well as clinical and other areas.

Inspection of kitchens and other catering establishments should be carried out regularly (at least every 12 months) by the ICD or their representative, in collaboration with the CCDC and the local authority environmental health officer.

Information and advice may be given by the ICD informally or at meetings of the Trust Board, Medical Staff Committee, ICC or Directorate Managers. However, if any immediate action is required, the ICD or Chairman of the ICC (see below) should be empowered to take whatever steps may be necessary without prior reference to the ICC. He or she should have ready access to the Chief Executive, Director of Operations, directors of clinical services and laboratory facilities, and work closely with the ICN and also the CCDC, especially

on notifiable infectious diseases. Some of the duties of the ICD may be delegated to other staff (e.g. the microbiology registrar, ICN or ICP, or biomedical
scientist, as appropriate).

Infection Control Nurse

The ICN should be a registered nurse with a broad range of clinical nursing
experience. They should be experienced in communicating with all grades and
disciplines, and be able to balance conflicting issues while maintaining the
individual patient's care needs.

The ICN is the only member of the ICT with a full-time responsibility for
infection control, enabling him or her to maintain a clinical input within wards
and departments and always to be accessible for advice and support. The nurse
responsible for infection control within a Trust should be graded as a Clinical
Nurse Specialist or Senior Nurse Manager, and have access and links across all
clinical directorates. Grading should depend on areas of responsibility and
should be reviewed within the Trust's corporate plan. It is recommended that,
for the induction of newly appointed ICNs, attendance for a short period at a
centre in which there are experienced ICNs working within an established ICT
should be included. The principles of hospital microbiology and laboratory
procedures, such as specimen collection, should be taught in the new ICN's
own hospital to enable development of essential links with laboratory personnel. It is expected that all nurses will complete one of the specialist training
courses for ICNs, for example, English National Board (ENB) 329 in the UK or
the equivalent at diploma or university degree level. Many Trusts within the
UK normally stipulate that all clinical nurse specialists should be able to function at degree level. The structure of these courses ensures that the ICN will
remain within his or her Trust, and that he or she will be able to reflect on the
knowledge gained and on practice within the clinical areas.

The attendance of ICNs at the annual conference of the Infection Prevention
Society (IPS) and other related specialist conferences (e.g. those of the Hospital
Infection Society) should be considered as part of their training, and as
mandatory updating required by the United Kingdom Central Council for
Nursing, Midwifery and Health Visiting (UKCC; 1995). Failure to provide a
career structure for ICNs leads to difficulties in recruitment and retention of
trained and experienced nurses within the health service.

The ICN is managerially accountable to the ICD and professionally accountable to the Director of Nursing Practice, who should be responsible for advising
on attendance by the ICN at conferences, courses and other relevant meetings.
If a person other than a nurse is appointed to take on some of these duties, he
or she should be on the laboratory staff and may be described, for example, as
an 'Infection Control Microbiologist', 'Infection Control Scientific Officer' or
'Infection Control Practitioner'. The appointment is usually in addition to that

of a nurse, although in the USA, the Infection Control Practitioner (Professional) is usually a nurse equivalent to an ICN in the UK.

The functions of the ICN are described below. These cover the whole field of infection control and involve cooperation with all of the departments mentioned in the section on the ICC, and particularly with the occupational health department. The ICN is a member of, and shares responsibility with, the Infection Control Team. The nurse should visit all wards regularly and discuss any problems with the staff. The laboratory should be visited every morning by the ICN. Instruction of nurses and other grades of staff in the practice of infection control is one of the major responsibilities, and should be treated as a priority.

The day-to-day activities of an infection control nurse include the following:

- identifying as promptly as possible potential infection hazards in patients, staff or equipment;
- compiling records of infected patients from ward notifications, case notes, laboratory reports and information collected during routine visits and discussions;
- arranging prompt isolation of infected patients (in cooperation with the ward manager and consultant who have initial responsibility) in accordance with hospital policy, and ensuring that there are adequate facilities for isolating patients, as well as introducing other measures as necessary to prevent the spread of infection or organisms that are highly resistant to antibiotics;
- regular audits of relevant wards in units to ensure that infection control and aseptic procedures are being carried out in accordance with hospital policy (see p. 51);
- liaison between laboratory and ward staff; informing heads of departments and giving advice on infection control problems;
- collaboration with occupational health staff in maintaining records of infection in medical, nursing, catering, domestic and other grades of staff; ensuring that clearance specimens are received before infected staff return to duty;
- collaborating with and advising community nurses on problems of infection;
- promptly supplying information about notifiable diseases by telephone to the public health medical officer (CCDC);
- informing other hospitals, general practitioners and other healthcare providers when infected patients are discharged from hospital or transferred elsewhere, and receiving relevant information from other hospitals or from the community where appropriate;
- participation in teaching and practical demonstrations of techniques for control of infection to medical, nursing, auxiliary, domestic, catering and other professions allied to medicine;

- informing the Director of Nursing and/or Directorate Nurse Managers of practical problems and difficulties in carrying out routine procedures related to nursing aspects of infection control;
- attending relevant committees, usually Control of Infection, Nursing Procedures, Clinical Audit, Risk Management, Equipment Purchase Groups, Health and Safety, Re-Use of Single-Use item Committees, etc.;
- produce and update infection control policies and guidelines;
- offer advice on purchase and decontamination of equipment, and on planning and capital projects;
- conferring with the sterile services manager about the management of equipment used by patients with certain infections in hospital (e.g. hepatitis B virus).

Much of the ICN's time will be spent providing advice to members of staff on infection control problems.

The nurse will collaborate with other members of the team in investigating outbreaks, conducting surveys, visiting kitchen and catering establishments, monitoring special units, collecting microbiological samples, preparing reports for the ICC, clinicians and Trust management, and assisting in research projects.

Infection Control Link (Liaison) Nurse

The development of an Infection Control Link Nurse within acute hospital, community and mental health Trusts initially caused concern with regard to the role of such a person. Key to any such role is the responsibility of the link or liaison nurse to a qualified ICN. Ongoing support and education of the link nurses is critical to enable them to be effective communicators and 'agents of change' at ward or department level. Further research is required to identify whether the increased education and knowledge of link nurses results in an improvement in practice throughout the clinical area in which they work. This has to be balanced against the time commitment required by the qualified ICN. Possible considerations could include stability of the workforce within a Trust and the number of ICNs. Link nurses may be particularly useful in specialist departments (e.g. intensive-care units and outlying or non-acute hospitals). Although their role is developing, they should report to the ICN early evidence of outbreaks or infection problems, and any changes in practice and in the use of new equipment relevant to infection control. It is recommended that the link nurse's role should be clearly defined in order to meet local needs, and the placing of excessive demands on individuals should be avoided.

In some hospitals or departments, particularly in developing countries, a Link Doctor could also be useful, but this post has not yet been developed in the UK.

Consultant in Communicable Disease Control

Consultants in Communicable Disease Control are employed by the HPA and are responsible for the surveillance, prevention and control of all communicable disease and infection in a specific geographical area. They are basically qualified in public health and/or medical microbiology, and are specifically trained for the post. The duties of the CCDC and ICD in the hospital overlap, and close collaboration between them is essential. The CCDC may advise the PCT and SHA on contractual requirements for infection control services and monitoring in the Trusts within the district. It also liaises with the ICT in the management of outbreaks of infection in hospital and the community, and liaises with adjacent health districts and provides epidemiological advice when required. The CCDC is a member of the ICT and Major Outbreak Committee, and if the latter involves the community, he or she may be appointed chairman of the committee.

INFECTION CONTROL COMMITTEE

The committee of a large hospital Trust should have representatives from all of the major departments concerned with control of infection (e.g. medical, nursing, occupational health, engineering, pharmacy, supplies, domestic, SSD, catering, microbiology, administration and community health), as well as from the ICT. The chairman of the committee may be the DIPC or the ICD, but could be a clinician with an interest in infection control (e.g. infectious diseases consultant or surgeon, or a senior ICN). Some hospital Trusts may prefer to appoint a small committee consisting of the ICT, the CCDC, a senior nurse, clinician and senior manager, and to co-opt others as necessary. The main advantages of a large committee are educational and to ensure adequate communication between the different departments. However, major decisions on hospital problems will be made by the ICT and possibly by a small executive committee as described above.

Meetings should be held 1–12 times a year depending on requirements, but three to four meetings should be adequate for most Trusts, and yearly meetings for small hospitals where problems tend to arise sporadically. The committee should:

- discuss any problems brought to them by the ICD, ICN or other members of the committee and provide support for decisions made by the ICT;
- take responsibility for major decisions;
- be given reports on current problems, and on the incidence of infection and evaluate other reports involving infection risk (e.g. kitchen inspections);
- arrange interdepartmental coordination and education in control of infection (it is therefore advantageous to have representation of members with various interests);

- introduce, maintain and, when necessary, modify policies (e.g. disinfectant, antibiotic, isolation);
- advise on the selection of equipment for the prevention of infection (e.g. sharps disposal boxes, etc.);
- make recommendations to other committees and departments on infection control techniques;
- advise Trusts on all aspects of infection control and make recommendations for use of resources.

Implementation of Committee recommendations

If the committee or team is to be effective, the results of the investigations and records of infection must be sent to the relevant authorities and recommendations rapidly implemented, especially when the safety of patients or staff is involved. Although the ICT has an overall advisory responsibility to the Trust or hospital, other members of the committee should ensure that recommendations within their own areas of responsibility are carried out as considered necessary by the committee. Heads of departments (e.g. catering, laundry), if they are not members of the committee, should be invited to attend committee meetings when problems concerning their own departments are to be discussed. The ICC should be a subcommittee of the Trust Board or equivalent and regular reports should be made to the Trust Board. The DIPC should have direct access to the Chief Executive, who may also be a member of the committee or team. All recommendations, instructions or procedures involving any aspect of infection in the hospital issued by the Directorates, other committees, the Health and Safety Executive (HSE), environmental health officers or CCDC should be referred for approval to the DIPC.

Objectives of the infection control department and implementation of policies

The main objective of the ICT is to reduce preventable infection to the lowest possible level at acceptable cost, and Health Authorities increasingly require evidence that infection control techniques are cost effective. Although costs can be measured, effectiveness is more difficult to assess, as patients vary in age and other characteristics, as well as undergoing different treatments. Hospitals vary in design and availability of facilities. Comparisons between infection rates in different hospitals or during different periods in the same hospital are of doubtful validity, and require a considerable amount of time for the collection of data. Even if the data can be collected, the numbers of infections over a year in a single hospital are not usually sufficient to provide statistical evidence of efficacy of measures (see Chapter 3). In addition, it is not possible to estimate the infections that might have occurred if early preventative measures had not been implemented.

It is therefore difficult to assess the infection control measures in terms of outcome (e.g. reduced infection rates), but it may be possible to infer the outcome from process measurements. The Study of Efficacy of Nosocomial Infection Control (SENIC) project conducted in the USA showed that a 'reduction in infection rates of about one-third could be obtained by intensive surveillance and control methods, the appointment of a physician with expertise in infection control and one Infection Control Nurse to 250 beds' (Haley *et al.*, 1985). It is inferred that, if the SENIC criteria are met, a reduction in infection rate will be achieved. However, it is unlikely that the appointment of more Infection Control Nurses will be possible in most hospitals around the world in the foreseeable future, and maintaining a comprehensive clinical surveillance system will often not represent optimal use of the nurse's time. However, the infection control staff should be able to demonstrate to the Trust Board that certain objectives have been achieved. Essential surveillance reports could be presented to the ICC, as well as evidence of audits of policies and appropriate infection control techniques which have proven value. Priorities can be defined and unnecessary rituals eliminated (e.g. wearing of caps and overshoes in intensive care units, and unnecessary washing of operating-theatre walls).

ACTION DURING AN OUTBREAK OF INFECTION

When an outbreak occurs (e.g. owing to the sudden appearance of an increasing incidence of one type of infection in a ward), immediate action is needed to prevent further spread to patients and staff. This action will vary according to the nature and severity of the infection, but certain general principles apply. The ICD or ICN must be notified, and they should take immediate steps (e.g. isolation of suspected cases) in consultation with the microbiologist (if not the same person) and the clinicians and nursing manager whose patients are involved. The CCDC responsible for communicable diseases should be informed if the outbreak is of a notifiable disease or involves the community. If a major outbreak occurs, a meeting of the 'emergencies' or 'outbreak' committee should immediately be arranged by the Chairman of the ICC or ICD and the Hospital Operations Manager or his or her representative. Other members of this committee include the ICT, the clinician responsible for affected patients, a senior nurse, the occupational health team and the CCDC. The CCDC has legal responsibility for controlling infection and may prefer to chair the committee himself or herself.

A major outbreak is difficult to define in terms of the numbers of patients and staff involved. Numbers of cases (e.g. '20 salmonella infections') have been suggested, but two cases – or even one – of a hazardous infection (e.g. diphtheria) might be considered to be a major outbreak. The decision should be made by the ICD, based on factors such as the severity and communicability of infections, the necessity of closing the ward, the need to prevent transfer of staff to other wards, to provide additional staff, to provide additional supplies, linen, etc., or to open an isolation ward.

The ICD (or chairman of the Infection Committee) will usually be responsible for coordinating infection control arrangements in the hospital. The following steps are suggested.

- Arrangements should be made for the clinical care of patients.
- Adequate channels of communication should be set up and a decision made as to who will be responsible for communication with the media.
- An assessment of the situation should be made – details of the patients with infection should be recorded, including date of admission and first symptoms, and the nature of the disease; bacteriological samples should be examined and, when possible, pathogens typed (or kept on suitable medium for typing) in the hospital or reference laboratory (in the UK, this would usually be a HPA laboratory).
- Isolation of infected patients (for appropriate methods, see Chapter 13).
- Introduction of additional techniques for control of infection in affected wards (e.g. alcoholic hand disinfection); closure of one or more wards (this is rarely required, but may be necessary if the outbreak is extensive, and particularly if the infection involves a hazard of severe illness or even death in some patients); the ward should be closed to further admissions, and thoroughly cleaned after discharge of the last patient before reopening; such a procedure may also apply to an operating-theatre or other affected area.
- The allocation of beds (e.g. the entire isolation unit, side wards, or possibly a larger ward) for care and management of infected patients may be required.
- An epidemiological survey should be undertaken, where appropriate, in order to provide evidence of the time and place where infection was acquired, including enquiry about the possible admission of patients incubating infection.
- Surveillance of contacts (who may be incubating the disease) is sometimes necessary, and this includes clinical surveillance and laboratory screening.
- Bacteriological search for the source of infection; examination of all staff and patients for carriage to see whether, for example, the same phage type of *Staphylococcus aureus* is isolated from all infections; search for the infecting strain in the inanimate environment (e.g. fluids if the organism is *Pseudomonas aeruginosa* or other Gram-negative bacilli, or food if the illness is gastroenteritis of possible food origin).
- Survey of methods, equipment and buildings – such a survey could include dressing technique, theatre discipline, kitchen hygiene – for evidence of lapses and the 'personal factor', and also for effectiveness of sterilizers,

ventilation systems, disinfection, and protection against recontamination of sterilized objects and solutions.

- The ICN or Occupational Health Nurse will discuss the situation with heads of departments (e.g. catering, SSD, laundry and domestic departments) to relieve anxieties and identify any necessary procedures.
- The requirement for assistance should be assessed at each meeting and advice sought as necessary (e.g. from the HPA, Division of Hospital Infection, Colindale, or other specialist physicians or units, such as the Infectious Diseases Physician, Hospital Infection Research Laboratory, Birmingham, or the Communicable Disease Surveillance Centre, Colindale).

Checklists of practices should be prepared for investigation of infection arising in surgical, maternity and general medical wards and in special departments (e.g. operating suites, kitchens, laundries, SSD; e.g. Williams *et al.*, 1966).

LEGAL ASPECTS OF INFECTION CONTROL

Legal regulations have increased considerably in recent years and have had a major impact on infection control staff. Many of these are the consequence of European Directives and Standards, and particularly apply to medical devices, waste disposal and the health and safety of staff. A key piece of legislation in the UK is the Health Act 2006 identifying a code of practice, which, by law, must be followed by all healthcare organizations. The requirements of the code of practice include appropriate management structures as well as clinical care protocols. National guidelines and standards have also been produced to improve quality of patient care, and all hospitals must have written policies and procedures for reducing healthcare-associated infections (this is a requirement under the Health Act).

Statutes and statutory regulations (i.e. Acts of Parliament and subsidiary regulations) may be used as a basis for either civil or criminal prosecution. They are usually less detailed than guidelines or standards, which are often used to add specific detail to the regulations. For example, the guidance produced by the Health Services Advisory Committee interprets and expands upon the Controlled Waste Regulations 1992 and the Environmental Protection Act 1990 for disposal of clinical waste. Other important Acts and Regulations are the Health and Safety Act (1974) and the Control of Substances Hazardous to Health Regulations (COSHH) Act of Parliament (1988).

However, medical negligence is often dealt with by common law based on previous court judgements. Medical negligence due to failure in the duty of care owed to patients usually involves a civil action unless the negligence is gross (e.g. if it is responsible for the death of a patient), and might then be associated with a criminal prosecution.

Guidelines, standards and policies

Guidelines and standards produced by national professional organizations, health departments and government agencies are usually advisory and not legally enforceable (Hurwitz, 1995). Nevertheless, they are frequently used as a basis for a civil action in claims of negligence, and when produced by a government agency may be used as a basis for criminal prosecution. Any deviation from national guidelines or standards requires careful consideration, although it must be accepted that a consensus decision reached by a group of experts does not always arrive at the only or necessarily the correct solution (see p. **31**). National standards produced by professional organizations or the British Standards Institute tend to be stronger in their requirements than guidelines, but usually allow some local deviations. For instance, the standards on 'Infection Control in Hospitals', prepared by four national organizations, mainly include managerial requirements and state that 'the proposed standards might be used as a point of reference in discussions between the Infection Control Team and managers about the arrangements needed to deliver a high quality infection control service' (Infection Control Working Party, 1993).

Clinical guidelines have been defined as 'systematically developed statements which assist healthcare staff and patients in making decisions about appropriate treatment or courses of action for specific conditions or procedures (modified from *Clinical Guidelines*, NHS Executive 1996). Wherever possible, these (as well as legal requirements, standards and policies) should be evidence based. The NHS Executive describes three categories of evidence:

1 randomized controlled trials;
2 other robust experimental or observational studies;
3 more limited evidence, but the advice relies on expert opinion and is endorsed by respected authorities.

For many years, the control of infection has, whenever possible, been based on scientific evidence. The Centers for Disease Control have produced guidelines on most infection control procedures and categorize them as follows (Garner, 1996):

1A strongly recommended for all hospitals, and strongly supported by well-designed experimental or epidemiologic studies;
1B strongly recommended for all hospitals, and reviewed as effective by experts in the field and consensus of the Hospital Infection Control Practices Advisory Committee (HICPAC), based on strong rationale and suggestive evidence, even though definitive scientific studies have not been performed;
2 suggested for implementation in many hospitals; recommendations may be supported by suggestive clinical or epidemiologic studies, a strong

theoretical rationale or definitive studies applicable to some, but not all, hospitals;

3   no recommendation – unresolved issue; practices for which insufficient evidence or consensus regarding efficacy exists.

Those responsible for preparing national guidelines should take into account variations in structure, resources and particular problems of individual hospitals, and should ensure that recommendations are practicable, reasonable and achievable. The guidelines should not inhibit advances made by practitioners who are prepared to take some risks, but deviations should be backed by research if possible. The same requirements apply to local guidelines and policies. Hospital policies should be included in an infection control manual available on all hospital wards and units. Manuals and policies or guidelines have been published and can be used as a guide to reduce the amount of work in an individual hospital (Damani, 1997; Ward et al., 1997). The recommendations in the manual should be implemented, and should be subject to regular audit and review. If a Health Authority or NHS Trust is sued for negligence, local guidelines and policies will be closely examined even if they are not legally enforceable. However, 'courts are unlikely to adopt standards of care advocated in clinical guidelines as "gold standards" because the mere fact that a guideline exists does not of itself establish that compliance with it is reasonable in the circumstances, or that non-compliance is negligent' (Hurwitz, 1999).

Failure to follow legal regulations, national guidelines or standards may be associated with the following:

• healthcare purchasers (i.e. Health Authorities in the UK) obtaining their medical services from another hospital (provider), or refusal by insurance companies to fund treatment in a particular private hospital;
• sanctions against the hospital by the NHS Executive or appropriate government authority;
• civil proceedings against the hospital Trust concerned for medical negligence;
• criminal proceedings against the hospital or healthcare worker taken by national or local government agencies because of failure to comply with official regulations, or in the event of possible gross negligence.

Legal responsibilities of hospital authorities, staff and patients

The legal responsibilities of hospital authorities and staff, visitors and patients depend upon the application of general common law principles and some statute law to the particular circumstances of each case.

Under the Occupiers Liability Act (1957), hospital authorities must provide safe premises, so that if patients are admitted to wards or hospitals where there is a known outbreak of infection, the hospital authorities might be made responsible for the death of a patient or for injury suffered by a patient as a result of such infection. Nursing and medical staff, therefore, have a duty to report such infection at the earliest possible opportunity when it is discovered, and the ICD or Team must decide immediately what steps should be taken to prevent a spread of the infection. There is a further duty of the hospital authorities to ensure that no staff are employed at the hospital who may transmit serious infection to others. If it becomes known to the hospital authorities that a particular member of staff is a carrier of organisms that may cause a dangerous infectious disease, then the hospital authorities must take steps either to terminate that person's employment (if appropriate) or to deploy him or her where there is minimal risk of infection to other members of staff or to patients. These restrictions must not be applied in the case of less dangerous organisms (e.g. *Staphylococcus aureus*), which are often carried by healthy persons. However, special precautions should be taken when these apparently less dangerous organisms cause an outbreak of clinical infection, but routine screening for symptomless carriers is not usually recommended.

In the case of tuberculosis, tuberculin testing of staff should be carried out routinely and BCG (bacille Calmette–Guérin) should be given if necessary when there is a possibility of nursing and other staff coming into contact with patients suffering from the disease. If this is not done, the hospital may be sued by a nurse or other member of staff who contracts tuberculosis, on the grounds that the hospital is not providing a safe system of work. Immunization against hepatitis B should similarly be offered to all staff involved with the use of invasive procedures or the handling of materials contaminated with blood or body fluids. Immunization against other diseases which can be prevented in this way should, in some circumstances, be offered.

A patient in a hospital cannot be held liable either for introducing infection or for spreading it in the hospital, but it is clear that the hospital authorities must take care, by all reasonable precautions, including some kind of isolation if necessary, to prevent the spread of infection. Similarly, a claim against the hospital authorities in respect of infection caused by a member of the hospital staff, either to another member of the staff or to a patient or visitor, would only be likely to succeed if the hospital had known (or should have known) about it and had failed to take any appropriate action.

If it is known that a visitor is suffering from an infection that he or she is likely to communicate to hospital staff or patients, there might be a responsibility upon the hospital to stop the visiting, but the hospital authorities cannot really be held responsible for every infection which may be either caused or spread by a visitor. A hospital authority can be, and has been, held legally responsible when a patient was discharged from a hospital suffering from a specific infectious disease that he subsequently communicated to another person. In that case it was held there was negligence on the part of the hospital authorities in discharging someone into the community who was likely to infect other members of that community. Such a patient should have been kept in hospital and isolated until he was judged to be no longer infectious (see section on balance of risks on p. **31**).

When a patient becomes infected through some error in aseptic techniques or hospital hygiene, the hospital authorities may be held responsible. For example, if it could be demonstrated that it was the accepted practice to sterilize certain containers (e.g. of saline solutions) and the hospital fails to sterilize and maintain sterility of the fluid in the bottle before distribution to patients, then the hospital authorities may be held liable if contamination of the fluid has taken place at any time before it is actually used. On the other hand, if a practice is not universally adopted (e.g. provision of 'ultraclean' air systems for total hip replacement operations) and the hip becomes infected, it could be argued that the hospital authorities should not be liable, as their failure to provide such an enclosure (if antibiotic prophylaxis was used) did not constitute a failure to provide a reasonable standard of care in the treatment of the patient in accordance with current practice in this country.

Health and Safety at Work Act (1974)

Under this Act responsibilities are placed upon health authorities to provide and maintain plant and systems of work that are, so far as is reasonably practicable, safe and without risks to the health of employees and to arrange to ensure, as far as is reasonably practicable, safety and absence of risks to health of employees in connection with the use, handling, storage and transport of articles and substances. Safety representatives may be appointed by staff and, if staff require this, hospital authorities must establish safety committees under the Safety Representatives and Safety Committees Regulations (1977). If this has not been done, it should be undertaken immediately, as there are additional responsibilities on Health Authorities under the Act towards patients so that they are not exposed to risks to their health and safety. The Department of Health and Social Security Act (1974) circular HC(78)30 states that, in view of the liabilities imposed by the Act on health authorities and their employees, each authority should establish a general structure of responsibility which makes it clear who is responsible for the discharge of particular aspects of the general duties imposed by the Act. It also sets out the responsibilities of management to have advisers and safety officers for specialist departments, safety liaison officers and, where staff require them, safety committees.

Control of Substances Hazardous to Health (COSHH) Regulations (1988)

These regulations have been in force since October 1989 and introduce a framework for controlling exposure of personnel to hazardous substances arising from work activity (Department of Health, 1989a; Harrison, 1991). It includes micro-organisms as well as toxic substances. The employer is responsible for assessing the health risks created by the work, and the substance, and the measures required to protect the health of the workers. These regulations are particularly relevant to infection control staff, and are likely to involve such hazards as glutaraldehyde in endoscopy units, ethylene oxide sterilizers in the SSD, disinfectants and detergents, transport of laboratory specimens, and protection of staff against bloodborne infection, tuberculosis and Legionnaire's disease. The regulations will obviously have a major application in hospital laboratories. Most hospitals will already have guidelines for the control of infection which should be adequate for the regulations involving infection in the clinical units, but there is a continual need for risk assessments.

European regulations and medical devices

At present, European regulations do not usually directly involve the clinical aspects of control of infection, but they may cover some associated aspects, such as consumer safety, environmental hygiene, medical devices, tests for disinfection and sterilization, pharmaceuticals, use of toxic agents and laboratory diagnostic tests. European regulations are issued in the form of Directives. A European Council Directive must be incorporated into the national legislation of all countries in the European Community within a defined period of time. The Directives provide a framework only and, if met, products can be identified with a CE mark that allows them to be sold throughout the European Community.

The Directives are expanded into standards produced by Comité Européen de Normalisation (CEN). Member countries of CEN are bound to comply with CEN/CENELEC International Regulations, which stipulate conditions for giving the standard the status of a national standard. A CEN standard in the UK replaces the national standard (i.e. British Standard). The CEN standard would usually have to be met for a manufacturer to use the CE mark, although a different but equivalent standard could still meet the requirements of the European Directive. The effects of these standard requirements in individual hospitals often remain unclear. Sterile services departments are technically manufacturers, but do not usually 'sell' their products to their own hospital, and would not require a CE mark. However, if they 'sell' products to another hospital Trust or general practitioner, they will have to meet the requirements of the Directive (Medical Devices Directive 93/42/EEC) and obtain a CE mark for these products (Medical Devices Agency, 1999; see also SSDs, Chapter 4). The Directive does not apply to other hospitals or health centres in the same Trust, but nevertheless every effort should be made by processing departments to reach the standards of *Good Manufacturing Practice* or its replacement European Guidance documents for all sterile products. However, this may not be possible, or even necessary, in small health centres or doctors' surgeries, carrying out their own processing of basic surgical instruments, provided that the procedures are safe. It is important that drafts of European standards are widely distributed for comment, so that problems, which are often peculiar to individual countries, can be detected at an early stage. Whenever possible, recommendations in standards should be based on evidence of effectiveness as discussed for national guidelines.

The European Community Directive on liability for unsafe products resulted in the Consumer Protection Act 1987 in the UK. Under this Act, a supplier of goods, including dressings, drugs, devices or servicing contractor, can be sued for negligence if a patient dies or suffers a personal injury from the item concerned. This applies to a hospital reprocessing a reusable item which is not legally covered by the Medical Devices Directive, or reprocessing an item labelled 'single-use'. Legal liability is transferred from the manufacturer to the hospital if an item labelled 'single-use' is reprocessed, but the responsibility for safe reprocessing is the same for the hospital as for any reusable item. However, an item marked 'single-use' would require particular care if it was reprocessed, as in some instances there may be a genuine reason for the 'single-use' label. The decision to reprocess single-use items should be taken by a hospital Devices Assessment Group (Central Sterilizing Club, 1999), and the requirements of the Medical Devices Agency (2006) should be followed. The manufacturer of a reusable item is responsible for providing instructions on reprocessing that are effective and that do not affect the performance of the device (Medical Devices Agency, 1999). The legal liability remains complex.

Medical negligence

Patients now have a greater expectation from treatment than previously, and are often unwilling to accept any risk at all from medical procedures or treatment. Media publicity (e.g. articles on 'superbugs') may influence their actions and therefore increase their willingness to make claims. It is important that patients are informed of risks prior to treatment (e.g. that wound infection rates are normally 5–10 per cent, depending on the operation, and that an operation always carries some risk).

Medical negligence is dealt with in the civil courts, unless the degree of negligence amounts to a criminal offence and the standard of proof depends on the balance of probabilities (i.e. whether it is more likely that there was negligence which caused a particular injury).

To demonstrate negligence, proof of all of the following must be obtained:

- the practitioner (doctor, nurse or other healthcare worker) owed the patient a *duty of care*;
- the defendant was negligent by breaching that duty of care and the plaintiff *suffered an injury*;
- the negligence actually *caused* the injury.

The standard of care required is the duty to exercise reasonable skill and care in the treatment of a patient. The standard of reasonable skill would be that of a competent practitioner in that speciality, for example, an ICD (consultant microbiologist) would be expected to exercise greater skills in the management of an infection control problem than a junior doctor.

Negligence is usually due to the following:

• outdated knowledge and skills;
• failure to adopt safety measures that are known to be necessary.

It is not always necessary to follow national guidelines (Hurwitz, 1995, 1999; NHS Executive, 1996; British Medical Association, 1997). In the Bolam case, it was stated:

> that a doctor is not guilty of negligence if he has acted in accordance with a practice accepted as proper by a responsible body of opinion of medical men skilled in that particular art; a doctor is not negligent if he is acting in accordance with such a practice merely because there is body of opinion that takes a contrary view.

However, the opinion held by a responsible body must be a logical one.

In the UK it is a requirement of the Health Act 2006 to have appropriate policies (ideally based on national guidance). Even where the existence of such policies is not a legal requirement, it is advisable to have them collated either electronically or in paper form, and to follow these wherever possible. It is also important to ensure that all relevant comments and recommendations are written in the patients' and ward records; for example, doses of antibiotics and times of starting and completing courses of treatment, or measures taken in a ward to combat a methicillin-resistant *Staphylococcus aureus* (MRSA) outbreak if the patient becomes infected or colonized with MRSA. The procedures introduced for the infected patient (e.g. isolation, nasal or skin treatment) should be written in the patient's records.

RISK ASSESSMENT AND MANAGEMENT

Balance of risks

Assessment of risk of spread should be based as far as possible on scientific evidence. A source, a route of spread and a portal of entry of sufficient numbers of organisms to a susceptible host are required for an infection to occur. If these conditions are not met, spread is not possible. For example, a surgical dressing from a patient with a human immunodeficiency virus (HIV) infection is not a risk if it is sealed in a plastic bag or handled with gloves. If the HIV seropositive rate in a hospital is low (e.g. 0.1 per cent), the risk of acquiring infection is extremely low. Only 0.4 per cent of personnel who receive a needlestick injury from a known HIV-infected person will acquire infection, and even less from exposure of mucous membrane or skin.

Measures to control infection can be expensive and time-wasting for staff and patients, and should not be introduced unless evidence of their potential value is available or there is consensus agreement by experts.

The application of the Health and Safety at Work Act to infection in hospitals may create problems that are not present in factories or in the general community. The interpretation of the Act in terms of infection in patients is sometimes uncertain, as it is not intended to interfere with the clinical responsibility of medical or nursing staff. The interpretation 'as far as is reasonably practicable' is difficult to define. Hospitals are establishments for treating sick people, many of whom are admitted with an existing infection or will acquire an infection during their stay. The diagnosis of an infection may take several days, and non-infective conditions can closely mimic infection. Susceptibility of the patient and techniques of treatment are important factors in the emergence of infection. Most hospital infections are unlikely to be transferred to staff, and the incidence of acquired infection in staff is usually very low (if the common upper respiratory infections are excluded). Although every effort is made to minimize risks, staff should accept that a high standard of personal hygiene is necessary, and they must also acknowledge that there is some risk of acquiring an infection during the course of their normal duties.

It is important that infected patients, irrespective of the infection (e.g. acquired immunodeficiency syndrome; AIDS), receive the best possible treatment and that this is not impaired because of their infection. The spread of infection between patients and staff cannot be eliminated, but it can be reduced by simple methods such as handwashing. Expensive measures involving uneconomic use of staff and resources may in fact achieve little more than do these simple basic measures. All grades of hospital staff are responsible for adopting measures to reduce the likelihood of spread of infection, and this personal responsibility cannot necessarily be passed on to the employing authority. Some departments (e.g. intensive care or isolation units) may be potentially more hazardous to patients and staff than others owing to the types of patient treated and the methods of treatment required. All patients and equipment should be considered to be potentially infective and require a basic standard of care or treatment to prevent transmission of infection.

Special measures may be recommended by infection control staff for known transmissible infections. The increased risks of infection should also be recognized by visitors and, where appropriate, visitors should be made aware of these possible hazards. Decisions on the measures that are required in a particular situation must be made in terms of possible benefit to patients, benefit to the hospital community and the cost of the measures. Cost benefit is obviously not a term to be used lightly when considering infection in patients or staff, but it is unfortunately a necessity. The occasional failure of soundly based, commonly accepted measures is not necessarily due to negligence. Some infections in hospitals are inevitable irrespective of preventative measures, and there is an irreducible minimum (Ayliffe, 1986). If legal or other authorities criticize staff in the absence of well-founded evidence, infection control staff are likely to adopt a defensive approach which is detrimental both to patient care and to the NHS as a whole. Some examples of difficult decisions for infection control staff are described below.

A common problem is the management of a chronic salmonella carrier – either a member of staff or a patient. Person-to-person spread of salmonella is rare except in infant nurseries. The staff carrier can still, with reasonable safety, return to work after the cessation of symptoms provided that he or she does not handle food or drugs, and is conscientious in matters of personal hygiene (Pether and Scott, 1982). A patient can with reasonable safety be sent home or to a long-term care unit while still excreting salmonella if he or she is otherwise fit to be discharged, and provided that suitable instructions about personal hygiene are given. If spread of infection occurs in either of these situations, the hospital could be held legally responsible, but the risk assessed as low and any other course of action would have been unrealistic.

Staphylococcus aureus is the commonest cause of infection of clean operation wounds and it is carried in the noses of 20 per cent of healthy individuals. Most of these strains are sensitive to antibiotics (except usually to penicillin) and rarely cause infection, but strains that cause infections in hospitals are often resistant to several antibiotics, which may include methicillin. Strains of MRSA have been present in hospitals worldwide for many years, and are not usually more virulent than antibiotic-sensitive strains. They are usually resistant to several antibiotics, including the penicillinase-resistant penicillins and cephalosporins, but most infections are still treatable (see Chapter 12). Some strains tend to spread more easily than antibiotic-sensitive strains, but they present little risk to the families and friends of infected patients. Patients are exposed to them in most hospitals, and they are not 'superbugs'. MRSA strains are often present in the noses of patients and staff without causing any symptoms, and they should be treated like any other multi-resistant organism. Efforts to eradicate them from hospitals in most countries have been unsuccessful without considerable use of resources. Although every effort should be made to prevent their spread in high-risk wards (e.g. intensive care), established preventative measures are not always successful (Joint Working Party of the British Society for Antimicrobial Chemotherapy, Hospital Infection Society and Infection Control Nurses Association, 2006; see also Chapter 12). However, full preventative measures may not be cost-effective if many wards are affected (i.e. if MRSA strains are endemic in the hospital). Staff should always make every reasonable effort to prevent the spread of MRSA (and other antibiotic-resistant strains) by handwashing and good hygiene, but the detection and isolation of all symptomless carriers in general hospital wards is rarely cost-effective or realistic, and failure to achieve this does not constitute negligence by the hospital. The acquisition of MRSA is one of the risks taken by patients in hospital today, and should be explained to all patients on admission. It should also be explained to the relatives of patients infected with MRSA.

Another of the major risk decisions is the deployment of staff carriers of hepatitis B or C virus, and HIV (see Chapter 9). The incidence of carriage is generally low and transmission is rare, so routine screening of staff is therefore not indicated. However, carriers of hepatitis B e antigen (HBeAg) have transmitted infection when performing certain invasive procedures, but risks of transfer from a hepatitis B surface antigen (HBsAg) carrier are very low, and the carrier who is e-antigen negative should be able to continue with normal work. The direct transmission of HIV infection from an infected health service staff member during a procedure has not been reported in the UK, and infected health staff members should also be able to continue with normal work. These low risks may still be unacceptable to the public, and patients might expect to be informed and to make their own choice. It is therefore important that the staff carrier receives impartial advice on these problems in line with national guidelines (e.g. UK Health Departments, 1998).

Routine screening of staff involves keeping them unnecessarily off duty without evidence that the organisms they are carrying are likely to infect others. A large proportion of the staff will, if screened, be found to carry *Staphylococcus aureus* in their noses, and a much smaller proportion may be found to carry Group A/β-haemolytic streptococci in the throat or salmonella in the faeces. However, most of them are unlikely to cause clinical infection in patients with whom they have contact.

The inanimate environment is not a major factor in the spread of infection, and structural alterations can be costly. Care should be taken not to embark on expensive structural changes on the basis of infection hazard because of an apparent requirement in a guidance document, rather than on the basis of evidence of efficacy in the prevention of infection. A good selective surveillance system is likely to be more cost effective in the prevention of infection than routine environmental monitoring, or routine screening of the faeces of catering staff or the noses of theatre staff. Routine monitoring of air or surfaces in operating-theatres, pharmacies or SSD clean rooms is an example of a test method which is not related to the risk of infection.

The risks of acquiring an infection caused by a spore-bearing organism from a properly cleaned and disinfected operative endoscope are small, despite the fact that spores are not killed by routine disinfection processes. Disinfection should therefore be considered a reasonable process even if a case of tetanus has occurred, as a chemical 'sterilization' process (e.g. exposure to glutaraldehyde for 3–10 hours) is not a practical possibility for routine decontamination, and in itself may pose an unnecessarily high risk to the healthcare worker who would be exposed to higher levels of the substance.

Risk management

Risk management is described as a practical approach to prevention of the possibility of incurring risk (incurring misfortune or loss). Within the context of the NHS, this is reflected in the management of potential financial loss, personal injury, loss of life, staff availability, buildings, equipment and reputation.

Risk management requires consideration of the activities of the organization by, for example:

• identifying the risks that exist;
• assessing their potential frequency and severity;
• eliminating risks if possible;
• reducing the risks that cannot be eliminated and putting in place financial mechanisms to absorb the financial consequences of the risks that remain.

The NHS Management Executive (Department of Health, 1993) have stated that effective infection control is vital for the successful operation of all healthcare premises, and discusses the following four specific sections:

• organization, policies and information;
• training and awareness;
• food;
• separating 'clean' and 'dirty' matter.

It includes the following action points:

• Policies and procedures for infection control must be known to all staff.
• Staff must be aware of whom they should approach for advice on infection control issues.
• All staff should receive appropriate training on infection control.
• All staff should be made aware of the importance of good hygiene in the handling and storage of food.
• There should be clear guidance to staff on the separation of clean and dirty materials and adequate facilities to put this into practice.

Although the above requirements are important, the main infection risks involve the management of patients, which often requires balancing risks against necessary treatment.

QUALITY, AND CLINICAL AND INFECTION CONTROL AUDIT

Since the introduction of the NHS, the need to provide a high-quality, cost-effective service has been evident. Measurements of quality in healthcare provision are still evolving. Today, in pursuit of quality, healthcare organizations are actively encouraged to monitor and critically evaluate the practices and resources used, through audit and resource management (Baggot, 1994). This has resulted in purchasing or commissioning authorities stipulating predetermined or negotiated standards of service. Providers, as part of the contractual process for patient services, should, in response to internal standard-setting, adhere to agreed quality standards. The adoption and internalization of the audit process should be viewed as essential activities in providing a quality service.

Independent bodies such as the National Audit Office (1986), the British Standards Institute, the Healthcare Commission and the King's Fund Centre all have reputations as experts in the audit of healthcare systems. British Standards are used throughout the UK as markers of quality, and many of them are being replaced by European Standards. Within healthcare organizations, particularly infection control, the British Standards Institute is recognized in several areas, including the disposal of sharps, and medical electrical equipment and sterilizers. The standards on infection control in hospitals produced for national organizations have been discussed above (see p. 25).

The King's Fund Organization Audit (KFOA) aims to stimulate good practice and innovations in healthcare management through service and organizational development, education, policy analysis and organizational audit (King's Fund Centre, 1988). The Organizational Audit project was launched in 1989, one week prior to the Government's White Paper entitled *Working for Patients* (Department of Health, 1989b), to determine whether a national approach to standard-setting in healthcare was appropriate. Although we have seen a change of government and the introduction of a new White Paper, *The New NHS: Modern, Dependable* (Department of Health, 1997), the focus is still on quality, with government directives aimed at providing a high-quality service for patients. The setting of 'National Standards of Excellence' and the introduction of 'Clinical Governance' is aimed at providing new incentives and imposing new sanctions on healthcare organizations to improve quality and efficiency whilst also defining clear boundaries of responsibility.

'Clinical governance' is a term which encompasses many of the fundamental elements used to improve quality (Department of Health, 1999). The principles behind clinical governance can be seen as a tool by which infection control teams provide a quality-led service to the patient, since many of the principles of clinical governance, such as 'evidence-based practice', audit and risk assessment, are essentially those already underpinning the role of Infection Control Teams.

For decades the aim of ICTs has been to provide a service which is based on good-quality practices and employs credible surveillance systems. Audit tools have been devised and used in various guises both to identify problem areas and to provide evidence for improvement of practice (Millward et al., 1993; Ward, 1995). The audit tool described by Millward and colleagues assesses compliance with infection control practice against specified standards which embody the basic principles of infection control. This tool has been used widely and effectively as a benchmark for good practice, enabling ICTs to identify and focus on problem areas. However, although audit tools are a valuable means of monitoring quality, Mehtar (1995) suggests that for surveillance to be effective it needs to be relevant, with findings relayed back to all personnel. Both Millward *et al.* (1993) and Ward (1995) reinforce this view, stating that audit tools should have a strong educational element.

In an attempt to improve quality and provide an efficient, cost-effective service, ICTs involved in clinical audit should be concerned with the processes which are likely to influence the acquisition of infection. The use and monitoring of infection control practices is an obvious requirement for the prevention and control of infection. However, although monitoring infection rates throughout the hospital is regarded by many as a means of audit, it is not generally perceived as practicable or necessarily cost-effective, as many variables exist (e.g. length of stay, type of operation and associated risk factors), which have the potential to introduce bias and impair the accuracy of data (see Chapter 3).

With the increasing demand for ICTs to produce data, especially on infection rates, there should be clear predefined aims and objectives with regard to the value and use of the audit data. To ensure accurate collection and analysis of data, the approach needs to be logical and consistent to enable standardization of results. Equally, when information is formalized, it is essential that all the relevant data collated include any complications within the clinical audit. However, because of the potential inconsistencies, it would be more appropriate if the data presented by infection control teams focused on specific elements such as infections in high-risk or other targeted areas, isolation of alert organisms and efficiency measures taken to control infections (see Chapter 3). Equally, for ICTs to disseminate the knowledge gained, they should participate in internal audit sessions to gain an insight into other practices being undertaken across healthcare organizations which have infection control implications.

When assessing the need for audit, it is important to take other influences into consideration. A report from the House of Lords focuses awareness on the emergence of multi-resistant organisms, highlighting the need for ICTs to audit antibiotic usage within Trusts, with a view to controlling the dispensing of inappropriate antibiotics (Select Committee on Science and Technology Report, House of Lords, 1998).

Information technology should be used as a tool to implement audit. The UK Government White Paper entitled *Information for Health* (Department of Health, 1998) aims to improve communication between hospitals and the community by forming strong computer links. If ICTs are engaging in audit, the links between hospitals and the community should be fully utilized in order to enable more accurate collection of data (e.g. the computerization of patient records and results and post-discharge complications such as wound infections). However, it is essential that, prior to the input of data, there are clearly defined criteria in place to allow standardization of results (see Chapter 3).

The following audit procedures should therefore be considered by the ICT:

- surveillance of infections (see Chapter 3);
- measurement of compliance with infection control policies and practices (e.g. handwashing, clinical practices, the environment, sharps safety and clinical waste). (These assessments should both allow identification of areas with good practice and target areas for improvement, enabling the ICNs to focus on problem areas. The ICT's involvement in the audit of policies and practice should be structured and concerned with processes likely to influence the acquisition of infection and not irrelevant testing, such as routine air-sampling of operating-theatres and SSD clean rooms.)
- taking part in audits of departments with an infection component, e.g. laundries, SSDs and catering establishments;
- attendance at clinical audit sessions on a regular basis to discuss infections with clinicians;
- audit of the ICT's own techniques (e.g. speed of response and efficacy of control of an outbreak).

NOTIFICATION OF INFECTIOUS DISEASES

Some diseases are notifiable by law to the CCDC. The doctor who diagnoses the infection is responsible for the notification. Although there is no statutory obligation to notify the detection of symptom-free carriers of bacteria that cause notifiable disease, it is recommended that persistent carriers of typhoid bacilli and other salmonellae should be reported to the CCDC.

REFERENCES

Act of Parliament (1988) *Control of Substances Hazardous to Health Regulations.* London: HMSO.

Ayliffe GAJ (1986) Nosocomial infection and the irreducible minimum. *Infection Control* 7(Suppl), 92.

Baggot R (1994) *Health and healthcare in Britain.* London: St Martin's Press.

British Medical Association (1997) Medical decisions must be logically defensible. *British Medical Journal* 315, 1327.

Central Sterilizing Club (1999) Reprocessing of single-use medical devices in hospitals. *Zentral Sterilization* 7, 37.

Damani NM (1997) *Hospital infection control.* London: Greenwich Medical Media Ltd.

Department of Health (1989a) *The control of substances hazardous to health: guidance for the initial assessment in hospitals.* London: HMSO.

Department of Health (1989b) *Working for patients. Medical audit.* Working paper no. 6. London: HMSO.

Department of Health (1993) *Risk management in the NHS.* London: Health Publications Unit.

Department of Health (1995) *Hospital infection control. Guidance on the control of infection in hospitals.* Paper prepared by the Hospital Infection Working Group of the Department of Health Public Health Laboratory Service. London: Department of Health and HMSO.

Department of Health (1997) *The new NHS: modern, dependable.* London: HMSO.

Department of Health (1998) *Information for Health.* London: HMSO.

Department of Health (1999) *Clinical governance: quality in the new NHS.* London: Department of Health.

Department of Health (2006) *The Health Act: code of practice for the prevention and control of health care associated infections.* London: Department of Health.

Garner JS (1996) Guidelines for isolation precautions in hospitals. *Infection Control and Hospital Epidemiology* **17**, 53.

Haley RW, Culver DH, White JW *et al.* (1985) The efficacy of infection surveillance and control programs in preventing nosocomial infection in US hospitals. *American Journal of Epidemiology* **121**, 182.

Harrison DI. (1991) Control of substances hazardous to health (COSHH). Regulations and hospital infection. *Journal of Hospital Infection* **17**(Suppl A), 530.

Hurwitz B (1995) Clinical guidelines and the law. What is the status of guidelines? *British Medical Journal* **311**, 1517.

Hurwitz B (1999) Legal and practical considerations of clinical practice guidelines. *British Medical Journal* **318**, 661.

Infection Control Working Party (1993) *Standards in infection control in hospitals,* London: HMSO.

Joint Working Party of the British Society for Antimicrobial Chemotherapy, Hospital Infection Society and Infection Control Nurses Association (2006) Guidelines for the control and prevention of methicillin-resistant *Staphylococcus aureus* (MRSA) in healthcare facilities. *Journal of Hospital Infection* **63S**, S1–S44.

King's Fund Centre (1988) *Health services accreditation.* London: Kings Fund.

Medical Devices Agency (1999) *Guidance on decontamination from the Microbiological Advisory Committee. Part 3. Procedures. Section 1.* London: Department of Health.

Mehtar S (1995) Infection control programmes – are they cost-effective? *Journal of Hospital Infection* **30**(Suppl), 26.

Millward S, Barnett J and Thomlinson D (1993) A clinical infection control audit programme: evaluation of an audit tool used by infection control nurses to monitor standards and assess effective staff training. *Journal of Hospital Infection* **24**, 219.

National Audit Office (1986) *Value for money: developments in the NHS.* London: HMSO.

NHS Executive (1996) *Clinical guidelines.* London: Department of Health.

Pether JVS and Scott RJD (1982) Salmonella carriers. Are they dangerous? Study to identify finger contamination with salmonella by convalescent carriers. *Journal of Infection* **5**, 81.

Select Committee on Science and Technology Report, House of Lords (1998) *Resistance to antibiotics and other antimicrobial agents.* London: HMSO.

United Kingdom Central Council for Nursing, Midwifery and Health Visiting (UKCC) (1995) *Post-registration education and practice (PREP).* London: UKCC.

UK Health Departments (1998) *Guidance for Clinical Health Care Workers: protection against infection with blood-borne viruses.* London: Department of Health.

Ward KA (1995) Education and infection control audit. *Journal of Hospital Infection.* **30**(Suppl), 248.

Ward V, Wilson J, Taylor L *et al.* (1997) Preventing hospital-acquired infection. *Clinical guidelines.* London: Public Health Laboratory Service.

Williams REO, Blowers R, Garrod LP and Shooter RA (1966) *Hospital infection: causes and prevention,* 2nd edn. London: Lloyd Luke.

3 SURVEILLANCE, AUDIT, RECORDS AND REPORTS

Peter Wilson

SURVEILLANCE

The definition of surveillance in the context of healthcare-associated infection is the ongoing systematic collection and analysis of data about a disease (or organism) that can lead to *action being taken* to control or prevent the disease.

The role of surveillance

The first step towards solving a problem is recognizing it, and surveillance provides this first step. Surveillance will then be beneficial in the following ways.

- It can indicate when there is a change in the pattern of disease providing an alert at the earliest opportunity of the existence of an (impending) outbreak, and/or identify the appearance and spread of a virulent organism.
- The database can be used to observe and judge the efficacy of measures taken to control the spread of an outbreak.
- The efficacy of the routine/regular measures used in infection control can be observed and judged.
- The planning process (whether architectural/structural design or planning the use/allocation of resources) can be supported.
- The effects of targeted measures on the rates of avoidable infection, possibly by the introduction of selective measures can be monitored.
- It will reduce nosocomial (hospital acquired) infection rates.

In the UK, it is recognised that surveillance is underdeveloped and under-utilized. That surveillance is a vital component of infection control has been recognized in the scientific community (Haley, 1995). Four components to a successful infection control programme have been described:

- surveillance (including feedback to the clinical staff);
- control/monitoring/auditing of practice;
- having an Infection Control Nurse (ICN) in post to deal with the surveillance and control;
- having in post a physician/microbiologist actively involved in the programme.

A very large project (The SENIC Project; Haley *et al.*, 1980) was set up to evaluate the implementation of Infection Surveillance and Control

Programmes by seeing their effect on nosocomial infections. This project was a nationwide study across the USA involving initially 6586 hospitals. They reported that at least 2.1 million nosocomial infections occurred annually among 37.7 million admissions in US hospitals, and considered 77 000 deaths to be associated with nosocomial infections. They also showed that the rates of infection in their hospitals could be *reduced* by 32 per cent by intensive surveillance programmes (Haley *et al.*, 1985). This reduced the rates of nosocomial urinary tract infection, surgical wound infection, pneumonia and bacteraemia. They also demonstrated that hospitals without effective programmes had *increases* in their infection rates. From Table 3.1 it can be seen that, in every case, surveillance provides the foundation for infection control, and it can achieve improvements of between 15 and 38 per cent.

Table 3.1 Percentage of nosocomial infections prevented by the most effective surveillance and control programmes (Haley *et al.*, 1985)

Type of infection	Components of the most effective programmes	% prevented
Surgical wound infection (SWI)	An organized hospital-wide programme with: intensive surveillance and control reporting SWI rates to surgeons plus an effective physician with special interest in infection control	20 35
Urinary tract infection	An organized hospital-wide programme with: intensive surveillance in operation for at least a year one full-time equivalent Infection Control Nurse (ICN) per 250 beds	38
Nosocomial bacteraemia	An organized hospital-wide programme with: intensive control alone plus: moderately intensive surveillance in operation for at least a year one full time equivalent ICN per 250 beds an infection control physician/microbiologist	15 35

The importance of surveillance has also been recognized by various government departments. In the words of the Chief Medical Officer of the Department of Health for England (Department of Health, 2000):

Good surveillance is the cornerstone of a system to control infectious diseases in the population. Without it, tracking disease trends, identifying new infectious disease threats, designing effective vaccines, spotting serious outbreaks and monitoring control measures would all be impossible.

Types of surveillance

Laboratory based

This is usually simple and straightforward to set up and is based on the provision of information based around 'alert' organisms. The 'alert' organisms are those which are likely to be of interest to the Infection Control Team (ICT), in other words those that have the potential to cause outbreaks. The list should be flexible and should be able to reflect local needs (e.g. particular resistance problems). A laboratory system alone is valuable but will need supporting information from the wards (e.g. a patient admitted with meningitis). The types of organism that are 'alert' organisms fall into different categories (see Box 3.1).

Box 3.1 Surveillance information for the Infection Control Team

ALERT ORGANISMS

- *Community-acquired alert organisms:* particularly pathogenic organisms (e.g. salmonella, *Shigella, Mycobacterium tuberculosis, Neisseria meningitidis, Streptococcus pyogenes,* etc.)
- *Hospital-acquired alert organisms:* generally those organisms that have resistance to a range of antibiotics and are capable of spreading (e.g. methicillin-resistant *Staphylococcus aureus,* Gram-negative rods resistant to gentamicin, extended-spectrum beta-lactamases, glycopeptide-resistant enterococci, etc.)
- *Positive clinical isolates from sterile sites* (e.g. isolates from blood culture, cerebrospinal fluid, etc.)
- *All positive clinical isolates from high-risk areas* (intensive care unit, special care baby unit, etc.)
- *Alert organism-positive patients:* all results from being identified as an alert-positive patient onwards
- *Positive clinical isolates from sites of interest to the infection control team:* (e.g. catheter-related infections [urinary and intravascular], operative samples [removed prostheses – heart valves, artificial joints, etc.])

An example of a daily report generated by the laboratory for the ICT is shown in Table 3.2.

The laboratory-based system will be able to give information such as the percentage of *Staphylococcus aureus* that are methicillin resistant and/or the percentage of wound swabs showing *S. aureus,* but it falls short of the more significant information of how many methicillin-resistant *Staphylococcus aureus* (MRSA) wound infections per 1000 bed days or per 1000 admissions. It is important to have access to clinical information (in particular the working diagnoses) as well as administrative information, such as knowing the bed number

Table 3.2 Example of a daily laboratory surveillance report (for the 5th April). The names used in the table are entirely fictional

Organism	Antibiogram	Patient	CNN	Date of birth	M/F	Sample	Date of sample	Ward	Consultant
S. aureus	**R** p,t,e	J Smith	376493	25/05/1935	M	N/swab	2 April	B	Iles
S. aureus (MRSA)	**R** p,t,e,f,m	F Silk	331675	01/03/1940	M	N/swab	2 April	B	Ramasammy
Grp A Strep	Fully sens	H Patel	834322	21/09/1923	F	W/swab	3 April	T	Littlejohns
S. typhi	**R** a, chlor, **S** ctrx cip	R Ali	887905	18/03/1957	M	Blood	3 April	D	Joans
Pneumo	**S** p	N Eydman	537690	04/10/1935	M	CSF	4 April	C	Littlejohns
Acinetobacter	**S** mer, col, tig	F Saddler	102039	30/12/1925	F	Swab	2 April	ITU	Defreighter

the patient is admitted to, so that if they acquire an infection from the bed next to them, there is a record. This information may be needed when an outbreak occurs and/or for medico-legal reasons. A link to the hospital patient administration computer system is therefore vital, so that this additional clinical information can be acquired. This additional information may be on an individual patient, or the data become useful for collation into local, regional or national databases, thus benefiting national surveillance.

Local data must include 'details' of wards and consultants. This is essential for the 'ownership' of the data, as well as the competitive element that is introduced by the inclusion of such data. The data need to be analysed promptly and sent to the ward/clinician as a weekly report, and must have local credibility. The responsibility for infection control is ultimately with the clinical staff and the way they carry out their clinical duties. Figure 3.1 shows the cycle of surveillance and demonstrates that surveillance is an ongoing process.

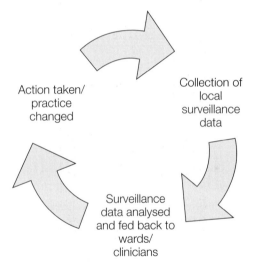

Action taken/
practice
changed

Collection of
local
surveillance
data

Surveillance
data analysed
and fed back to
wards/
clinicians

Figure 3.1 The surveillance cycle.

Post-discharge surveillance

This is an important area that so far has received inadequate support and attention. At least half and possibly as many as 70 per cent of surgical wound infections do not show themselves until after discharge from hospital (Reilly *et al.*, 2006). As hospital stays become shorter, this figure is under constant pressure to increase. The appearance of an infection after discharge does not mean that the infection was acquired at home. In particular, the more prosthetic items are inserted by surgeons, the more infections reveal themselves even years after the original surgery. This is often related to low-grade pathogens such as coagulase-negative staphylococci, which are probably introduced at the time of the operation, but 'hide' on the prosthesis for extended periods without apparently doing any harm, only eventually showing the destruction of which they are capable.

To complete this section of the surveillance is important but labour intensive. Extra staff may be required to facilitate this service. The data can be collated from various sources, for example:

- community nurses;
- general practitioners;
- the patient;
- outpatient clinics;
- telephones.

Targeted surveillance

This is surveillance that provides data that are not routinely captured. It focuses on a particular issue by case mix, by ward or unit or by site of infection. It will often take place in response to a particular problem, or a desire to know more about a particular issue.

Sentinel surveillance

This is surveillance by a specialized small group of people, which captures sufficient data to create meaningful collections (e.g. genitourinary clinics for sexually transmissible diseases, or neurologists for Creutzfeldt–Jakob disease).

Surveillance of staff

This is generally the domain of the Occupational Health Department, but there may be the occasional situation where the immunity status of staff needs to be checked, or where the MRSA status of a group of staff needs to be ascertained. If staff need to be removed from duty, they are considered 'off duty for medical reasons' rather than 'off sick'. Occasionally, members of staff will present with chronic skin problems that lead to them becoming chronic carriers and dispersers of staphylococci. Such situations will require referral to the Occupational Health Department and a consultant dermatologist.

Surveillance and resistance

Surveillance is the only way we can gain an understanding of how resistant organisms are spreading, and to what extent they are replacing more sensitive strains. Antimicrobial policies should be informed by local surveillance data. Guidance for the empirical treatment of infections must state the time and place to which it refers; if either of these factors change, the guidance may be different. This can be illustrated by penicillin-resistant pneumococci. At a time when the resistance rate was running at about 1 or 2 per cent nationally, it was running at 11 per cent in one locality (Wilson et al., 1996). Similarly when the national recommendations were to continue using trimethoprim for urinary tract infections, local data indicated an unacceptably high rate of resistance to this drug; thus cephalexin, as judged by local data, was a clear recommendation for first-line treatment.

Linking the surveillance computing system with the pharmacy system can be beneficial for both prescribers and microbiologists:

- for prescribers, it will provide an alert if they prescribe an agent to which there is considerable resistance or that is not in accordance with the local antibiotic policy;
- for microbiologists, it will provide data on prescribing habits.

Surveillance can also be useful for research purposes; for example, a trial on the use of peri-operative mupirocin examined not just the numbers of post-operative infections, but also showed that there was no increase in the rate of mupirocin resistance (Wilcox *et al.*, 2003).

Regional surveillance

Surveillance on a regional basis, summarized and distributed as a weekly report is a useful system. E-mail distribution facilitates this style of report. It can provide alerts as to which diseases to watch out for, or seeks further information (e.g. it informs us about an outbreak of food poisoning at a certain location and asks for other cases to be reported to a responsible individual). It can also act as a reminder of seasonal variations (e.g. mycoplasma) or provide warnings about outbreaks (e.g. multi-drug resistant tuberculosis). Frequent reports (e.g. weekly) ensure that the information is current.

National surveillance

The Health Protection Agency (HPA) in the UK has a role that includes continuous surveillance (sometimes supplemented by snapshot surveys) on a national basis. The HPA manages the mandatory reporting scheme for MRSA bacteraemia, glycopeptide-resistant enterococci and *Clostridium difficile*.

National data are made up from local data in many different Trusts. These data must be comparable if they are to be collated. A recent illustration of this concerns MRSA bacteraemia rates. If some Trusts are submitting data on *all* MRSA-positive blood cultures while others are only providing details if the cultures are hospital acquired, then the collated data become meaningless.

Such surveillance often creates 'league tables', where performances of different Trusts are collated together and compared. These tables frequently provoke discussion and many more questions are raised than have been answered. Nevertheless, the basic trends in the growth and spread of resistant organisms on a national basis have been recorded.

The guidelines for the prophylaxis and treatment of MRSA infections in the UK (Gemmel *et al.*, 2006) are evidence-based guidelines and use the results of surveillance as the basis for their recommendations.

International surveillance

International surveillance, by its very scale and complexity, is difficult to manage and the use of comparable data (as illustrated above) is critical; however, the data generated this way can be very valuable.

Sometimes point prevalence surveys are used, which are repeated at intervals to build up a picture.

Which computer system?

The use of technology rather than a manual system should enable data to be analysed more easily and should be encouraged. Various computer packages are available. These should be compatible with the clinical laboratory system and integrate with the hospital information technology patient management system in order to obtain meaningful data with a minimum of effort.

Outbreaks

Organisms that are indistinguishable from each other may be involved in an outbreak. When the outbreak is first detected, typing of the isolates will not yet be available. However, if they are isolates with the same identification and the same antibiogram, then they should be considered as indistinguishable. If there is a difference in the antibiograms of only one antibiotic, then the organisms can still be considered as indistinguishable. The next task is to establish if and how the isolates are linked in time and space. This is most easily achieved by drawing a time/space bar chart. This can be done by hand, but for clarity of presentation and ease of updating, it is better to use a spreadsheet. A worksheet can be used to represent the 'calendar' of events. Examples of worksheets are illustrated in Figures 3.2–3.4.

It can be seen that patient 1 was admitted to the ward on 6 July, swabbed on 9 July and the results of the swabbing were positive. Patient 2 was admitted to the ward on 11 July, swabbed on 14 July and the results of the swabbing were positive. Patient 3 was admitted to the ward on 12 July, swabbed on 15 July and the results of the swabbing were positive. Patient 1 was transferred from T ward to B ward on 17 July, while still (as far as is known) positive. Patient 1 was re-swabbed on 19 July and the results were negative. Patients 2 and 3 were discharged on 19 July and Patient 1 on 21 July. It can be easily seen that all three patients are linked in time and space while on T ward, and direct transfer of the organism is possible, or indirect via temporary carriage on the hands or via fomites. Patient 1 is the index case. It is also possible for a member of staff to be a carrier, who, when on duty, transmits the organism to a patient.

Figure 3.3 illustrates an 'explosive' outbreak in that many patients suddenly acquire an infection. An example would be when a member of staff, who is a food-handler, is also a carrier of salmonella and, with lapses of hygiene, is able

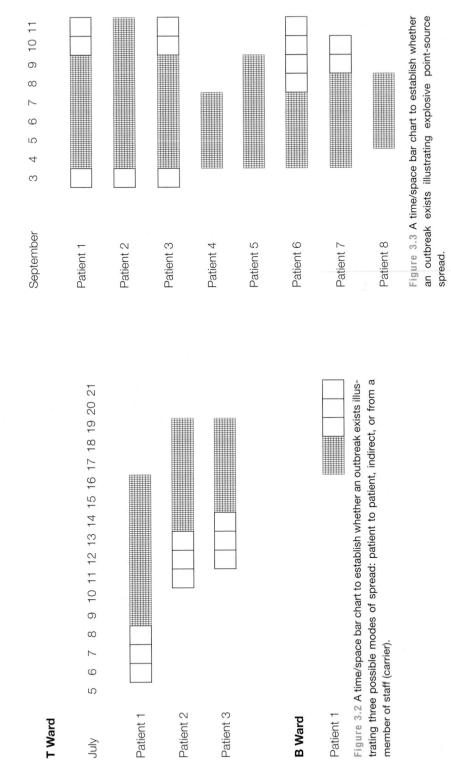

T Ward

July   5   6   7   8   9   10   11   12   13   14   15   16   17   18   19   20   21

Patient 1

Patient 2

Patient 3

B Ward

Patient 1

Figure 3.2 A time/space bar chart to establish whether an outbreak exists illustrating three possible modes of spread: patient to patient, indirect, or from a member of staff (carrier).

T Ward

September   3   4   5   6   7   8   9   10   11

Patient 1

Patient 2

Patient 3

Patient 4

Patient 5

Patient 6

Patient 7

Patient 8

Figure 3.3 A time/space bar chart to establish whether an outbreak exists illustrating explosive point-source spread.

ITU

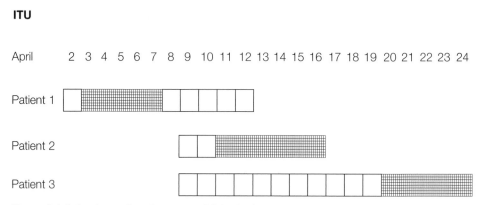

Figure 3.4 A time/space bar chart to establish whether an outbreak exists illustrating persistence in the environment, hence indirect spread.

to infect a number of patients on one ward all at the same time. If this pattern is repeated across the hospital, the point source is likely to be in the kitchens. 'Explosive' outbreaks can occur with Salmonellae, norovirus and *Legionella* when there is a point source that infects many individuals at the same time.

Figure 3.4 illustrates an outbreak where there is survival of the organism in the environment. The index case is Patient 1, and the surveillance system flagged the organism to the ICT because it was a drug-resistant *Acinetobacter baumanii*. The patient had been in the hospital for 3 weeks, had deteriorated and was transferred to the intensive care unit (ICU) on 2 April. The next day, blood cultures were taken; these were positive for the *Acinetobacter*. This organism was also later grown from sputum samples. Treatment was rapidly initiated and he was apparently free of the organism on 8 April. He remained on the ICU until 12 April. On 9 April, a time when Patient 1 is apparently free of *Acinetobacter*, Patient 2 was admitted to ICU from the general wards. An indwelling line removed on 11 April was cultured and grew the same *Acineto-bacter*. The surveillance system flagged this isolate to the attention of the ICT. Survival in the environment enabled Patient 2 to acquire the infection, and likewise Patient 3. Indeed, the patients do not even need to be in the ward at the same time: *Acinetobacter* is capable of surviving for 2 or 3 months, and so quite prolonged periods of the environment being apparently free of the organism (as judged by clinical samples) are possible.

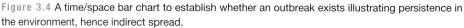

Place of acquisition of post-operative infection

There are times when deducing at what stage the infection was acquired will be helpful in guiding the next steps of the investigation.

Infection acquired in theatres

This will be apparent in the early post-operative period, a maximum of 3 post-operative days. Questions may be asked regarding whether additional patients who have developed post-operative infection have the same surgeon or the same theatre suite in common, as well as whether an organism is indistinguishable from another. Infection is usually present as a deep rather than superficial wound infection.

Infection acquired in the ward

These are usually relatively superficial, occurring more than 3 days after the operation. Questions may be asked concerning other patients on the same ward with the same organism.

It is important to remember that the 'dirtier' the field of surgery, the greater the chances of a post-operative infection. For example, an infection rate of 2 per cent may cause concern in orthopaedics, but an infection rate of 5 per cent may be of no concern in colorectal surgery. Operations can be formally classified as shown in the following.

Types of operation

1 *Clean* (e.g. hernia repair, breast surgery): this is an operation carried out where there is no known apparent risk of infection. It is not carried out in an area where there is any inflammatory reaction or in an area known to be inhabited by bacteria (i.e. not transecting gastrointestinal tract, urinary tract or upper respiratory tract).
2 *Clean/contaminated* (e.g. operation on the gall bladder): bacterial contamination is possible but not overwhelming, and there is no macroscopic evidence of contamination.
3 *Contaminated* (e.g. operations on the colon): bacteria are known to be present and abundant.

An additional category of 'dirty' may also be included when there is macroscopic contamination (e.g. faecal spillage).

AUDIT

What is audit? What to audit

There is enormous scope for audit in infection control. Clinical audit examines the actual situation and compares it to the written policy or other known standard or yardstick/benchmark. The whole point of audit is the improvement of the service because audit provides a blame-free mechanism for changes in practice to occur without any scalp-hunting exercises. The results of the audit should be fed back as soon as possible and any changes made, and then a

re-audit is required to show the improvement (or otherwise; see Figure 3.5).
Audit tools are now commonly referred to as 'quality improvement tools'.

Initially, it is probably worth selecting a small number of areas to audit,
preferably those that are important to the organization and probably better
dealt with 'little and often'. For example, handwashing is probably the most
important issue; it can be audited and all concerned require constant
reminders. A rapid audit cycle plan can be completed in a few days and the
results fed back very rapidly (Figure 3.6).

It is not necessary to audit the whole hospital. If 2 hours are spent collecting
the data for the audit, the results can then be analysed and fed back to the relevant departments. The new data along with the previous results of the same
ward/department, as well as comparisons between wards, can be presented.
Graphs and pictorial representations can be used and praise given when
deserved.

Audit of the environment should usually be carried out in conjunction with
the domestic staff. There is a standard data set which can be used (National
Patient Safety Agency, 2007). Environmental swabs are rarely taken but in
some circumstances they can provide a useful support (e.g. when dealing with
an outbreak of an organism that survives well in the environment). There
may be a benefit in having some audits without the domestic staff on an
'unannounced' basis.

Audits of indwelling lines and urinary catheters should involve discussion
with clinical and nursing staff as well as seeing the patient. The quality of the
documentation will also be subject to audit. This can be improved by providing
a standard format. Repeated quick audits in these areas should generate
improvements, which can be identified in the audits.

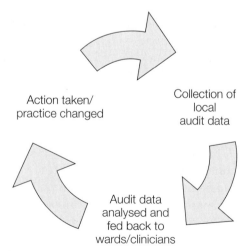

Action taken/
practice changed

Collection of
local
audit data

Audit data
analysed and
fed back to
wards/clinicians

Figure 3.5 The audit cycle.

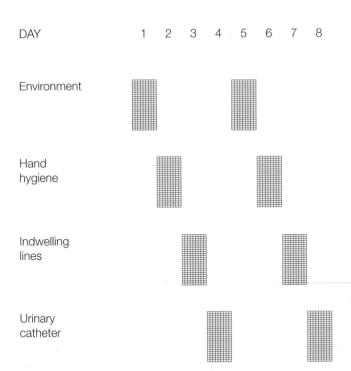

Figure 3.6 A rapid cycle audit plan.

This approach can be modified to local needs. It is a good idea *not* to have a rigid routine, such as hand hygiene on Mondays, indwelling lines on Tuesdays, etc. for the following reasons:

- staff will become used to the idea they only need to perform on a certain day;
- this may result in re-auditing a small number of staff repeatedly, if the staffing rota is also based on a weekly cycle;
- the demands on the staff may vary according to the weekly timetable (e.g. on a surgical ward, there may be three lists on a Thursday, so staff will be very busy on Thursdays).

As well as the rapid cycle plan, an annual plan is also required (Figure 3.7). The results of each audit should be presented on an annual basis. The plan should have enough flexibility to allow for occasional in year 'ad hoc' audits.

The annual audit plan is made up of audits that will not occur very frequently. The plan described allocates a 3-month slot for surgical site infections, which recognizes the extra demands on staff to comply with the mandatory surveillance (e.g. in orthopaedics). Audit of compliance with the MRSA admission screening policy is to be carried out twice during the year. Likewise sharps will be audited twice during the year. All the other topics will receive an audit

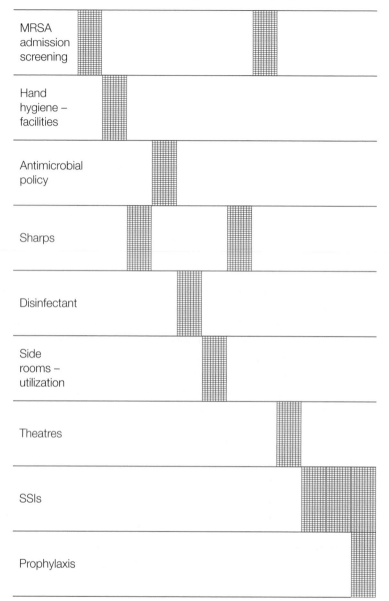

Figure 3.7 An example of an annual audit plan. MRSA, methicillin-resistant *Staphylococcus aureus*; SSI, surgical site infection.

only once. This is with the assumption that the facilities for hand hygiene do not change with great speed, that the antimicrobial policy (and therefore also prophylaxis) receives attention from the microbiology service and so practice is reasonably reflective of the policies, and that theatres and the use of disinfectants are not subject to rapid change. In this example side-room utilization can only be audited once during the year. Since there may be seasonal variation, this single audit may not be adequate.

Why audit?

The principal aim of auditing is to improve the service.

When to audit

Auditing should be carried out at regular intervals and at every opportunity.

How to audit

Areas of good and bad practice should be audited. Even the good areas can be improved. The audits should be reported to the Trust Board in the Annual Report and so it is important that the Trust Board members are given an insight into the priority areas that need improvement as well as the areas that are performing well. If there are some areas that can be audited more than once within the year, then so much the better. It is the second and subsequent audits that will demonstrate improvements (or deterioration). It is important to be clear what is being audited and therefore what data to collect. The value of collecting data just in case it may be of interest is doubtful.

A data collection sheet/check list will be required for each audit so that the approach is standardized. Figure 3.8 shows an example based on national standards of cleanliness to be used when the cleanliness of the environment is being audited (National Patient Safety Agency, 2007).

There may not be readily available 'off the shelf' scoring sheets for everything that needs to be audited but, if such sheets are available, it may be best to use them. Alternatively, it may be necessary to modify an existing score sheet. It is important to consider what the issues are and how they can be measured. The environmental audit sheet given as an example breaks down the environment into its components. Each component can then be scored as satisfactory or not, and the scores can be added up and compared to other areas or can demonstrate changes over time.

RECORDING

Record-keeping and documentation in day-to-day practice

It is important to document all advice at the time it is given. This will avoid the possibility of being misunderstood or mis-recording advice. When giving advice, it is important to obtain the following information:

AUDIT SHEET

Area being audited .... Weighting ....

Auditors .... Audit date ....

Sub-areas audited

Element	Acceptable/ unacceptable	Comments	Action time frame	Action taken Yes	Action taken No
External features, fire exits, stairwells					
Walls, skirtings, ceilings					
Windows					
Doors					
Hard floors					
Soft floors					
Ducts, grills, vents					
Electrical					
Kitchen appliances					
Toilets bathroom					
Furnishings fixtures					
Patient equipment					
Odour control					
General tidiness					
TOTAL SCORE	SCORE%				

Acceptable = 1   Unacceptable = 0   Not applicable = n/a   Signature ....

Figure 3.8 Audit of the environment – cleanliness.

- a clinical summary – the patient's history and examination details;
- significant investigation results;
- a working diagnosis;
- treatment details;
- microbiological findings;
- the advice given with the reasoning behind the advice.

It is not worth taking notes unless they are retrievable when needed, perhaps some considerable time later. They can be kept chronologically, as a 'diary', which is probably the simplest, or they can be filed by the patient's name. If the latter system is used, there should be an awareness that family names and given names can be mistakenly swapped over. If the former is used, each patient's notes should be kept separate, in loose-leaf style, to avoid conflicts of confidentiality.

Records should be kept for at least 8 years. Where children are involved, the records should be kept at least until the child's 21st birthday.

'Chain of evidence'

National guidance has been issued by the Royal College of Pathologists (2005) relating to suspected sexually transmitted infections in children, for medico-legal purposes. The form supports the legal concept of an unbroken chain from its source to providing evidence in the court. This means that each person handling the sample is a link in that chain, and they need to sign for their involvement, along with the date and time. The form needs to have the support of a Standard Operating Procedure (SOP), and can be modified for local use. An example is shown in Figure 3.9.

Miscellaneous records

Contractors/outside work force

It should always be absolutely clear whether an item of equipment, a room or whatever is in clinical use or has been 'handed over' to the contractors. To assist this process, the contractor should be given a certificate confirming that it is safe for them to proceed. When the contractor has finished, there should be a formal 'handing back' for clinical use. Contractors should not 'work around' the patient(s) or allow continued use of the equipment.

REPORTING

Weekly reports

These reports provide rapid feedback on current issues while they are still fresh. They are designed to improve performance. The reports should contain

Please complete a separate LCOEF for each specimen

Staple LCOEF to request form

Date taken	Time taken	Doctor's name

Patient's details		Doctor's signature
Name:	Number:	
Date of Birth:	Sex (circle): Male/Female	

Specimen type	Urethral	Cervical	Vaginal	Urine	Other (please state)
Please circle/state					

Test(s) requested	Microscopy	Bacterial culture	Chlamydia detection	Virus culture	Serology (please state type)
Please circle/state					

ALL NAMES MUST BE ACCOMPANIED BY A SIGNATURE				
Procedure	Name	Signature	Date	Time
Specimen taken by			/ /	:
Specimen delivered to laboratory by			/ /	:
Received by BMS (on-call? Yes/No)			/ /	:
BMS 3/4 Check at receipt			/ /	:
BMS 3/4 check on completion			/ /	:
Medical staff check on completion			/ /	:

Figure 3.9 Laboratory 'chain of evidence' form (LCOEF). BMS, biomedical scientist.

information on alert organisms and infectious patients. They are generated by the ICNs and sent to the wards, departments and clinicians. They are rapid and functional, and should include simple graphs.

Monthly reports

Monthly reports should include the following sections.

- *Surveillance*: findings should be summarized using graphs, explaining both good and the bad results. Copies of the mandatory surveillance data should be included and a report should be made on the advice given. Targets and trends should be clear and any outbreaks reported.
- *Audit*: results of audit should be presented (both those conducted by the ICT and those conducted by the wards in liaison with the ICT), such as use of side rooms, handwashing compliance, etc., and summaries of the weekly reports.
- *Education and training*: there should have been a minimum of two training sessions each month, but more typically four. Details of these sessions should be included.
- *Consultation*: those issues on which the ICT has been consulted (e.g. capital planning, purchase of equipment, new policies, revision of existing policies, etc.) should be noted. Nil returns are important.
- *Targets*: achievements of the targets from the annual plan should be reported, or any difficulties encountered which may prevent achievements.
- *Other*: there may be other issues to report.

The reports are sent to all members of the ICT within two or three days of the new calendar month. If this is not possible, the team is not managing its data satisfactorily.

An example of a monthly report for surgical wards for June is shown in Box 3.2.

Quarterly reports

These reports are for the infection control quarterly meetings. They are formal reports and include recommendations to management. The reports are copied to the Chief Executive.

Education data on who attends the sessions should be included. The attendance of members of the ICT at meetings (e.g. capital planning, policy reviews, etc.) to represent the team should also be reported.

Annual reports

The annual report is intended for the Trust Board. It should be written in a style that the intelligent lay person can understand. This report is important to

Box 3.2 Monthly report for June – surgical wards

SURVEILLANCE

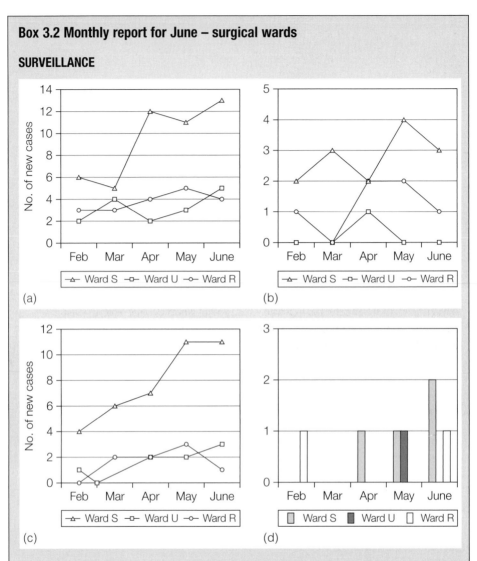

Figure B3.1 Numbers of new cases for: (a) methicillin-resistant *Staphylococcus aureus* (MRSA; all new cases); (b) MRSA (blood); (c) *Clostridium difficile*; (e) *Acinetobacter*.

Action/advice given

In May, surgical wards were audited for compliance with hand hygiene by the Infection Control Team:

• Ward S scored 22% overall
• Ward U scored 46% overall
• Ward R scored 49% overall

In June, handwashing facilities were audited in S ward, and found to be satisfactory. Information on staffing levels, patient numbers and patient dependency scores has been requested.

Surgical site infections

No appointment has yet been made to the post which deals with these data. It is vital this is expedited.

AUDIT

The audit plan

The audit plan for June was for side-room utilization. This has been completed and the results are attached.

The rapid audit cycle

Ward S has been the subject of a series of audits during June involving handwashing, the environment, catheter care and indwelling lines; improvements have been demonstrated for all four issues. Congratulations to them on all their hard work but there is still more work to be done. See graphs below (Figs B3.2a–c).

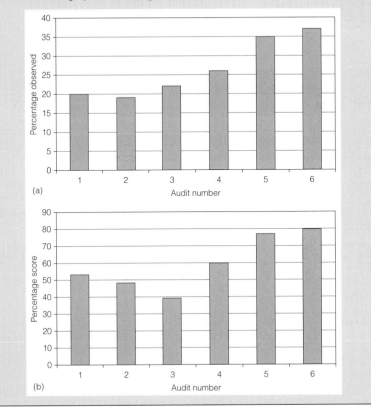

Box 3.2 Monthly report for June – surgical wards – *contd*

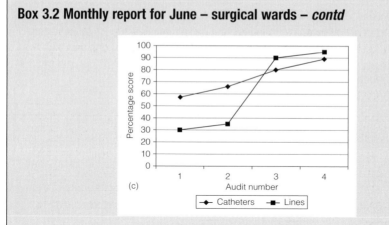

(c)

Figure B3.2 Results from a series of audits for S ward: (a) handwashing; (b) the environment; and (c) catheter and indwelling line care.

EDUCATION AND TRAINING (JUNE)

One session was organized for the physiotherapy staff for which there were 17 attendees. The maximum number expected was 23.

Two ad hoc teaching sessions were organized during May for the surgical nursing staff. These were attended by 3 staff from ward S, 12 from ward U and 14 from ward R.

CONSULTATIONS

The sharps policy is being reviewed and a new endoscopy washer is being considered.

TARGETS

The MRSA bacteraemia target total is 36 maximum at the end of the year (average 3 per month). In 5 months there were 21 bacteraemias (average 4.2 per month).

board members and should be comprehensive. The Trust is obliged to meet with the Code of Practice issued by the Department of Health (2008) and so this is an opportunity to make the Trust Board aware of how well (or badly) they measure up to that code. It would be helpful therefore to have a section where the structure of the report followed the layout of the code.

It may be worth including a glossary of terms. The authors' name and the date of writing should be clearly shown.

An example of an annual report is given in Box 3.3.

Box 3.3 Example of an annual report

(Sections in italics are presented as they would appear in the actual report, so as to illustrate an example. It is not intended to reproduce all of the report, as this may well exceed 100 pages.)

EXECUTIVE SUMMARY

Poorly controlled infection is costing the NHS about £1 billion per annum, costing the lives of about 5000 people, and adding to the misery of existing disease for countless others, extending hospital stays and necessitating additional operations. Investment in Hospital Infection Control gets the reward of savings, coupled with an assured quality of care.

This report details how the Infection Control Team (ICT) performed against the objectives which were set a year ago. It also provides data indicating the performance of the Trust as a whole.

Details of the performance of the Trust as a whole should include data on operations/day cases/admissions/beds, etc., so that the numbers of infections have a context. The aspects that are improving and those that are worsening should be indicated. Explanations should be offered for why this is occurring and whether additional resources are required. The case should be presented clearly, using exact figures as much as possible. If data are available (and if relevant), the Trust should be compared with other similar ones.

The number of admissions of notifiable diseases, patients who have methicillin-resistant *Staphylococcus aureus* (MRSA) on admission, and the average length of stay of patients who need isolation (such as those with tuberculosis), all help to paint the picture for the Trust Board member.

New problems encountered during the year (e.g. the first time a glycopeptide-resistant enterococcus is found in the Trust, and/or the appearance of a hypervirulent strain of *Clostridium difficile* for the first time) and the implications for the patient(s) and the Trust should be included. Then details of each 'alert' organism and how it has impacted on the Trust over the year need to be provided. Each organism will need to be introduced to the Board members, as illustrated below with MRSA.

SURVEILLANCE OF ALERT ORGANISMS

Staphylococcus aureus/*MRSA*

Staphylococcus aureus (S. aureus) *is one of the most common bacteria. In a reasonably average population of people about a third (or more) will be carrying* S. aureus *in their noses. This is a perfectly normal healthy situation.* S. aureus *on the other hand is capable of producing a range of diseases from minor skin infections and boils to deeper seated abscesses, food poisoning, post-operative wound infections, osteomyelitis, endocarditis, a life-threatening chest infection and septicaemia. In the 1940s, in the early days of penicillin, 95% of the isolates of* S. aureus *were sensitive to penicillin, but this figure was to change rapidly and today over 99% of* S. aureus *is resistant to penicillin.* S. aureus *is a*

Box 3.3 Example of an annual report – *contd*

good example to illustrate the enormous evolutionary potential that bacteria possess. Methicillin (and flucloxacillin) were developed as antibiotics that were still active against those S. aureus *strains that were resistant to penicillin. In the 1950s, penicillin-resistant* S. aureus *became widespread and so the development of methicillin, which was still active against these strains, was welcomed. However, not long after its introduction, methicillin-resistant* S. aureus *was described in 1961. In the 1970s 'MRSA' became a common organism and MRSA was understood to mean both resistance to methicillin and many other antibiotics (multi-drug resistant* S. aureus*).*

Graphs of mandatory data should be presented and any additional data included, such as details within the Trust identifying the major problems and the action taken to combat them. Obviously data from the quarterly reports, extended over a longer time scale, should be used. The extent of the problem is less important than the ability to show there has been constant improvement.

A similar approach to that for *C. difficile*, *Acinetobacter* and the other alert organisms should be used.

AUDIT

A summary should be provided of all the audits carried out and the resulting improvements (or changes), both the rapid cycle audits and those in the annual plan. This should be illustrated comprehensively with graphs.

EDUCATION AND TRAINING

A summary of the education given by the ICT, as illustrated below, should be included.

Educational events – infection control

Subject	Date	Tuition time (hours)	Attendance (actual)	Attendance (maximum)	Professional group
Induction	Feb	2	24	25	Junior doctors
Handwashing	Feb	1	8	9	Nursing
BBVs	Feb	1	9	10	Midwives
Infection control	Mar	6	27	30	Nursing
Instruments	Mar	1	10	12	Theatre staff
Isolating patients	Mar	1	3	8	Managers
MRSA	Mar	1	10	22	Domestics
etc.					

Then the continuing professional development of the ICT should be covered. At this point there is the opportunity of showing off the contribution of the ICT to medical science (i.e. papers published, research presented, invited lectures given, etc.).

CONSULTATION

This is perhaps best laid out as a month-by-month summary of the issues that have received formal consultation by the ICT members. If there have been outstanding omissions these should be noted.

LAST YEAR'S ACHIEVEMENTS AGAINST THE AGREED PLAN

This is important for continuity.

SCIENTIFIC/MEDICAL ADVANCES IN THE PAST YEAR

It is advisable to mention only those advances that will have an impact on practice. There should be an awareness of whether the changes will produce savings, or will need additional resources. Examples would include molecular screening for MRSA and how this could speed up the screening process, and the appearance of new organisms such as *C. difficile* 027.

COMPLIANCE WITH THE CODE OF PRACTICE

The Code of Practice has been laid down by the Department of Health (2008). The components of the Code of Practice should be itemized with an outline of how well or badly the Trust is fairing against each component.

REFERENCES

Department of Health (2002) Getting ahead of the curve: a strategy for combating infectious diseases. Available online at: http://www.dh.gov.uk/en/Publicationsand-statistics/Publications/PublicationsPolicyAndGuidance/Browsable/DH_4095398 (last accessed 19 November 2008).

Department of Health (2008) *The Health Act 2006. Code of practice for the prevention and control of healthcare associated infection.* Available online at: http://www.dh.gov.uk/en/Publicationsandstatistics/Publications/PublicationsPolicyAndGuidance/DH_081 927 (last accessed 19 November 2008).

Gemmell CG, Edwards DI, Fraise AP, Gould FK, Ridgway GL and Warren RE (2006) Guidelines for the prophylaxis and treatment of methicillin-resistant *Staphylococcus aureus* (MRSA) infections in the UK. *Journal of Antimicrobial Chemotherapy* **57**, 589.

Haley RW (1995) The scientific basis for using surveillance and risk factor data to reduce nosocomial infection rates. *Journal of Hospital Infection* **30**(Suppl), 3.

Haley RW, Quade D, Freeman HE, Bennett JV and the CDC SENIC Planning Committee (1980) The SENIC Project (Study on the Efficacy of Nosocomial Infection Control). Summary of study design. *American Journal of Epidemiology* **111**, 472.

Haley RW, Culver DH, White JW, Morgan WM, Emori TG, Munn VP and Hooton TM (1985) The efficacy of infection surveillance and control programs in preventing nosocomial infections in US hospitals. *American Journal of Epidemiology* **121**, 182.

National Patient Safety Agency (2007) The national specifications for cleanliness in the NHS: a framework for setting and measuring performance outcomes.

Available online at: http://www.npsa.nhs.uk/nrls/improvingpatientsafety/cleaning-and-nutrition/national-specifications-of-cleanliness/ (last accessed 19 November 2008).

Reilly J, Clift A, Johnston L, Noone A, Philips G, Rowley D and Sullivan F (2006) Post discharge surveillance of surgical site infection: a validation of patient self diagnosis. *Journal of Bone and Joint Surgery* **88B**(Suppl III), 400.

Royal College of Pathologists (2005) *National Guidelines on a standardised proforma for 'chain of evidence' specimen collection and on retention and storage of specimens relating to the management of suspected sexually transmitted infections in children and young people for medico-legal purposes.* May 2005. Available online at: http://www.rcpath.org/resources/pdf/ChainOfEvidence-June06.pdf (last accessed 19 November 2008).

Wilcox MH, Hall J, Pike H, Templeton PA, Fawley WN, Parnell P and Verity P (2003) Use of perioperative mupirocin to prevent methicillin-resistant *Staphylococcus aureus* (MRSA) orthopaedic surgical site infections. *Journal of Hospital Infection* **54**, 196.

Wilson P, Lewis D, Jenks P and Hoque S (1996) Prevalence of antibiotic resistance in pneumococci. *British Medical Journal* **313**, 819.

4 STERILIZATION

Peter Hooper

INTRODUCTION

Until recently, the sterilization of reusable medical devices was seen as the major stage in making them safe for reuse. Cleaning and disinfection were merely prior stages to sterilization, the purpose of which was to destroy bacterial spores. The challenge of new contaminants and a better understanding of the complete decontamination process have led to the cleaning stages sharing the importance of sterilization. While the emphasis may have changed, the fundamentals of the sterilization process remain of prior importance. Development of new processes and sterilants has only added to the need to understand these basic principles fully, enabling users to confirm the sterilization process as effective. Further constraints within European and International Standards require better definitions of sterilants and sterilization processes, and quality systems require full and comprehensive validation, testing and maintenance of sterilizing equipment. Indeed, the Medical Devices Directive (European Union, 1995) requires the user to confirm that medical devices undergo processes that are fully validated and monitored so that they do no harm to the patient.

DEFINITION

Most dictionaries will define 'sterilization' as a process that destroys or removes all living material. This definition is sensible, as it reflects the real purpose of the sterilization stage of the reprocessing of reusable medical devices. It reflects a residual contamination level of zero. While being acceptable in a philosophical manner, this definition presents problems when a protocol is to be produced to validate and routinely monitor the performance of any electro-mechanical or chemical sterilization process. The measurement of a zero residual can be achieved, if at all, only with great difficulty and will render the product becoming non-sterile by the test method itself. This paradox highlights two fundamentals of any sterilization process. First, the confirmation of a successful process must be via a practical definition capable of being challenged and tested. Second, the routine ongoing monitoring of the process must be an indirect protocol, which does not affect the product that has undergone the sterilization process.

While the latter of these points is discussed within Quality System Standards, the former is the subject of a European Standard. EN 556-1 (British Standards Institution, 2001) defines what must happen to a device, or collection of devices, during a sterilization process for the device(s) to be designated as 'sterile'. This definition is based on the probability of an organism surviving a sterilization process and reflects the way in which a sterilant achieves the aim of the process. The Standard requires a theoretical probability of survival of a viable micro-organism in or on the device equal to, or less than, one in a million. While the logic of the Standard's statement may be presented in different, seemingly conflicting ways, it may be clearly represented by the following.

While Figure 4.1 illustrates the exponential decay of survivors over a period of time, the linear characteristics can be seen when represented on a logarithmic scale (Figure 4.2). In both cases, an original contamination level of one million, 10^6, is shown. Figure 4.3 shows the extension of the logarithmic scale to extrapolate the process to achieve a survival probability of 10^{-6} that is required to meet EN 556-1. It should be noted that this will enable, for each sterilization process tested, the parameter values necessary for compliance with this Standard to be assessed. Zero survival would, in practice, be expected at anything over half-cycle exposure but is not sufficient for compliance. This representation is capable of being tested, either in the laboratory or in the field, and thus validation of the process can be achieved. This will allow simple definitions of parameter requirements in standard, repeatable cycles, or individual assessments to be made for special or ad-hoc sterilization processes. It thus defines what a sterilant must achieve and also allows validation and routine monitoring to be defined, performed and documented. This microbiological survival basis of a sterilization process can be used either to confirm the parameter values required, leading to a parametric release protocol, or for a definition of critical values, which may be monitored on a microbiological or other basis.

The application of EN 556-1 is based on the destruction of bacterial spores as a worst case. At present, a process meeting the requirements of this Standard may enable the goods being processed to be designated as 'sterile' even though it may not be capable of destroying, or deactivating, a more complex contaminant, such as prions or a bacterial endotoxin. Clearly alternative or additional methods or processes for destroying, deactivating or removing such contaminants must be made. A cleaning process that is validated as capable of removing proteinaceous contamination may suffice as may filtration or distillation of liquids to remove endotoxins.

STERILANTS AND STERILIZATION PROCESSES

It must be understood that there is no single, universal, sterilization cycle. Users – those responsible for the safe reprocessing of reusable medical devices –

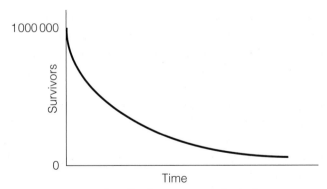

Figure 4.1 Survivor curve for a set of sterilization parameters (typical).

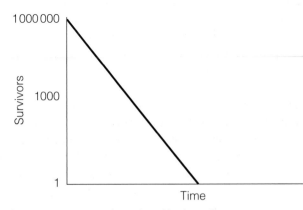

Figure 4.2 Survivor curve represented on a logarithmic scale.

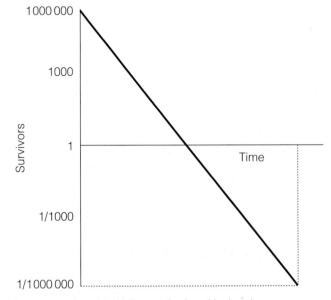

Figure 4.3 Survivor curve extrapolated into negative logarithmic values.

will have a number of options available, depending on the variety of instruments to be reprocessed, their construction and materials. Considerations of storage times and packaging materials will also increase the diversity of sterilization processes available. Some processes may be capable of meeting a variety of load types, materials and packaging, while others may be specifically designed for a small range of parameters.

While all sterilization processes must be capable of meeting the requirements of EN 556-1, they may not achieve this with equal efficacy. Processes will range in cycle time and the ease of meeting the Standard, and will possess a wide range of design and technical complexities. Engineering service and utility requirements will differ in quantity and quality, and some processes may require specific dedicated accessories and supplies. Choice of sterilants and sterilization processes must therefore be made in full knowledge of the variation in parameters of all devices being, or likely to be, processed. Major details to be considered include the following:

- sensitivity to temperature;
- sensitivity to moisture;
- sensitivity to pressure changes;
- sensitivity to chemicals;
- design considerations (e.g. solid, hollow or air-retentive);
- requirement to store, and hence package, before sterilization;
- complexity and cost of facilities;
- complexity and cost of processing.

The easiest, least complex, choice will be for those load items, which are solid and not susceptible to temperature, moisture or pressure changes. As this combination of properties covers the large majority of instruments to be reprocessed, the least complex equipment will be ubiquitous. However, the increasing complexity of both surgical procedures and the instrumentation required, has led to a greater need for less simple sterilization processes. It should be noted, however, that even the least complex sterilization process will possess its own degree of complexity with the subsequent need for understanding and diligence during use.

Steam

Steam has been formally used for sterilization for over 100 years, and remains the sterilant of choice because of its efficiency and relative simplicity. A steam sterilization process will utilize high temperature, moisture and wide pressure variations, but if the load items can withstand these parameters and if the required critical parameters are controlled properly, then the requirements of EN 556-1 will be easily met. Steam denatures the protein of contamination, allowing its thermal energy to destroy the residue. As the initial denaturing

requires the presence of moisture, the critical parameters of a steam sterilization cycle will be:

- moisture;
- thermal energy (indicated by temperature);
- sufficient exposure time for the required lethality.

   While it is possible to use steam at a continuum of relationships, the chosen
time/temperature relationships include the following:

- 134°C for 3 minutes;
- 126°C for 10 minutes;
- 121°C for 15 minutes.

   Steam is a highly complex vapour but its use as a sterilant is relatively crude.
Its raw material is water and the means of turning cold water into steam
involves two separate stages. Thermal energy first raises cold water to its boiling
point, the exact value of which is defined by the pressure acting on the surface
of the water. At atmospheric pressures this is 100°C, but increased pressure
within a boiler or steam generator requires the water to be raised to a higher
boiling point. Once boiling point is reached, further energy called latent energy
must be applied to reorganize the molecular construction into that of a vapour
free to escape the water's surface. It is this latent energy that is transferred to
the relatively cold load within the sterilizer chamber as condensation occurs.
The load is raised to steam temperature by this condensation and the subsequent energy transfer provides that required for sterilization. It is essential that
this condensation occurs over the complete surface area of the load. Any resistance to this will render the sterilization process ineffective even if all the critical parameters are met. In order for this to be achieved, all residual air in the
chamber, within and surrounding the load or packaging, must be removed. If
the load items are solid and unwrapped, then this air removal will be easier
than if the items are hollow, air-retentive and packaged for storage. Complete
air-removal should therefore be added as a fourth critical parameter and sterilizers should monitor their efficiency of air removal. This differential in air-
removal difficulty has thus led to the development of two types of steam
sterilizer: one for unwrapped solid items, and one for air-retentive (usually
referred to as porous) loads. These two types of steam sterilizer are vastly different in complexity, size and cost, although the operating principles are
similar. The porous-load sterilizer may be used for both solid, unwrapped
loads as well as air-retentive packaged items but the unwrapped instrument
sterilizer may be used only for unwrapped, solid, non air-retentive items.
Hence items from this latter type of sterilizer may not be stored and must be
used immediately.

   It can be seen that steam is being used merely as a transporter of thermal
energy from the boiler/steam generator to the load in the chamber. The water

produced by the required condensation is thus an unwanted by-product of the process and must be removed from the chamber. Any residual water or wetness present on a load is undesirable on unwrapped instruments, and unacceptable on or within packaged porous-loads. Drying can be performed by the creation of a negative pressure around the load sufficiently low and long enough for residual water to be changed into steam by virtue of its own residual energy to be removed by the vacuum creation system. The sterilizer will thus need to possess the ability to perform the following stages:

1 complete air-removal;
2 attainment and maintenance of the required steam temperature for the required time;
3 drying stage to remove residual water;
4 introduction of filtered air to equalize pressure (if vacuum drying is used).

All stages are automatically controlled and safety devices must ensure that only those cycles that achieve the required values of critical parameters will be indicated as successful cycles. These parameters should also be independently monitored and indicated so that untoward errors of the control system leading to the false indication of acceptability are avoided.

As well as existing in the two types – unwrapped instrument and porous-load – steam sterilizers vary in size. Those that can accommodate a load item 300 mm × 300 mm × 600 mm are known as 'large' sterilizers, while those that cannot are known as 'small' sterilizers. While large sterilizers can exist in exceedingly large sizes, this capacity differential is important when compliance to European and International Standards is concerned. Small steam sterilizers must meet the requirements of EN 13060 (British Standards Institution, 2004a), while large steam sterilizers are defined in EN 285 (British Standards Institution, 2006a). Whatever the size of the sterilizer, the ongoing monitoring and process control of any steam sterilizer is defined in ISO 17665 (British Standards Institution, 2006b).

Protocols for validation and routine testing may be within the content of these Standards but reference may be made to local documentation for further details of routine periodic testing. Within the UK, further advice may be found in health technical memoranda (HTMs): HTM 01 (Department of Health, 2006) replaces HTM 2010 (Department of Health, 1994), HTM 2030 (Department of Health, 1997a) and HTM 2031 (Department of Health, 1997b), bringing them in harmony with current and newly published EN and ISO Standards. Details of operational procedures and further discussion on test procedures can be found only within the HTMs and those responsible for reprocessing reusable medical devices are advised to seek guidance on the content and implementation of all relevant local (e.g. UK), European and International documentation.

Dry heat

While steam is the most popular process, it is not available to those loads that are susceptible to moisture. As long as the load remains temperature-tolerant, dry heat would be the process of choice. This is effectively steam sterilization without the moisture and hot air acts as the source of energy. Without the moisture, destruction is less efficient and the exposure times are necessarily longer, even though the operating temperature is higher than that used for steam. Likely choices include:

- 180°C for 30 minutes;
- 170°C for 60 minutes;
- 160°C for 120 minutes.

It is possible to use the higher parameter values to achieve depyrogenation. The dry heat sterilizer is not unlike a complex fan-assisted electric oven. Loading must ensure that circulation of air is not impeded and the use of packaging tolerant of high temperatures is essential.

Dry-heat cycles enabling heating up and cooling down are necessarily lengthy, owing to the poor thermal conductivity of air and the fact that typical load items contain non-aqueous liquids and oils. However, the use of dry heat in healthcare situations is probably limited to laboratories and, where necessary, pharmaceutical production units.

Low-temperature steam with formaldehyde

If the load items are sensitive to temperature, then a low-temperature process will be required. This process utilizes the properties and thermal effects of steam at a lower temperature. If temperatures below 100°C are required, then the process must be conducted below atmospheric pressure when the boiling temperature of water will be less than 100°C. As the ability of steam at these conditions is insufficient to perform sterilization, the addition of a chemical effect from formaldehyde gas may allow the requirements of EN 556-1 to be met. As with high-temperature steam sterilization, the presence of moisture is essential and thus this low-temperature variation will not be compatible with load items that are moisture-sensitive.

Although the parameter values can be predetermined and monitored, the use of a chemical for sterilization will indicate that routine monitoring should be performed with biological indicators. While there are moves to use a parametric monitoring protocol for chemical sterilization processes, the use of low-temperature steam and formaldehyde for sterilization has, like dry heat, dramatically reduced in recent years. It is possible, however, to find some sterile service departments still using this process for specific loads. Process temperatures are generally between 60 and 75°C. Reference should be made to EN 14180 (British Standards Institution, 2003) for construction requirements.

Ethylene oxide

Even lower process temperatures can be provided by ethylene oxide sterilization. This process relies on the chemical effect of the gas together with some thermal energy and humidity. This process is particularly effective for electronic components and load items with high-temperature sensitivity. Process temperatures of below 60°C are possible. Reference to EN 550 (British Standards Institution, 1994) and EN 1422 (British Standards Institution, 1997a) will define construction, performance and monitoring requirements. Some small ethylene oxide sterilizers remain with healthcare facilities but, in the main, this process is used under contract from an external supplier.

Irradiation

The sterilizing effect of irradiation has long been understood but has yet to be implemented in a practical sterilization process capable of installation in a healthcare facility. The process is universally available as a contracted external service only where commercial facilities will be sized for manufacturing quantities. Reference should be made to EN ISO 11137 (British Standards Institution, 2006c).

Hydrogen peroxide vapour

There is current development in the use of vaporized hydrogen peroxide, particularly for the fumigation or sterilization of closed rooms. It has been used both in terrorist situations and pharmaceutical production, but has yet to be applied in fixed units for medical devices.

Hydrogen peroxide gas plasma

Much development has been performed on the combination of exposure of devices to hydrogen peroxide vapour at very low pressures combined with the radiofrequency production of plasma surrounding the load items. Small sterilizers are able to expose compatible loads to the vapour, which is then subjected to the plasma production. This causes dissociation of the peroxide into aggressive radicals, which, in conjunction with the vapour stage, allow the requirements of EN 556-1 to be met. As with all low-temperature processes, the compatibility with load items is not universal but it is possible to validate successful cycles on a variety of loads, including some cannulated devices. Further progress may include multi-channel flexible endoscopes in this category, although at present compatibility is limited to single-channel endoscopes with limitations on length and diameter. However, this process is capable of providing sterilization on loads similar to those processed in steam and, in some cases, has the advantage that it may provide sterilization instead of previous processes, which were only capable of disinfection.

Liquid chemical sterilization

Many liquid chemicals routinely used for disinfection, especially for flexible endoscopes, may be capable of achieving the requirements of EN 556-1, if the exposure time is sufficiently long. However, the length of time required is usually excessively long, rendering the use of liquid chemical sterilization, in the main, impractical. However, liquid chemical sterilizers are available and, while the requirements of EN 556-1 must be met, there may not be an immediately relevant Standard for them. The recent publication of EN ISO 14937 (British Standards Institution, 2000), discussed further below, has resolved this problem.

MEDICAL DEVICES DIRECTIVE

This European Directive was first published in 1995, with a three-year lead-in period applicable in the UK. Its purpose was to ensure that the manufacture of medical devices was performed in a safe manner, and that any process used during the manufacturing process was capable of validation and presented no risk to the patient or any User. Devices that can be demonstrated to comply with this Directive are capable of bearing the CE mark. This enables purchasers to utilize the presence of this mark to purchase devices compliant with the Directive. While the text of the Directive describes devices being 'placed on the market', there was some discussion regarding its application to those instruments reprocessed within a healthcare facility. The danger of differing levels of compliance when comparing manufacturers and reprocessors has largely been avoided by an acceptance that the principles of the Directive should apply to any device and hence all cases of sterilization.

A difficulty of the Directive is that, while defining essential requirements of the manufacture/reprocessing of devices, it does not provide technical details that must be in place in order to demonstrate compliance. It is compliance with the Standards defined throughout this chapter that can be used to demonstrate this. An irony is that, while compliance with the Directive is a legal requirement, harmonized Standards are not in themselves legal documents, although the risks of sterilizing devices with processes clearly non-compliant with the Standards are so great that the Standards carry similar weight to the Directive.

The breadth of the essential requirements of the Directive means that there is a raft of Standards relevant to virtually every aspect of decontamination, including sterilization. They cover sterilizing equipment, their validation and routine monitoring, accessories and associated devices. Sterilizers themselves, like washer–disinfectors, are classified as medical devices and must similarly carry the CE mark. Additionally, the Directive requires a manufacturer of devices to provide decontamination instructions and this is reinforced in EN ISO 17664 (British Standards Institution, 2004b). Thus the purchaser of medical devices should possess all relevant information to choose the sterilization process, and the method of validating and routinely monitoring its protocol. Any deviations from this set of instructions and procedures should not be made lightly as they, and their effects on the decontamination process, will need to be justified.

STANDARDS

Reference has been made within this chapter to the relevant Standards for a sterilization process. It is usual to find a Standard for the sterilizing equipment and a separate Standard for the routine control and monitoring of that process. This pattern of documentation allows the person responsible for reprocessing to produce a written protocol to include operating procedures, validation, routine periodic testing and maintenance. There is thus a datum against which the use of such sterilizers can be judged for, say a Quality System accreditation.

New and revised versions of these Standards will reflect their application over wide regional and international perspectives. This is only possible if the freedom to apply a variety of monitoring procedures, techniques and devices allows a continuation of local differences while achieving a similar aim of confirming the safety of all reprocessed devices at the point of use. This eventual aim represents the implementation of the complete philosophy of sterilization, which may be represented by the following:

• Properly define the process.
• Purchase a sterilizer to achieve this.
• Fully understand the critical parameter values required.
• Monitor these parameters independently.
• Record all processes and data.
• Implement and fully document validation, testing and maintenance.
• Utilize all documentation for the purposes of product release and retain for inspection by others.

The production of these protocols is relatively easy for those sterilization processes for which there is a Standard, either for the sterilizing equipment or the routine control and monitoring of that process, or both. However, for those sterilization processes for which there is no longer a Standard, or where the process is so new that a Standard has not been produced, this may appear to be difficult. There is, however, a Standard for such situations. ISO 14937 is a generic Standard intended to apply to any sterilization process for which no current Standard exists. It requires the manufacturer/supplier of such a sterilizer to characterize the efficacy of the sterilant fully, this defining the critical process parameters. A validation protocol and routine monitoring protocol may be jointly produced by the manufacturer, the User and the manufacturer/supplier of the load items to be processed. Liaison between these three parties is thus essential to the ongoing acceptable use of such a sterilizer, and relies upon complete and full implementation of these protocols. The outcome of the publication of this Standard means that it is possible to define operating procedures for any sterilization process, new or old, in order to demonstrate compliance to the requirements of EN 556-1.

ASSOCIATED DOCUMENTATION

In addition to Standards, there might exist local or regional guidance documentation defining local best practice or acting as addenda to Standards. In the UK, the publication of Department of Health HTMs has assisted designers, planners and practitioners in a wide variety of engineering and technical fields. There are three HTMs relevant to decontamination with two, HTM 2010 'Sterilizers' and HTM 2031 'Clean steam for sterilization', particularly relevant to sterilizers, their use, operation and testing.

HTM 2010 was first published under the title of HTM 10 in the 1960s and was revised in 1968 (Department of Health, 1968) and 1980 (Department of Health, 1980) with the same designation. The revision in 1994 was the first to bear the title HTM 2010. The complexity of this HTM has increased at each revision and the 1994 version exists in six parts, strangely published in five volumes. It represented the policy changes required to associate itself fully with the European and international perspectives of the time. Its content was to form a larger extent of the UK input to the European Standards being developed at the time, and comparison between the 1994 edition of HTM 2010 and ENs 285 and 554 displays this heritage. The HTM continued the tradition of providing testing protocols for both validation and routine periodic testing.

The 1994 edition redefined the roles and responsibilities of those disciplines involved in sterilization and clearly placed the User – the person with day-to-day managerial responsibility for sterilizers – in the role with sole responsibility. In order to state that all sterilizers were fit-for-use, the User sought advice from a variety of others including Competent Persons. These performed relevant testing and maintenance duties as defined within the HTM and reported to the User on the results. The User's acceptance of their advice, signified by a signature on the testing/maintenance documentation, acted as this certification of fitness-for-use.

Because of the content of HTM 2010 and the heritage of European Standards, compliance with the HTM was seen as sufficient demonstration of best practice. Current work of Technical Committees and Working Groups within

the Comité Européen de Normalisation (CEN) and the International Organization for Standardization (ISO) means that many new or imminent Standards
are overtaking the current content of HTM 2010 and the Department of
Health has responded accordingly. The three decontamination HTMs are now
combined into a new document, HTM 01, acting as a single point of reference
for all decontamination issues. The content on sterilization has changed to
reflect the content of all the new sterilization Standards and cross-refers to the
relevant Standards where necessary instead of repeating – or possibly contra-
dicting – the content of that Standard. The implication is that all disciplines
involved in sterilization need to possess and be familiar with all European and
International Standards relevant to the processes in use and that these documents are the over-riding definition of technical requirements. Associated documentation, such as HTMs will thus act as guidance to the implementation of
the Standards. As new Standards are continually being discussed, withdrawn,
revised and published, there is a need to keep up-to-date.

PROVISION OF ENGINEERING SERVICES AND UTILITIES

In order to meet the requirements of EN 556-1, a sterilizer will need a control
system so that all critical process parameters can be obtained at the proper
stage of the cycle and maintained for the requisite period of time. As shown
above, these stages may include air-removal and drying as well as the sterilization hold period itself. In addition to machine design and control system functionality, the provision of engineering services and utilities will be of critical
importance to the successful operation of the sterilizer. Major services are considered below and advice on other services may be found in relevant Standards
and associated documentation.

Steam

As steam sterilization is the most popular, then the provision of steam is the
most important engineering service. This service must satisfy the following
requirements:

• sufficient quantity to fulfil the sterilizer's requirements;
• sufficient quality to enable the sterilization to occur;
• sufficient quality so that the devices are safe to use.

The generation of steam is not a simple process. The quality of the raw water
supply and the care with which it is turned into steam at defined temperature
will greatly affect the quantity and quality of steam delivered to the sterilizer
chamber. All raw water supplies will contain impurities and the degree of
impurity should be known so that steps can be taken to ensure that the steam
supplied is of an acceptable quality. The use of softening plant prior to the

boiler/generator will protect the boiler if the water hardness is high. Softening, however, will leave impurities within the water and excessive softening may lead to dissociation of some of these impurities within the boiler, leading to inert gases being driven off accompanying the steam.

The requirements within the sterilizer will include the following:

- steam containing a small quantity of water to enable protein denaturation to begin;
- steam containing few, if any, inert gases that could impede both the sterilizing process and the sterilizer's safety devices;
- steam with no impurities, that could be deposited on the devices and may thus be transferred to the patient.

The values of the steam wetness, content of inert non-condensable gases and chemical impurities can be found in either HTM 01 or the ISO 17665. The 1994 version of EN 285 contained acceptable impurity levels in Table B1. The response of the UK Department of Health was to provide its own advice in HTM 2031, 'Clean steam for sterilization'. However, the two reference tables in these documents are both included in ISO 17665, removing this dual standard.

The quality of steam, in all aspects described above, should be routinely tested and checked so that the User possesses full knowledge of the quality of the environment surrounding the devices during the sterilization process. It remains the responsibility of the designer/planner to ensure that the steam supply is sufficient to provide the amount of steam required to maintain full production of the sterilizers within a sterile services department. Note must be taken of the maximum flow requirements and the operating principles on which the department has been assessed. Simultaneous use or availability for use of all sterilizers will require a steam supply based on maximum simultaneous demand. Reductions in supply quantity may be acceptable only if any restrictions to sterilizer usage with the subsequent loss of productivity have been fully taken into account during the design and planning stages.

Water

Most sterilizers will use large quantities of water. In most cases, this water will not come into contact with the load items and thus its quality and composition is not an important factor. However, if contact is possible, even in failure situations, the quality may be relevant. Essentially, the water supply is a question of quantity. Condensers and vacuum pumps may function throughout a sterilizing cycle and the designer of the sterilizer and department must take these factors into account. Much of this water will be immediately wasted into the drainage system. As with supply systems, the removal systems must be capable of dealing with maximum flows but the subsequent waste of much thermal energy has been the impetus for a new approach to water consumption. Reuse of, or energy extraction from, waste water will necessarily make the sterilizer design more complex and expensive, but the reduction in use of services and utilities may well make up such costs in relatively short times. These design issues should be considered during the tendering process leading to choice of sterilizer supply.

Electricity

All sterilizers require an electrical supply. This supply will vary in quantity, voltage and phase depending upon the sterilizer's requirements and design. Much attention will be placed on the safety aspects of electrical supply where the safety of Users, Operators, and Competent Persons should be considered. Emergency cut-off devices should be fitted and should be clearly seen, easy to operate and fitted in a position where they can function properly. The precise details of these devices will depend upon local legislation. Specialist advice may need to be sought to clarify these requirements.

Compressed air

Many sterilizers will use compressed air for a variety of functions including valve opening/closing and door-seal operation. If the air carries no risk of coming into contact with the load, then the required quality will largely depend on the technical requirements for, say, a pneumatic system. When it is used for door-seal operation there is a risk of load contact if the seal is not good and thus medical-quality air may be required. Compressed air may be supplied by individual compressors dedicated to each sterilizer or a central system. Proper capacity planning must be performed for both options.

VALIDATION, ROUTINE PERIODIC TESTING AND MAINTENANCE

It is essential that these functions are not only carried out but fully understood. Their performance can be seen as a direct consequence of the Medical Devices Directive and their procedures are likely to be defined in the relevant Standard or associated documentation.

The purchase of a new sterilizer should be made via a specification defining not only the purchaser's requirements for the sterilizer, but also the roles and responsibilities for the performance of, and provision of test loads for, the validation. Validation is a sequential process of tests to confirm that the sterilizer meets the predetermined parameters defined within the relevant Standard and the specification. Once completed successfully, the validation report should be monitored by an external advisor and the machine may be handed over for use. The report should include those tests of the machine's installation – installation qualification or IQ – and tests of the operating cycle known as operational qualification or OQ. Test loads for OQ will consist of repeatable loads used for testing. Clearly, if these repeatable loads bear little or no resemblance to the process loads that the sterilizer will experience, then further validation tests on these department-specific loads will be required. These tests are defined as performance qualification, or PQ.

Once in use, the sterilizer should be checked at routine intervals in order to demonstrate that the cycles and parameters confirmed at OQ and PQ are still being met. The relevant Standard or associated document will provide a protocol of these periodic tests, which will vary in test frequency and test performance. The protocol may include daily tests such as a Bowie and Dick test performed by the Operator or more complex technical tests performed every 3 or 12 months by a suitably qualified Competent Person. It is usual, on an annual basis, for any PQ tests to be repeated but it should be noted that validation is not repeated in full. Clearly all test results should be compared to those results achieved at validation in order to confirm ongoing acceptable performance. The only reasons why validation should be repeated are where serious defects, subsequent repairs, renovation or re-siting may require the whole testing process to be repeated. All testing should be fully documented and the log books, in conjunction with the validation report and specification, act as a growing library of evidence of acceptable performance.

Throughout the sterilizer's working life, the machine should be serviced and maintained in accordance with the manufacturer's instructions. Servicing and maintenance do not confirm the performance aspects of the sterilizer: that is the function of routine periodic testing. Maintenance records should be provided and retained in a similar manner to testing log books. Quality system inspections will require these records to be provided. All documentation should, therefore, be available by the sterilizer rather than being stored elsewhere.

PROCESS MONITORING

In addition to the validation, routine periodic testing and maintenance of all sterilizers, an essential part of confirming acceptability of processed medical devices is the ability to monitor the sterilizer's performance on every occasion. While the control system may be sophisticated and complex, it is not unknown for such systems to make errors. The monitoring of each cycle externally from the control system ensures that the process is fully checked. While there may be discussion on whether this independent monitoring is performed by a second automated system or by a human being, its performance is essential and depends upon the fitting of monitoring systems, preferably at the construction stage.

In essence, the independent system will measure all the critical process parameters necessary to achieve not only sterilization but other aspects such as vacuum drying performance. The requirements are well defined in the relevant Standard but will include sensors, connectors and indicators separate from the control system to either independently assess the process or provide information for the Operator to determine acceptability of the process. Full knowledge of those parameters that are critical, together with their required values, must be present. Clearly there must be a stated acceptable deviation from the values achieved at validation and advice should be sought on the calculation of these acceptable deviations.

Alternatively, the process may be monitored with chemical or biological indicators. The prevalence of parametric, chemical or biological monitoring may depend upon local, national or regional traditions, and it is possible to make a good case for not only all three methods of monitoring but also a combination of one or more. Process challenge devices are a further method of indirectly indicating that proper parameters have been achieved.

Use of biological indicators must ensure that the indicator is compatible with the process and representative of the whole load and type of contamination likely to be met. The testing process is also a source of contamination and thus manufacturer's instructions should be properly followed in all cases. Monitoring by chemical indicators is possible but is more commonly seen as complementary to parametric or biological monitoring. Indeed the validation protocols defined in most Standards provides for this variety in monitoring techniques. There are, however, some basic principles that apply to all techniques.

The function of monitoring is to confirm that each process cycle has been performed in the way that the sterilizer was validated to perform. The monitoring method must be compatible with the validation method and thus, at least, proper correlation must be made so that the monitoring technique accurately challenges the validated cycle. Evidence of this correlation must be available at all times. A combination of monitoring techniques should be assessed so that there can be no contradictory information. Clearly the function of an air-detector and a Bowie and Dick test, essentially measuring the same achievement, should both give pass or failure indications in relevant circumstances. All monitoring should be capable of being recorded and retained. Not only does this information enable a decision on process acceptability to be made but its retention will act as evidence of successful processing at any later date.

TRACEABILITY

The final aspect of monitoring described above alludes to the requirements for the traceability of each sterilizing process. The data discussed above will act not only as monitoring information but as essential content of the traceability system. Terms such as 'traceability' and 'tracking' seem to have interchangeable definitions of different functions. For the purpose of this chapter, the term 'traceability' refers to the ability to trace from patient record or notes back to the individual sterilization cycles that made the devices safe for use during that patient's surgical procedure. This tracing will confirm, at any future date, that the decision to release the product for patient use was correct and that the sterilization cycle (in addition to any cleaning and disinfection stage included in the devices' decontamination) were performed to the parameters determined during validation, or within acceptable deviations of those values. This link sounds a relatively simple process but its success relies upon a number of issues.

First, the sterilizer must possess the monitoring system, together with recording or indicating facilities, discussed above. These data must include processing date, time and unique cycle number, and must be retained for whatever length of time that such traceability is required. This period will depend on local or national legislation, but may stretch in excess of 20 years. When despatched from the sterile services department, the packaging or instruments must carry a label including data necessary to link to the retained data. This label must be removed at the site of the surgical procedure and retained within the patient record. These records must be retained for a similar length of time to the process data.

When required, the patient record will link, via the unique cycle number within the label, back to the retained process data. The accuracy of these data will be confirmed by the periodic testing log book confirming the accuracy of the sterilizer's instrumentation. The validation report will confirm the initial setting of these together with the acceptable deviations. The maintenance and service records together with the sterilizer specification will complete the traceability trail. The trail suggests the retention of large quantities of paperwork over lengthy periods. This is unavoidable but the problem may be obviated with electronic storage. The acceptability of such methods should be checked before use.

ACCESSORIES

It should be remembered that the use of fully compliant sterilizers within compliant decontamination systems may be negated by the use of accessories that do not meet the rigours met by the sterilizer. The umbrella of Standards has been designed to apply to as many of these devices as possible. Their content will contain construction and performance constraints where relevant, and the manufacturer/supplier must supply full use instructions. There is a long list of accessories but the following are included:

- chemical indicators including Bowie and Dick test packs(see EN 867; British Standards Institution, 1997b);
- biological indicators (see EN 866; British Standards Institution, 1996);
- packaging, including paper, man-made materials and metal sterilization containers (see EN 868; British Standards Institution, 1999).

Current revisions and new documents mean that the currency of relevant Standards for accessories should be checked, advice may be sought.

SINGLE-USE DEVICES

Regional and national differences in the philosophy of decontamination have been alluded to within this chapter but the policy regarding single-use devices remains problematical. Medical devices may be classified as follows:

- single-use only (also implies single decontamination, including sterilization, only);
- single patient use (may be reused but only on the same patient);
- defined reuse (may be reprocessed a defined number of times);
- undefined reuse (may be reprocessed any number of times until it becomes unusable, unacceptable, ceases to function or is disposed of for any reason).

An implication of the Medical Devices Directive and relevant Standards is that, for the latter three categories, the manufacturer/supplier must supply decontamination instructions. For single-use devices, however, there is no need to provide such instructions as reprocessing is not required.

Single-use devices must be designated by bearing the symbol shown in Figure 4.4 either on the instrument or on its packaging. No designation is required for devices for single-patient use, although this designation will be made in the manufacturer's instructions.

There is often a temptation to reuse single-use devices. This may be based on cost, availability or other reasons, but must be avoided. When designating a device as single use, the manufacturer may be reflecting construction procedures or materials that may be impaired or destroyed by any subsequent decon-

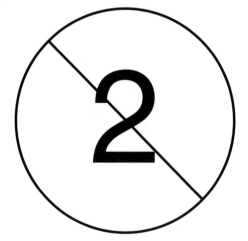

Figure 4.4 Designation of a single-use device, seen on a device or packaging.

tamination/sterilization process. The single-use designation effectively states that the item is not suitable for reprocessing, even if it appears to be capable of withstanding those sterilization processes available to the User. Should the User ignore the designation and decide to reuse and hence reprocess the device, then the lack of decontamination instructions will imply that the reprocessing is performed in total ignorance of its effect. Such reprocessing may create a risk or danger to the patient, immediately contravening the requirements of the Medical Devices Directive. Evidence is available of the effects that can arise from such procedure. The User would be solely responsible for any such untoward events of reprocessing single-use devices. For these reasons, the Department of Health in the UK (Medicines and Healthcare Products Regulatory Agency, 2006) has stated that single-use devices shall not, in any circumstances, be reused. This was reiterated in UK Health Circular 179 (Department of Health, 1999). Elsewhere, where local guidance makes no such statement and reuse occurs, the User must be aware not only of the subsequent responsibilities being taken but also that the Medical Devices Directive is being contravened. A thorough risk assessment must be undertaken if reuse of a single-use device is being considered taking into account the risk of infection, device integrity, etc.

SUMMARY CHECKLIST

It can be seen that sterilization is a multi-faceted subject, not merely a discussion of the sterilizer alone. The sterilizer should be seen as one link in a chain of items involving a number of individuals in differing roles and disciplines. The chapter can be summarized in the following checklist:

• Purchase the sterilizer against a comprehensive specification.
• Ensure the specification cross-refers to all relevant Standards.
• Ensure the specification fully defines the roles and responsibilities for performing validation protocols.
• Ensure the engineering services/utilities of the right quantity and quality are available.
• Ensure the sterilizer includes the required levels of independent monitoring equipment.
• Ensure full validation is completed and results are acceptable prior to handover.
• Ensure the validation report is independently audited.
• Ensure all operators, maintainers and testers are fully trained in their roles and responsibilities.
• Ensure the values of critical parameters demonstrated at validation are understood by all relevant technicians and that acceptable deviations from those values have been defined.

- Ensure the documentation system recording process data is fully functional from sterilizer to Patient Record.
- Ensure the sterilizer is only used for those items for which the cycle is applicable.
- Ensure the loads and loading patterns do not exceed the repeatable validation loads or specific PQ loads.
- Ensure the sterilizer is maintained and serviced to the manufacturer's instructions throughout its working life.
- Ensure routine periodic testing is performed in compliance with the protocol in the relevant Standard/local documentation.
- Ensure all loads subjected to PQ testing are retested on an annual basis.
- Ensure all maintenance and testing records are retained in the vicinity of the sterilizer.
- Ensure the User certifies acceptable performance by routinely signing testing log sheets.
- Ensure all documentation is checked annually by an independent audit.
- Ensure all technicians are kept up-to-date with revisions to Standards and relevant associated documentation.
- Ensure the engineering services are checked for quality/purity at the frequency defined in relevant Standards or associated documentation.
- Ensure all involved in using, collecting, delivering and reprocessing medical devices are fully aware of the requirements of, and their role in, traceability.
- Ensure all accessories used in conjunction with the sterilizer are compatible and comply with all relevant Standards.
- Ensure all operation, service, maintenance, testing, component replacement, breakdowns and repairs are fully documented in chronological order.
- Continually review the operating system encompassing the sterilizer and respond to changes in Standards and associated documentation.

If this checklist is fully implemented, then the User will be well on the way to demonstrate not only compliance with all relevant Standards and guidance documentation, but will be able to demonstrate current best practice. If all the principles of sterilization are understood, then similar systems may be applied to the cleaning and disinfection stages of the decontamination cycle.

REFERENCES

British Standards Institution (1994) EN 550:1994 *Sterilization of medical devices: validation and routine control of ethylene oxide sterilization.* Milton Keynes: British Standards Institution.

British Standards Institution (1996) EN 866:1996–1999 *Biological systems for testing sterilizers and sterilization processes.* Milton Keynes: British Standards Institution.

British Standards Institution (1997a) EN 1422:1997 *Sterilizers for medical purposes – Ethylene oxide sterilizers – Requirements and testing.* Milton Keynes: British Standards Institution.

British Standards Institution (1997b) EN 867:1997–2001 *Non-biological systems for use in sterilizers.* Milton Keynes: British Standards Institution.

British Standards Institution (1999) EN 868:1999–2001 *Packaging materials and systems for medical devices which are to be sterilized.* Milton Keynes: British Standards Institution.

British Standards Institution (2000) EN ISO 14937:2000 *Sterilization of health care products: General requirements for characterization of a sterilizing agent and the development, validation and routine control of a sterilization process for medical devices.* Milton Keynes: British Standards Institution.

British Standards Institution (2001) EN 556-1:2001 *Sterilization of medical devices: requirements for medical devices to be designated 'STERILE' – Part 1: Requirements for terminally sterilized medical devices.* Milton Keynes: British Standards Institution.

British Standards Institution (2003) EN 14180:2003 *Sterilizers for medical purposes – Low temperature steam and formaldehyde sterilizers – Requirements and test methods.* Milton Keynes: British Standards Institution.

British Standards Institution (2004a) EN 13060:2004 *Small steam sterilizers.* Milton Keynes: British Standards Institution.

British Standards Institution (2004b) EN ISO 17664:2004 *Sterilization of medical devices – information to be provided by the manufacturer for the processing of resterilizable medical devices.* Milton Keynes: British Standards Institution.

British Standards Institution (2006a) EN 285:2006 *Sterilization – Steam sterilizers – Large sterilizers.* Milton Keynes: British Standards Institution.

British Standards Institution (2006b) prEN 17665:2006 *Sterilization of health care products – Moist heat.* Milton Keynes: British Standards Institution.

British Standards Institution (2006c) EN ISO 11137:2006 *Sterilization of health care products – Radiation.* Milton Keynes: British Standards Institution.

Department of Health (1968) HTM 10 *Pressure steam sterilizers.* London: Department of Health.

Department of Health (1980) HTM 10 *Sterilizers.* London: Department of Health.

Department of Health (1994) HTM 2010 *Sterilizers.* London: Department of Health.

Department of Health (1997a) HTM 2030 *Washer disinfectors.* London: Department of Health.

Department of Health (1997b) HTM 2031 *Clean steam for sterilization.* London: Department of Health.

Department of Health (1999) HSC 1999 179 *Controls assurance in infection control: decontamination of medical devices.* London: Department of Health.

Department of Health (2006) HTM 01-01 *Decontamination.* London: Department of Health.

European Union (1995) 93/42/EEC *Council Directive, Medical Devices Directive.* Brussels: European Union.

Medicines and Healthcare Products Regulatory Agency (2006) *Single use medical devices: implications and consequences of reuse,* CB 2006(04). London: Medicines and Healthcare Products Regulatory Agency.

5 PHYSICAL AND CHEMICAL DISINFECTION

Christina Bradley

Disinfection can be achieved using moist heat or chemicals. The applications for each method are described in Chapter 6. Wherever possible, heat should be used for the decontamination of instruments and equipment. However, if this is not possible owing to the thermal tolerance of the item, the time available or the accessibility/availability of processing equipment, chemical disinfectants may be used.

PHYSICAL DISINFECTION

Exposure to moist heat is probably the most effective and controllable method for the disinfection of heat-tolerant items. This method is widely used for respiratory/anaesthetic equipment, surgical instruments and trays, bedpans, urine bottles, linen, crockery and cutlery.

Process times and temperatures

These vary between 65°C and 100°C, but generally, the higher the processing temperature, the shorter the processing time. The recommended times and temperatures in the UK (Medicines and Healthcare Products Regulatory Agency (MHRA) 2005) are shown in Table 5.1.

Boilers

The use of boilers has largely been discouraged owing to the lack of process control and the risk of scalding. However, they may still be used in the

Table 5.1 Recommended process times and temperatures in the UK (MHRA, 2005)*

	Temperature (°C)	Time
Instrument boiler	100	10 min
Automated washer–disinfectors[a] for medical equipment, including bedpans and urine bottles	71 80 90	3 min 1 min 1 s[b]
Linen	65 71	10 min 3 min

*Reproduced with permission. © 2005 Crown Copyright.

[a]Lower temperatures are used in washer–disinfectors as cleansing accompanies the decontamination process.

[b]1 s is difficult to measure, so 12 s is recommended.

community and small clinics for instruments such as proctoscopes and other non-invasive medical equipment. Very few boilers have thermal interlocks, so it is possible to remove items before they have been effectively disinfected. If they are used correctly and items are added to boiling water and maintained for at least 10 min, therefore achieving 5 min at 100°C, boilers can disinfect reliably. Small bench-top washer–disinfectors, which are relatively inexpensive and now widely available, provide a far more reliable decontamination process that can be more easily validated.

Thermal washer–disinfectors

These are used for automatic cleaning and thermal disinfection of surgical instruments and trays, holloware, respiratory/anaesthetic equipment and receptacles for human waste. They have the advantage of cleaning items, in addition to thermally disinfecting them, thereby reducing staff handling of contaminated instruments and equipment.

Washer–disinfectors are widely used in hospital sterile service departments (SSD) for the decontamination of used instruments and equipment from operating-theatres and other departments. Their use at the recommended temperatures for thermal disinfection has not been adopted for flexible endoscopes owing to the damage sustained by these instruments. However, they are suitable for non-invasive heat-tolerant rigid endoscopes if sterilization by autoclaving is not possible and disinfection is acceptable. Washer–disinfectors vary in design from large conveyor/cabinet machines, which have a rapid throughput and are widely used in SSDs, to smaller cabinet machines that are used in small departments and clinics. They may be a suitable alternative to chemical disinfectants (e.g. clear soluble phenolics) for instruments used in post-mortem rooms.

Users/purchasers should ensure that the equipment complies with national guidelines/recommendations. In the UK this would be EN 15883 (British Standards Institution, 2006b), and HTM 2030 (NHS Estates, 1997). These documents describe design considerations and test methods for the assessment of cycle parameters such as cleansing efficacy, temperature compliance and drying. Other European and international standards are currently under discussion. It is recommended that machines are tested on commissioning, after changing the programme or detergent, on the advice of the infection control team/committee or if a problem associated with the washer–disinfector is highlighted. EN 15883 and HTM-01 describe a schedule of tests that should be carried out at regular intervals. If the washer–disinfector is functioning correctly, it should render processed items free from infection risk and safe for patient reuse. If organic material is not removed from surfaces, it may become baked or fixed onto them during subsequent heat or chemical sterilization, it may cause friction in moving parts (causing accelerated wear) and it may lead to blockages in lumens.

A typical cycle consists of a low-temperature flush/rinse at a temperature which will not fix or bake organic material (usually <35°C), and a main wash at >55°C followed by a disinfection rinse at the appropriate temperature as stated in Table 5.1. Optional stages include a final rinse and a drying stage.

The management of decontamination equipment including thermal washer–disinfectors is described in HTM 01-01 Part A (Department of Health, 2007).

CHEMICAL DISINFECTION – TYPES OF CHEMICAL DISINFECTANTS (see Hoffman, 2004)

Most healthcare facilities have produced their own policy for the use of disinfectants, but it is still possible to find inappropriate disinfectants being used at inadequate or inappropriate concentrations. Expensive and ineffective disinfectants are still in use when cheaper or more effective agents are available, or when a disinfectant is not required at all. There remains a need for some degree of regional (if not national) standardization. A sound disinfectant policy should considerably increase the cost effectiveness of disinfection in hospitals.

Phenolics

Phenols and cresols are mainly derived from the distillation of coal tar, but mixtures of synthetic phenols may be used. Chlorinated fractions and petroleum residues may also be added.

Black and white fluids

These are crude coal-tar derivatives. Black fluids (e.g. 'Jeyes fluid') are solubilized in soap and toxic and irritating to the skin. White fluids (e.g. 'Izal') are emulsified suspensions and tend to precipitate on surfaces, making subsequent cleaning more difficult. These disinfectants, especially white fluids, are sometimes used for environmental disinfection in hospitals, but have been largely replaced by alternative agents.

Clear soluble phenolics (e.g. Stericol, Hycolin, Clearsol)

Like other phenolics, these compounds are active against a wide range of bacteria, including *Pseudomonas aeruginosa* and *Mycobacterium tuberculosis*. They are fungicidal, but have limited virucidal activity and poor activity against bacterial spores. They are relatively cheap, stable and are not readily inactivated by organic matter. However, they often contain a compatible detergent, so precleaning of the surface is not necessary.

However, in the UK as a result of the European Union (EU) Biocidal Products Regulations (2001), products containing 2,4,6-trichlorophenol and xylenol have been withdrawn from the market. This includes the clear soluble phenolics Hycolin, Clearsol and Stericol.

Uses are mainly confined to environmental disinfection, particularly in the presence of faeces or sputum, as they are too corrosive for many instruments and too toxic to be applied to the skin. These and other phenolics should not be used in food preparation areas as they taint food, or on equipment that is likely to be in contact with skin or mucous membranes. Their use has decreased as a result of the growing need for a virucidal disinfectant for blood-borne viruses, and they have been largely replaced by chlorine-releasing agents. However, they are still widely used for instruments in post-mortem rooms when thermal decontamination methods are not available. They are also widely used in microbiological laboratories handling mycobacteria. Owing to their withdrawal a suitable alternative should be used.

Chloroxylenols (e.g. Dettol and Ibcol)

These are non-irritant but are readily inactivated by a wide range of materials, including organic matter and hard water, and high concentrations are required (2.5–5 per cent). Chloroxylenols are effective against Gram-positive bacteria but poorly active against Gram-negative bacteria. The addition of a chelating agent (ethylenediamine tetra-acetic acid; EDTA) increases the activity of chloroxylenols against Gram-negative bacilli. They are non-corrosive and non-irritant. However, they are not suitable for environmental or instrument use in hospitals.

Pine oil disinfectants

These compounds are non-toxic and non-irritant, but are relatively ineffective against many organisms, especially *Pseudomonas aeruginosa*. They should not be used in hospitals.

Halogens (compounds or solutions that release chlorine or iodine)

Chlorine-releasing agents

These are cheap and effective disinfectants which act by releasing available chlorine. They are rapidly effective against viruses, fungi, bacteria and spores, and particularly recommended for use where special hazards of viral infection exist (e.g. hepatitis B virus [HBV] or human immunodeficiency virus [HIV]) and *Clostridium difficile* where sporicidal activity is required. Solutions are unstable at use concentration, so dilutions should be prepared daily. They are readily inactivated by organic matter (e.g. pus, dirt, blood, etc.) and may damage certain materials (e.g. plastics, rubber, some metals and fabrics). Chlorine-releasing agents are not compatible with some detergents, and should not be mixed with acids, including acidic body fluids, such as urine, as the free chlorine produced may be harmful, particularly in a confined space. Solutions may be stabilized with alkali or sodium chloride. Chlorine-releasing agents at low concentrations are non-toxic and are particularly useful for water treatment, babies' feeding bottles and food-preparation areas, and may also have other uses in the hospital environment. Their uses and recommended concentrations are shown in Table 5.2.

Preparations of chlorine-releasing agents include the following.

- Strong alkaline hypochlorite solutions (e.g. Chloros, Domestos) containing approximately 10 per cent (100 000) ppm available chlorine (av Cl_2). Similar solutions in the USA are supplied at 5 per cent (50 000 ppm av Cl_2). The concentrated solutions are corrosive and should be handled with care. Dilute solutions may be used with a compatible detergent, but will only reliably disinfect clean surfaces.
- Hypochlorite solutions containing 1 per cent (10 000 ppm av Cl_2) and stabilized with sodium chloride (e.g. Milton or a preparation with comparable properties). These solutions are usually diluted 1:80 (125 ppm av Cl_2) for the disinfection of infant feeding bottles and catering equipment and surfaces. The low chlorine content is inactivated by very small amounts of organic matter, and in-use solutions have a much narrower margin of safety.
- Hypochlorite/hypobromite powders (e.g. Diversol BX). Solutions of these powders (0.5–1.0 per cent) are used in the same way as other hypochlorite preparations, and are rather less corrosive. The powder may be used for cleaning baths and sinks where an abrasive preparation is undesirable.
- Abrasive powders containing hypochlorites (e.g. hospital scouring powder, Vim, Ajax, etc.)

Table 5.2 Concentrations of chlorine-releasing agents in use

Uses	Available chlorine (mg/L) (ppm)[a]
Blood spillage from patient with HIV or HBV infection	10 000
Laboratory discard jars	2 500
General environmental disinfection	1 000
Disinfection of clean instruments	500
Infant feeding bottles and teats	125
Food-preparation areas and catering equipment	
Eradication of *Legionella* from water supply system, depending on exposure time	5–50
Hydrotherapy pools	
Routine	1.5–3
If contaminated	6–10
Routine water treatment	0.5–1

[a]Undiluted commercial hypochlorite solution contains approximately 100 000 ppm available chlorine.

HBV, hepatitis B virus; HIV, human immunodeficiency virus.

- Non-abrasive powders (e.g. Titan, Diversey Detergent Sanitizer) containing hypochlorites are now usually preferred to abrasive powders for cleaning and disinfection of hospital baths and sinks.
- Other chlorine-releasing compounds include sodium dichloroisocyanurate (NaDCC; e.g. Sanichlor, Haztab, Presept) tablets, powders or granules. These compounds are growing in popularity as the tablets/powders are stable during storage, and solutions can be prepared more conveniently and accurately. However, the stability of prepared solutions is similar to that of sodium hypochlorite solutions. They tend to be slightly more effective and less corrosive than hypochlorite solutions, but care is still necessary with metals. The cost of preparing solutions with a low concentration (e.g. 100–200 ppm av Cl_2) is comparable to that of liquid hypochlorite preparations, but the use of tablets for preparing high concentrations (e.g. 10 000 ppm av Cl_2) may be slightly more expensive.

NaDCC powders or granules may be applied directly to spillage of blood or body fluids from patients with suspected HBV or HIV, and are convenient and effective alternatives to solutions (Coates, 1988; Bloomfield and Miller, 1989). However, their use may not be suitable for large spills (>30 mL), when disposable cloths, or a mop and bucket with a solution of disinfectant may be more appropriate.

Chlorine dioxide (e.g. Tristel)

This has been used for many years for the treatment of drinking and waste water and for slime control, but products are now available for disinfection of heat-sensitive instruments, for example, flexible endoscopes (Babb and Bradley, 1995). Chlorine dioxide is a highly effective compound, which is rapidly bactericidal – including activity against mycobacteria (Griffiths *et al.*, 1999) – virucidal and sporicidal, achieving high-level disinfection within 5 min and sporicidal activity within 10 min. The product is supplied at several concentrations, which will affect the stability/use-life. This compound may be suitable for the decontamination of heat-labile equipment (e.g. endoscopes) provided that user acceptance and instrument and processor compatibility have been established (see Chapter 6).

Iodine and iodophors

A 1 per cent solution of iodine in 70 per cent alcohol is an effective preoperative skin antiseptic. Skin reactions may occur in some individuals, and for this reason 0.5 per cent alcoholic chlorhexidine or an alcoholic iodophor solution is usually preferred.

Iodophors are complexes of iodine and 'solubilizers', which possess the same activity as iodine, but are non-irritant and do not stain the skin. Iodophors are mainly used for hand disinfection, for example, povidone-iodine (PVP-I;

Betadine, Disadine, Videne) detergent preparations or 'surgical scrubs'. These contain 7.5 per cent PVP-I (equivalent to 0.7 per cent available iodine) and are effective for this purpose. Alcoholic preparations containing 10 per cent PVP-I (1 per cent available iodine) are suitable for pre-operative preparation of the skin at the operation site. Some iodophors may also be used for disinfection of the environment, but they are expensive and cannot be recommended for general disinfection in hospital.

Iodine is the only antiseptic which has been shown to have a useful sporicidal action on the skin. When applied as an iodophor, it can be left on the skin long enough to remove a large proportion of *Clostridium perfringens* spores when these are present, but this property is of uncertain clinical value (see Chapter 12).

Superoxidized/electrolysed water (e.g. Sterilox)

This is used for the decontamination of flexible endoscopes. The solution is produced by electrolysing a salt solution and collecting the solution produced at the anode (anolyte). A generator produces the solution at the point of use and pipes it to existing washer–disinfectors (provided that they are compatible). The solution is used once only and then discarded. Freshly generated Sterilox is rapidly sporicidal (Selkon *et al.*, 1999) and mycobactericidal (Selkon *et al.*, 1999; Shetty *et al.*, 1999), provided that generation criteria are fulfilled. These criteria are the redox potential (>950 mV), pH (5.0–6.5) and current (9 A). Sterilox is affected by organic matter, so items need to be scrupulously clean, and it is also very unstable. Only freshly generated solutions should be used, and the pipework should be purged to remove 'dead' solution if left for a period of time. This product may be suitable for the decontamination of heat-labile equipment (e.g. flexible endoscopes) provided that compatibility between instrument and processor has been established. Other superoxidized/electrolysed (acid) water systems with varying pH are under development, which may also prove useful for the decontamination of endoscopes.

Quaternary ammonium compounds such as benzalkonium chloride

These are relatively non-toxic antibacterial compounds with detergent properties. They are active against Gram-positive organisms but much less active against Gram-negative bacilli, and are readily inactivated by soap, anionic detergents and organic matter. Quaternary ammonium compounds (QACs) at higher dilutions inhibit the growth of organisms (i.e. they are 'bacteriostatic') but do not necessarily kill them (i.e. they do not show a 'bactericidal' effect). For this reason, their effectiveness has often been exaggerated. Their use in hospitals is limited because of their narrow spectrum of activity, but they may be useful for cleansing dirty wounds (e.g. cetrimide). Apart from possible uses in food-preparation areas, QACs are not widely used in the UK for environmental disinfection. Contamination of a weak solution of a QAC with

Gram-negative bacilli is a possible hazard, which can be prevented by avoidance of cork closures or of 'topping-up' stock bottles. Incorporating a chelating agent enhances the activity of QACs against Gram-negative bacilli. However, QACs are ineffective against HBV, tubercle bacilli and spores, and show variable activity against HIV. More recently, some QAC mixtures have been introduced that show activity against *Pseudomonas aeruginosa* and other Gram-negative bacilli, some viruses and mycobacteria.

Chlorhexidine

This useful skin antiseptic is highly active against vegetative Gram-positive organisms, but less active against Gram-negative bacilli. It also has good fungicidal activity, but shows little or no activity against tubercle bacilli, enveloped viruses and bacterial spores. It is relatively non-toxic, but is inactivated by soaps. Its use in hospitals should be restricted as much as possible to procedures involving contact with skin or mucous membranes. It is too expensive for environmental use and has limited value.

Detergent solutions containing 4 per cent chlorhexidine gluconate are available (e.g. Hibiscrub, Hibiclens). These have been found to be highly effective for the disinfection of surgeons' hands prior to operating, and they have a good persistent effect owing to residuals left on the skin after rinsing and drying. Some alternative preparations show inadequate bactericidal effects and may be irritant to the skin. Trials are necessary before new products are introduced even if they contain similar concentrations of chlorhexidine gluconate. Cosmetic acceptability is an important factor when a disinfectant is being selected for the skin, particularly that of the hands.

Savlon is a mixture of chlorhexidine and cetrimide. The hospital concentrate contains 15 per cent cetrimide and 1.5 per cent chlorhexidine. It is usually used at a concentration of 1 per cent. At this concentration the antimicrobial activity of the chlorhexidine is poor. However, cetrimide is a good cleansing agent and enhances the activity of chlorhexidine. Savlon is expensive and, if used, should be reserved for clinical procedures, such as cleansing dirty wounds, and not used for instruments or environmental disinfection.

Low concentrations of antiseptics are likely to become contaminated during use. The provision of pre-sterilized single-use sachets (Hibidil, Savlodil) reduces this risk.

Hibisol is a 0.5 per cent solution of chlorhexidine in 70 per cent isopropanol, used for disinfection of clean intact skin (e.g. that of the hands); 0.5 per cent chlorhexidine gluconate in 70 per cent ethanol (or isopropanol) is used for disinfection of the operation site. A 2 per cent solution of chlorhexidine in 70 per cent isopropyl alcohol is now available which is recommended for disinfection of the skin prior to insertion of central venous devices (Pratt *et al.*, 2007).

Hexachlorophane

This compound is highly active against Gram-positive organisms but less active against Gram-negative ones. It is relatively insoluble in water, but can be incorporated in soap or detergent solutions without loss of activity. It has a good residual effect on the skin. These solutions are prone to contamination with Gram-negative bacteria unless a preservative is included in the formulation. Potentially neurotoxic levels may occur in the blood if emulsions or other preparations of hexachlorophane are repeatedly and extensively applied to the body surface of babies. This product, although very effective, is now infrequently used for skin disinfection in hospitals, and can only be obtained for use on medical advice. It may be used for handwashing by staff during staphylococcal outbreaks or for surgical hand disinfection. Toxic levels are not approached when a hexachlorophane dusting powder is used on the umbilical stump of neonates, and this method, which has been found to be highly effective in the control of staphylococcal infection, may still be considered to have a role in hospital practice. It may also be applied to the groin and buttock regions of methicillin-resistant *Staphylococcus aureus* (MRSA) carriers.

Triclosan

Triclosan-containing products have properties and a spectrum of activity similar to those of hexachlorophane, but they show no toxicity to neonates. They are now widely used as an alternative to hexachlorophane in hand rubs, soaps and bath concentrates. In-use concentrations are in the range 0.3–2.0 per cent. Antimicrobial tests and trials for tolerance are required before the use of individual products, as these are variable and generally less effective than chlorhexidine preparations. Triclosan-containing products are often used for the treatment of MRSA carriers, as they are better tolerated than some other antiseptic-containing detergents.

Alcohols

Ethyl alcohol 70 per cent (ethanol) and 60 per cent isopropyl alcohol (isopropanol) are effective and rapidly acting disinfectants and antiseptics, with the additional advantage that they evaporate, leaving the treated surfaces dry, but they have poor penetrative powers and should only be used on clean surfaces. They are active against mycobacteria but not against spores. Their activity against viruses is variable, and non-enveloped viruses (e.g. poliovirus) tend to be more resistant, particularly to isopropanol (Tyler *et al.*, 1990). The recommended concentrations of ethanol (70 per cent) and isopropanol (60 per cent) are optimal *in vitro* for killing organisms and are more effective than absolute alcohol. Alcohol or alcohol-impregnated wipes may be used for the rapid disinfection of smooth clean surfaces (e.g. trolley tops, thermometers, probes and electrical/electronic equipment), which cannot be safely immersed in aqueous disinfectants. They are also useful for irrigating the lumens of bronchoscopes after rinsing, if the microbiological quality of the rinse water cannot be guaranteed to eradicate atypical mycobacteria. If the item is contaminated with blood or secretions, prior cleaning is advised. Owing to the fixative properties of alcohol, it should not be used on soiled surfaces and where there is a risk of transmission of transmissible spongiform encephalopathies.

Alcohol is commonly used for skin disinfection (e.g. without additives for treating skin prior to injection). With the addition of 1 per cent glycerol or other suitable emollients, 60–70 per cent alcohol rubbed on until the skin is dry is an effective agent for the rapid disinfection of physically clean hands, especially if handwashing facilities are unsuitable or not readily available. The addition of other bactericides to alcohol does not appreciably increase its immediate effect as a skin antiseptic, but the repeated use of alcohol solutions may lead to lower equilibrium levels of bacteria on the skin. The addition of non-volatile antiseptics (e.g. chlorhexidine, povidone iodine and triclosan) may provide a residual antiseptic action on the skin.

Aldehydes – formaldehyde, glutaraldehyde and succine dialdehyde

Although formaldehyde is required in extreme circumstances, for example, for fumigation of rooms following care of a patient with a viral haemorrhagic fever (Advisory Committee on Dangerous Pathogens, 1997) or disinfection of a ventilator not protected by a bacteria-retaining filter, and may achieve sterilization if used with sub-atmospheric steam, solutions of formaldehyde are too irritant for use as general disinfectants. However, formaldehyde is still recommended for the fumigation of laboratory safety cabinets (Advisory Committee on Dangerous Pathogens, 2001; Health and Safety Executive, 2003).

Glutaraldehyde is generally used as a 2 per cent activated alkaline solution at room temperature, and is recommended for heat-sensitive items, particularly flexible endoscopes. It is non-damaging to metals, plastics and rubber, and is effective against vegetative organisms, viruses (including HBV and HIV) and fungi. Its activity against *Mycobacterium tuberculosis* is relatively slow (i.e. 20 min of exposure time may be required; Griffiths *et al.*, 1999), as is its sporicidal activity (>60 min; Babb *et al.*, 1980). Glutaraldehyde may be irritating to the eyes, skin and respiratory tract, and can cause sensitization, including occupational asthma and contact dermatitis (Cowan *et al.*, 1993). Its use should be restricted to areas where adequate provision has been made for the extraction/total containment of aldehyde vapour and personal protective equipment (e.g. gloves, apron, goggles, respiratory masks) is available in the event of a spillage. In the UK, glutaraldeyhde is no longer used owing to health and safety issues and its fixative properties. Alkaline solutions require activation and, once activated, they remain stable for 2–4 weeks depending on the preparation. However, they may become diluted during use, particularly in automated washers, and may require a more frequent exchange. To ensure sporicidal activity, an exposure period of at least 3 hours is required, although shorter times may be sufficient to kill some pathogenic spores (e.g. *Clostridium* difficile; Dyas and Das, 1985; Rutala *et al.*, 1993).

Acid solutions of glutaraldehyde are more stable and do not require activation, but usually have a slower sporicidal effect. They may be more suitable for the occasional or small user. Their activity is improved by use at a temperature of 50–60°C, although this can be associated with an increase in vapour levels and possible damage to instruments. Lower concentrations of aldehydes (0.125–2 per cent) have been used at an elevated temperature (45–60°C) within an automated endoscope washer–disinfector. Other aldehydes (e.g. succine dialdehyde) have similar properties to glutaraldehyde. The addition of a phenolic compound to 2 per cent glutaraldehyde improves the sporicidal action but the advantages are marginal for routine disinfection.

Ortho-phthalaldehyde (OPA) has more recently been introduced for the decontamination of flexible endoscopes. It is efficacious against bacteria, including mycobacteria and viruses, but no claims for sporicidal activity have been made. It is compatible with flexible endoscopes and is available at use-dilution or in a concentrated form for use in washer–disinfectors. A safety warning was issued in 2004 by the MHRA in the UK recommending that OPA is not used for flexible cystoscopes owing to residuals possibly causing post-procedural sensitization in some individuals.

Hydrogen peroxide

Hydrogen peroxide (3 or 6 per cent) is infrequently used as a hospital disinfectant in the UK compared to the USA. It is used for the disinfection of tonometers and soft contact lenses, and also for ventilators not protected by filters. It has also been added to urinary drainage bags. Frequent use has been associated with corrosion of certain metals. However, it is now being used in dedicated systems for room fumigation/disinfection.

Peroxygen compounds (e.g. Virkon) have variable virucidal activity (Tyler *et al.*, 1990) and little or no activity against mycobacteria (Broadley *et al.*, 1993; Holton *et al.*, 1995; Griffiths *et al.*, 1999). They are less corrosive than hypochlorites, so they may have a role in the disinfection of laboratory equipment and environmental surfaces, where the infection risk is low and compatibility with the surface has been established. Virkon powder may be used as a less corrosive alternative for decontamination of spillage (e.g. on carpets).

Peracetic acid

Peracetic acid has been used for the disinfection of certain types of equipment (e.g. patient isolators and, more recently, for the decontamination of endoscopes). It is rapidly bactericidal, virucidal, mycobactericidal and sporicidal, and is claimed to be relatively non-toxic and non-corrosive at the concentrations used. There are various products on the market and contact times vary from, for example, 5 to 20 min depending on the concentration pH and target organism. Users should check with the manufacturers to ensure the correct concentration and contact time is used. Some products are reusable solutions and others are used once only. Steris contains 0.2 per cent peracetic acid solution and has to be used in a dedicated processing machine (i.e. a Steris System 1 Endoscope Processor at an elevated temperature of 45°C; Bradley *et al.*, 1995). The disinfectant is supplied as a concentrate, which is diluted within the machine and discarded to waste after use. It is important to establish compatibility with instruments and processing equipment before use.

Other antimicrobial compounds

Many other antimicrobial compounds have been used. Among these are the acridine and triphenyl methane (crystal violet and brilliant green) dyes, which were once widely used as antiseptics for skin and for wounds. Silver nitrate and other silver compounds (e.g. silver sulphadiazine) have a valuable place as topical antiseptics in prophylaxis against infection of burns. 8-Hydroxyquinoline has been found to be effective as a fungicide. Mercurial compounds have poor bactericidal powers, but they are strongly bacteriostatic. Phenyl mercuric nitrate has been used as an effective preservative for ophthalmic solutions.

Other compounds have been described by Block (1991) and Fraise *et al.* (2004).

THE FORMULATION OF A DISINFECTION POLICY

The general principles for formulation of a policy are summarized below (Hoffman *et al.*, 2004). The infection control committee should prepare the disinfectant policy and decide on the types of disinfectants to be used. This requires consultation between the microbiologist, infection control doctor, infection control nurse, pharmacist, supplies officer and representatives of medical, nursing and domestic staff. Demands for disinfectants come from many departments of the hospital, and there are many sources of supply. All requests for disinfectants should be approved by the hospital pharmacist, who can check whether they are in agreement with the hospital policy.

The selection of a disinfectant depends on many factors (Fraise, 1999), including the following:

- intended use of the disinfectant – medical equipment, environment, skin and mucous membranes;
- range of activity;
- speed of action;
- inactivation by organic material;
- compatibility with items processed and processing equipment;
- user safety;
- stability;
- cost.

Principles

1 List all of the purposes for which disinfectants are used, then check requisitions and orders to ensure that the list is complete.

2 Eliminate the use of chemical disinfectants when heat can reasonably be used as an alternative, when sterilization is required, when thorough cleaning alone is adequate, or if single-use equipment can be used economically. There should be few remaining uses for chemical disinfectants.

3 Select the smallest practicable number of disinfectants for the remaining uses, that is, one routine disinfectant for each field of use (the environment, skin and equipment), plus an alternative for use if patients or staff are sensitive to the routine disinfectants, for instruments which may be damaged by the disinfectant, and for use when the routine disinfectant is either unavailable or inappropriate for a particular purpose.

4 Arrange for the distribution of disinfectants chosen at the correct use-dilution, or supply equipment and personal protective equipment for preparing and measuring disinfectants at the site of use.

5 All potential users of disinfectants should receive adequate instruction in their preparation and use. This should include information on the following:
   (a) the correct disinfectant and concentration to be used for each task;
   (b) the shelf-life of the disinfectant at the concentration supplied, the type of container to be used, and the frequency with which the solution should be changed;
   (c) substances or materials which will react with or neutralize the disinfectant;
   (d) an assessment of toxic or other risks to employees using the disinfectant or detergent is needed, together with the measures required for protection of employees [Control of Substances Hazardous to Health (COSHH) Regulations, 1988]. Personal safety measures should be addressed, for example, whether rubber gloves should be worn, how the product can be safely opened and prepared, how the disinfectant should be disposed of, what action is required if the product comes into contact with the skin or eye.

6 The policy should be monitored to ensure that it is effective and continues to be so.

Selection of disinfectants

Antimicrobial properties

Where this is compatible with other requirements, the disinfectants used should be bactericidal rather than bacteriostatic, active against a wide range of microbes, and not readily inactivated. The manufacturer should supply information on the properties of the disinfectant, but independent antimicrobial tests are also required. The EU has now introduced European Norm (EN) tests to which all newly marketed disinfectants should be subjected. These will take the form of a standardized suspension test and surface/carrier tests using relevant test organisms and, in the future, more practical 'in-use' tests. The Association of Official Analytical Chemists (AOAC) surface test in the USA has been criticized on account of its lack of reproducibility and it is hoped that some international standardization of tests will be possible in the future. Manufacturers should also provide Material Safety Data Sheets to enable the user to carry out COSHH assessments, as well as information on material compatibility and instructions for use.

Other properties

The properties of the disinfectants chosen should be considered in terms of acceptability as well as antibacterial activity. Stability, toxicity and corrosiveness/compatibility should be assessed with the aid of relevant information obtained from the manufacturers. Acceptability and cleaning properties should also be assessed. Cost is clearly important, and a regional contract for one or two generally acceptable disinfectants should considerably reduce costs. A trial period (possibly of 3 months) might be introduced, and an assessment of all relevant factors should be made before the policy is permanently implemented. COSHH assessments should be performed on all chemical disinfectants.

Review of policy

This should be considered annually. Defects of the current system should be noted and changes introduced where necessary.

RECOMMENDED DISINFECTANTS AND USE-DILUTIONS

Environment

A chlorine-releasing agent and a phenolic disinfectant should be sufficient for most environmental hospital requirements.

Hypochlorites and other chlorine-releasing agents (see Table 5.2, p. **92**) have the properties already mentioned. They may be incorporated in a powder (abrasive or non-abrasive) for cleaning baths, toilets and washbasins. Solutions (1000 ppm av Cl_2) may be used for disinfecting clean surfaces and, when necessary, for food-preparation areas. Chlorine-releasing agents should be used if disinfection of virus-contaminated material is required. However, routine or too frequent use can cause expensive corrosion and damage to equipment and some surfaces, in which case other less corrosive antiviral agents are required. Higher concentrations of chlorine (i.e. 10 000 ppm) are recommended in the presence of organic material (e.g. blood/body-fluid spillages).

A clear soluble phenolic disinfectant (e.g. Stericol, Hycolin, Clearsol) is often chosen as one of the disinfectants for routine use, especially where contamination with mycobacterial species is known or suspected. However, these products are no longer available in the UK. Other agents are available, including chlorine-releasing agents, which do have demonstrable mycobactericidal efficacy.

After thorough cleansing with detergent and water, items may be immersed in alcohol or cleaned and disinfected using a disposable alcohol-impregnated wipe. This is preferable to the use of glutaraldehyde, peracetic acid or chlorine dioxide. NaDCC compounds tend to be less corrosive than hypochlorites.

Instruments

If possible, heat-tolerant instruments should be purchased. However, for heat-labile instruments glutaraldehyde may be used provided that total containment/extraction of vapour is in place. Other alternative agents include peracetic acid and chlorine dioxide, but users are advised to establish instrument and processing equipment compatibility and to ascertain what personal protective equipment is required in relation to COSHH.

Skin

Antiseptics containing chlorhexidine, povidone iodine or triclosan are widely used for the disinfection of the skin (i.e. hands and operation site). Alcohol is also widely used for the hands, especially where handwashing facilities are either unavailable or unsuitable. Cosmetic acceptability is an important factor when selecting agents for the skin, particularly the hands. In most instances, soap and water are sufficient (see Chapter 6).

Dilution and distribution of disinfectants

Ineffective cleaning and too low a concentration are the commonest causes of failure of a disinfectant to kill organisms, and survival of contaminants in the disinfectant is unlikely if it is at the recommended use-dilution. It is therefore preferable for the pharmacist to supply departments with containers of disinfectant already prepared at the correct use-dilution, or for departments to prepare their own solutions. Containers should be labelled with the date of issue and the date after which the disinfectant should not be used (e.g. 1 week after issue); they should be clearly labelled with an instruction such as 'do not dilute' or 'use undiluted' and any relevant safety information. Containers should ideally be single-use but, if reusable, should be thoroughly washed and preferably disinfected by heat before refilling. If heating is not possible, thorough drying after washing should be adequate, as this will kill most of the bacteria that are likely to be present. Corks must not be used; containers should have plastic closures, which can be easily cleaned.

The main disadvantage of this method of dispensing is the transport of large quantities of fluid (mainly water), particularly if large amounts of disinfectants are used, and because some disinfectants (e.g. chlorine-releasing agents) are unstable when diluted. The alternative method is to supply undiluted disinfectant to the department where dilutions are prepared when required. A suitable and relatively foolproof measuring system is required for both disinfectant and water. A measuring device attached to the container is commonly used, but unless staff are well trained, dilutions will be inaccurate. A measured amount of undiluted disinfectant in a bottle, tablet or sachet is an alternative, but the water must also be measured. The strong disinfectant solution requires careful handling and appropriate personal protective equipment in order to avoid damage to the skin or the eyes of the operator. Gloves and a plastic apron should be worn and eye protection is necessary if splashing is likely.

Training and staff instruction

Whichever system of supplying disinfectants is used, all personnel handling or using them must be adequately trained, supervised and regularly updated. Training should include preparation and use of the disinfectant, with particular emphasis placed on accuracy of preparation, safe use and the COSHH regulations.

DISINFECTANT TESTING

In Europe, standards have now been published for establishing the efficacy of chemical disinfectants. The standards are made up of three phases as follows.

- *Phase 1*: a simple suspension test to establish basic bactericidal activity against *Pseudomonas aeruginosa* and *Staphylococcus aureus*. The test is carried out in the absence of organic material and a 5 $\log_{10}$ reduction is required in 60 min to pass the test.
- *Phase 2*: tests designed to simulate practical in-use conditions. Tests are carried out in the presence of low and high levels of soiling (albumin and

Table 5.3 EN 14385 (British Standards Institution, 2006a) Standard test methods to be used to substantiate claims. (Reproduced from British Standards Institution [2006a] EN 14385:2006 Chemical disinfectants and antiseptics – application of European Standards for chemical disinfectants and antiseptics)

Type and/or purpose of product	Phase step	Activity claims							
		Bactericidal	Fungicidal	Yeasticidal	Mycobactericidal	Tuberculocidal	Virucidal	Sporicidal	Legionella
Hygienic handwash	2.1	*	***	**	***	***	EN 14476	***	
	2.2	EN 1499	***	***	***	***	***	***	
Hygienic handrub	2.1	*	***	**	***	***	EN 14476	***	
	2.2	EN 1500	***	***	***	***	***	***	
Surgical hand disinfection (handrub and handwash)	2.1	*	***	**	***	***	EN 14476	***	
	2.2	EN 12791	***	***	***	***	***	***	
Surface disinfection clean and dirty conditions	2.1	**	**	**	EN 14348	EN 14348	EN 14476	**	
	2.2	**	**	**	**	**	*	**	
Instrument disinfection clean and dirty conditions	2.1	EN 13727	EN 13624	EN 13624	EN 14348	EN 14348	EN 14776	*	
	2.2	EN 14561	EN 14562	EN 14562	EN 14563	EN 14563	*	*	
Water treatment	2.1	***	***	***	***	***	***	***	*

* Work item approved.

** No work items are yet approved but relevant standards may become available in the future.

*** No intention to develop a test.

sheep erythrocytes) and include tests against bacteria, fungi/yeasts, viruses and mycobacteria. This phase of testing is subdivided into Phase 2 Step 1 (i.e. suspension tests) and Phase 2 Step 2 (i.e. surface tests).

• *Phase 3*: field tests under practical conditions. The methodology for these tests has not yet been established.

EN 14385 (British Standards Institution, 2006a) summarizes the tests available for different applications (i.e. medical, food, veterinary and domestic use), the test strains, the organic load and the requirements for passing the test. The requirements for disinfectants used in the medical area are shown in Table 5.3.

Other countries (e.g. the USA and Australia) also have standard test methods for establishing the efficacy of chemical disinfectants. The advantage of having standard test methods is that users can compare efficacy between products in the knowledge that the same test method was used by different test agencies. Standards can give clear guidance on what is required to validate efficacy claims.

REFERENCES

Advisory Committee on Dangerous Pathogens (1997). *Management and control of viral haemorrhagic fevers.* London: HMSO.

Advisory Committee on Dangerous Pathogens (2001) *Categorisation of biological agents according to hazard and categories of containment,* 4th edn. London: HMSO.

Babb JR and Bradley CR (1995) A review of glutaraldehyde alternatives. *British Journal of Theatre Nursing* **5**, 20.

Babb JR, Bradley CR and Ayliffe GAJ (1980) Sporicidal activity of glutaraldehyde and hypochlorite and other factors influencing their selection for the treatment of medical equipment. *Journal of Hospital Infection* **1**, 63.

Biocidal Products Regulations (2001) *Statutory instrument 2001 no. 880.* Available online at: http://www.opsi.gov.uk/si/si2001/20010880.htm (last accessed 27 November 2008).

Block SS (1991) *Disinfection, sterilization and preservation,* 4th edn. Philadelphia, PA: Lea & Febiger.

Bloomfield SF and Miller EA (1989) A comparison of hypochlorite and phenolic disinfectants for disinfection of clean and soiled surfaces and blood spillages. *Journal of Hospital Infection* **13**, 231.

Bradley CR, Babb JR and Ayliffe GAJ (1995) Evaluation of the Steris System 1 peracetic acid endoscope processor. *Journal of Hospital Infection* **29**, 143.

British Standards Institution (2006a) EN 14385:2006 *Chemical disinfectants and antiseptics – application of European Standards for chemical disinfectants and antiseptics.* Milton Keynes: British Standards Institution.

British Standards Institution (2006b) EN ISO 15883:2006 *Washer disinfectors, Parts 1–4.* Milton Keynes: British Standards Institution.

Broadley SJ, Furr JR, Jenkins PA and Russell AD (1993) Antimycobacterial activity of 'Virkon'. *Journal of Hospital Infection* **23**, 189.

Coates D (1988) Comparison of sodium hypochlorite and sodium dichloroisocyanurate disinfectants. Neutralization by serum. *Journal of Hospital Infection* **11**, 60.

Control of Substances Hazardous to Health Regulations (1988). London: HMSO.

Cowan RE, Manning AP, Ayliffe GAJ *et al.* (1993) Aldehyde disinfectants and health in endoscopy units. *Gut* **34**, 1641.

Department of Health (2007) HTM 01-01 Part A: Decontamination of Medical Devices. London: Department of Health.

Dyas A and Das BC (1985) The activity of glutaraldehyde against *Clostridium difficile*. *Journal of Hospital Infection* **6**, 41.

Fraise AP (1999) Choosing disinfectants. *Journal of Hospital Infection* **43**, 255.

Fraise AP, Lambert PA and Maillard J-Y (2004) *Principles and practice of disinfection, sterilization and preservation*, 4th edn. Oxford: Blackwell Publishing.

Griffiths PA, Babb JR and Fraise AP (1999) Mycobactericidal activity of selected disinfectants using a quantitative suspension test. *Journal of Hospital Infection* **41**, 111.

Health and Safety Executive (2003) *Health Services Advisory Committee. Safe working and the prevention of infection in clinical laboratories and similar facilities*. London: HMSO.

Hoffman PN, Bradley CR, Ayliffe GAJ (2004) *Disinfection in healthcare*, 3rd edn. London: Health Protection Agency/Oxford: Blackwell Publishing.

Holton J, Nye P and McDonald V (1995) Efficacy of selected disinfectants against mycobacteria and cryptosporidia. *Journal of Hospital Infection* **31**, 235.

http://www.mhra.gov.uk/Safetyinformation/Generalsafetyinformationandadvice/Technicalinformation/Decontaminationandinfectioncontrol/CON019632 (Last accessed 8 September 2008).

Medicines and Healthcare Products Regulatory Agency (2005) *Sterilization, disinfection and cleaning of medical equipment: guidance on decontamination from the Microbiology Advisory Committee. Part 2 Protocols*. London: Department of Health.

NHS Estates (1997) *Health Technical Memorandum 2030. Washer disinfectors: design considerations*. Leeds: NHS Estates.

Pratt RJ, Pellowe CM, Wilson JA *et al.* (2007) epic2: national evidence based guidelines for preventing healthcare associated infections in UK hospitals. *Journal of Hospital Infection* **65S**, S1.

Rutala WA, Gergen MF and Weber DJ (1993) Inactivation of *Clostridium difficile* spores by disinfectants. *Infection Control and Hospital Epidemiology* **14**, 36.

Selkon JB, Babb JR and Morris R (1999) Evaluation of the antimicrobial activity of a new super-oxidised water, Sterilox™, for the disinfection of endoscopes. *Journal of Hospital Infection* **41**, 59.

Shetty N, Srinivasan S, Holton J and Ridgway GL (1999) Evaluation of microbicidal activity of a new disinfectant: Sterilox™ 2500, against *Clostridium difficile* spores, *Helicobacter pylori*, vancomycin-resistant *Enterococcus* species, *Candida albicans* and several *Mycobacterium* species. *Journal of Hospital Infection* **41**, 101.

Tyler R, Ayliffe GAJ and Bradley CR (1990) Virucidal activity of disinfectants: studies with the poliovirus. *Journal of Hospital Infection* **15**, 339.

6 DECONTAMINATION OF EQUIPMENT, THE ENVIRONMENT AND THE SKIN

Adam Fraise and Christina Bradley

The choice of method of decontamination (i.e. cleaning, disinfection or sterilization) depends on many factors, but the initial choice can be based on infection risks to patients. These can be classified as high, intermediate, low and minimal risks (Hoffman *et al.*, 2004). However, there is an overlap between these categories and requirements for decontamination may vary within a category.

INFECTION RISKS TO PATIENTS FROM EQUIPMENT, MATERIALS AND THE ENVIRONMENT

High risk

For invasive items, those in close contact with a break in the skin or mucous membrane, or introduced into a sterile body area (e.g. surgical instruments, dressings, catheters and prosthetic devices; see p. 109), sterilization is required. If sterilization is not practically achievable, high-level disinfection, although not optimal, may be adequate.

Intermediate risk

For items in contact with intact mucous membranes, body fluids or contaminated with particularly virulent or readily transmissible organisms, or items to be used on highly susceptible patients or sites (e.g. gastrointestinal endoscopes, respiratory equipment), disinfection is required.

Low risk

For items in contact with normal and intact skin (e.g. washing bowls, toilets and bedding), cleaning and drying is usually adequate. Disinfection is needed if there is a known infection risk, for example, baths after washing a patient with methicillin-resistant *Staphylococcus aureus* (MRSA).

Minimal risk

Items not in close contact with patients or their immediate surroundings are in the minimal risk category. For surfaces that are unlikely to be contaminated with a significant number of pathogens or those transferred to a susceptible site (e.g. floors, walls, sinks), cleaning to remove organisms and drying is usually adequate.

DECONTAMINATION POLICY

All healthcare institutions should have a policy outlining the recommendation agreement of cleaning and decontaminating equipment and the environment. All levels of decontamination should be appropriate to the risk category of the item to be decontaminated. Cleansing alone will be sufficient for low-risk items, particularly floors, walls and ceilings. For intermediate-risk equipment, decontamination by heat is the preferred option but, if this is not practical, a risk assessment will be required. Single-use items in some instances may be preferable. Where single-use items are not appropriate and the equipment is heat labile, cleaning agents may be the most suitable choice and a range of alternative agents must be considered as part of the risk assessment.

MANAGEMENT OF DECONTAMINATION

In the UK Health Technical Memorandum (HTM) 01-01 Part A (Department of Health, 2007) describes the functional responsibilities for decontamination for key personnel within a healthcare organization. Every healthcare establishment must have an individual, preferably at Board level, who takes overall responsibility for decontamination. This person is usually referred to as the Decontamination Lead. Many hospitals are now appointing a Decontamination Manager/Advisor who is responsible for providing day-to-day technical guidance on all aspects of decontamination of medical devices. They will coordinate the formulation of policies and carry out audits of decontamination and be instrumental in staff training.

The User is the person designated by management to be responsible for the management of the decontamination process. The User could be the sterile services department (SSD) manager, theatre manager, endoscopy unit manager, general practitioner, dentist or other healthcare professional The User has the responsibility for ensuring the item is 'fit for purpose' (i.e. is suitable for processing all items of equipment intended for reuse within the department, for ensuring the equipment is subjected to periodic testing and for ensuring operators of the equipment have received training in operation of the equipment).

Other individuals involved are:

• *an authorizing engineer* (decontamination) who will provide independent auditing of validation reports and can advise on the purchase of new equipment and assist when problems occur;

- *an authorized person* (decontamination) who will manage the engineering aspects of decontamination and provide day-to-day operational management of decontamination equipment within a healthcare organization;
- *a competent person* (decontamination) who has undergone specific training on testing and maintenance of decontamination equipment;
- *the Infection Control Team*, who can advise on purchase and testing of equipment.

In the UK, the Medicines and Healthcare Products Regulatory Agency (MHRA) have published a Device Bulletin on the Management of Medical Devices (MHRA, 2006b). This recommends the formation of a medical devices committee to manage the formulation of decontamination policies, the purchase of medical devices and decontamination equipment, training in use and decontamination of medical devices and ensuring servicing and maintenance takes place.

It is important that all staff carrying out decontamination of medical devices should have received adequate training that includes, as a minimum, device construction, compatibility and the procedures to be followed.

EQUIPMENT PROCUREMENT

Procurement of equipment must take place using a process that considers decontamination issues as well as price and function.

Someone with knowledge of decontamination must be involved in the process to ensure that any newly purchased equipment can be decontaminated adequately. Equipment must fulfil the requirements of any relevant standard which in Europe is indicated by the presence of a CE mark, whereas in the USA adherence to the Food and Drugs Administration status is required. Reusable equipment should have a validated decontamination method identification in the manufacturer's literature and the manufacturer's advice should be sought to ensure that any decontamination processes are compatible for the equipment.

DECONTAMINATION OF MEDICAL EQUIPMENT

See also Appendix (p. **142**) and MHRA (2002/2005/2006).

High-risk items

Most of the items in this category (e.g. surgical instruments, prosthetic devices, dressings, surgical drapes and gowns, parenteral fluids, etc.) can be sterilized by steam at high temperatures. Dry heat can be used to sterilize some delicate sharp instruments used in ophthalmic and dental surgery, glass syringes, oils and powders. Single-use items (e.g. catheters, plastic syringes, needles, grafts and internal pacemakers) are usually sterilized by the manufacturer using ethylene oxide or irradiation. Inexpensive items, especially those which are heat sensitive and difficult to clean, should not be reused (MHRA, 2006a). All reprocessed equipment should be cleaned thoroughly before sterilization prior to reuse. Properly validated, automated washer–disinfectors are preferred (NHS Estates, 1997; MHRA, 2002; British Standards Institution, 2006). Under the Medical Devices Directive (European Union, 1995), manufacturers are required to state which methods of decontamination can be used for any reusable item of equipment. Non-disposable items should preferably be able to withstand autoclaving at 134°C (or at least 80°C). If items are damaged at these temperatures, or if they cannot be cleaned easily, their use should be discouraged. Some expensive items, such as flexible endoscopes, are heat sensitive and must be decontaminated by less effective methods, such as immersion in disinfectants. Aldehyde-based disinfectants (e.g. 2 per cent glutaraldehyde) have been used but in the UK increased levels of sensitization have led to them no longer being available. Other agents (e.g. peracetic acid and chlorine dioxide) are now more widely used (see Chapter 5).

Instruments, holloware, etc. for clinical procedures

These should be supplied packed and sterilized by the SSD. Sterilization or disinfection of instruments at ward level should rarely be required. In some circumstances, single use may be preferable. If it is necessary to sterilize instruments at the point of use, a bench-top washer–disinfector and autoclave should preferably be used in a dedicated decontamination area. Bench-top autoclaves with vacuum-assisted air removal should be used for packaged, lumened and porous items. Boiling-water baths do not sterilize but, if used correctly, they are a more reliable method of disinfection than most chemical agents. In an emergency, pre-cleaned instruments can be disinfected, but not sterilized, in boiling water for 5–10 min. Immersion of clean instruments in an effective chemical disinfectant will disinfect, but is not as reliably effective as hot water or steam. Instruments immersed in chemicals, with the exception of 70 per cent alcohol should be thoroughly rinsed in water in order to remove irritant residues before use. Sterile water should be used for invasive items. Disinfectants suitable for heat-sensitive items are available (e.g. peracetic acid, chlorine dioxide; see Chapter 5). Wiping with 70 per cent alcohol is a rapid but less certain method of disinfection of instruments such as scissors, but is particularly useful for electrical equipment and other items that cannot be immersed.

Used instruments should be placed in the original wrapping with the traceability label, and placed in a rigid container and returned without further treatment to the SSD. If a long delay is anticipated before processing, gross soiling with blood or other body fluids should be safely removed by manual cleaning, otherwise subsequent removal may prove difficult. Suitable protective clothing (e.g. gloves and apron) should be worn. Blood, body fluids and tissue are very difficult to remove if allowed to dry on to surfaces This is of particular concern in the UK because of the possible risk of transmission of prion-associated disease.

Operative endoscopes (e.g. arthroscopes, laparoscopes)

Since an increasing amount of operative surgery will be carried out in the future using an endoscope, autoclavable instruments and accessories are preferred (Ayliffe *et al.*, 1992; MHRA, 2002). However, many of the newer instruments are flexible and therefore damaged by heat. They should be cleaned thoroughly and, if possible, sterilized with ethylene oxide or an alternative low-temperature sterilization method. There may be limitations with some low-temperature methods with the length and diameter of the lumens. Advice should be sought from the sterilizer and instrument manufacturer. As these methods may be unavailable or impracticable, immersion in a sporicidal disinfectant (e.g. 2 per cent glutaraldehyde, peracetic acid, chlorine dioxide) is an acceptable alternative, but this method is less reliable owing to the possible presence of air bubbles and recontamination on subsequent rinsing. Shorter immersion times are usually used because of the limited availability of instruments. There is evidence that these short contact times are effective against some pathogenic spores (e.g. *Clostridium difficile*; Dyas and Das, 1985). This process is referred to as high-level disinfection; it is effective against vegetative bacteria, including *Mycobacterium tuberculosis* viruses and fungi, but not usually all bacterial spores or some atypical mycobacteria (Rutala, 1990). Provided that the endoscope is well cleaned before disinfection, the risk of infection is small, although the remote risk of infection due to spore-forming organisms cannot be excluded. All invasive endoscopes immersed in chemical disinfectants should be thoroughly rinsed in sterile or bacteria free (filtered $<0.22\,\mu m$) water to remove toxic residues prior to immediate reuse.

Two per cent activated alkaline glutaraldehyde has been the disinfectant of choice for flexible endoscopes for many years and is still widely used throughout the world. Although microbiologically effective, glutaraldehyde is an irritant to the skin, eyes and respiratory tract. Impermeable gloves (e.g. nitrile) and aprons should always be worn, as well as eye protection, if splashing is likely. Alternative agents that have a similar microbial spectrum of activity are now available (e.g. peracetic acid, chlorine dioxide, etc.; see Chapter 5). It is important to rinse thoroughly all items immersed in disinfectants.

Cystoscopes

Autoclaving is preferred for heat-tolerant rigid cystoscopes, but high-level disinfection is sometimes used (i.e. immersion in 2 per cent glutaraldehyde for

10 min; Cooke *et al.*, 1993) The longer exposure time of 20 min is required if an effect against *M. tuberculosis* is required (Best *et al.*, 1990; Griffiths *et al.*, 1999). Alternative agents such as peracetic acid and chlorine dioxide may be more rapidly effective. Pasteurization in a water bath at 70–80°C for 10 min is an alternative to chemical disinfection, but the manufacturer should be consulted on heat tolerance if hot water or steam is used. Thermal disinfection/ sterilization is unsuitable for flexible cystoscopes. Other disinfectants suitable for flexible endoscopes are available (e.g. peracetic acid or chlorine dioxide).

Miscellaneous high-risk items

Catheters

Single use is preferred. Some cardiac catheters are too expensive for single use, and reprocessing may therefore be necessary, although it is not usually recommended by regulating authorities in the wealthier countries (MHRA, 2006a). They may be re-sterilized with ethylene oxide provided that the cleaning process is efficient, and the structure and function remain unimpaired. Single-use items should be reused only if a risk assessment has been carried out and it is cost effective and safe to do so. The hospital or Trust must then take corporate legal responsibility for reprocessing and reuse. Single-use items must not be reused if suitable reusable items are available.

Grafts (heart valves, arterial grafts, joints and other implants)

These should be autoclaved if possible. If they are heat labile, use ethylene oxide. Sterilization of these items in the hospital should not usually be necessary.

Cryoprobes

These should be autoclaved if possible. If they are heat labile, use ethylene oxide or another low-temperature method of sterilization (e.g. gas plasma). Immersion in peracetic acid, chlorine dioxide, 2 per cent glutaraldehyde or 70 per cent alcohol may be necessary if cryoprobes are heat labile and gaseous sterilization facilities are not available. Single-use probes may be available.

Transducers and blood-monitoring equipment

These may be a source of infection. Single-use items are preferable, or else ethylene oxide or low temperature steam and formaldehyde should be used. High-level disinfection may sometimes be necessary.

Haemodialysis equipment

See Chapter 14 (Renal).

Intermediate-risk items

Non-invasive endoscopes (e.g. gastroscopes, colonoscopes, bronchoscopes and cystoscopes)

Many professional bodies have issued guidance on the decontamination of flexible endoscopes, for example, the British Society of Gastroenterology (2008), the British Thoracic Society (2001) and the Association of Practitioners in Infection Control (Alvarado and Reichelderfer, 2000).

Pseudomonas aeruginosa and other Gram-negative bacilli, including salmonella, have been transferred from one patient to another on inadequately decontaminated flexible fibreoptic endoscopes (Ayliffe, 1999). Reports on the transfer of mycobacteria and hepatitis B virus (HBV) are rare, and there has been no evidence of transfer of human immunodeficiency virus (HIV; Morris *et al.*, 2006). Nevertheless, care is necessary to avoid the possibility of spread of any infection by ineffective decontamination (Spach *et al.*, 1993). Endoscopic retrograde cholangiopancreatography (ERCP) is a particularly vulnerable procedure and severe Gram-negative infections have been reported. Thorough cleaning and disinfection are important with this procedure. Potential pathogens, such as the Gram-negative bacilli, can grow overnight in the channels of the endoscope, the water bottle and in processing equipment, and disinfection is required at the beginning of the list as well as after each patient. The time available for processing between patients is often short; therefore, the disinfectant chosen should be efficacious in the time available. Other factors to consider are compatibility with the endoscope, and the processing equipment and any health and safety issues. A variety of automatic cleaning and disinfection machines are available. Most of these are effective and protect the User from potentially toxic/irritant processing chemicals, but preliminary brushing of accessible channels (e.g. the suction/biopsy channel) and wiping of the insertion tube are still required. All channels should be cleaned and disinfected. If disinfectants are reused, the concentration may be reduced during repeated use, particularly in automated systems, and the solution should be changed regularly (e.g. after 20–40 procedures). The rinse water should also be changed after each instrument, in order to avoid any build-up of chemical residues. Infection has been reported from Gram-negative bacilli growing in the rinse-water tank. This should be routinely disinfected. Bacteria-free filtered (0.2–0.45 µm) or sterile water is recommended for invasive instruments and those used for ERCP, cystoscopy and bronchoscopy.

Before the method of decontamination (e.g. the chemicals or the washer–disinfector) is changed, it is advisable to consult the manufacturer and give them details of the method to be used. Some disinfectants are corrosive and may damage the endoscope. It should also be noted that low-temperature steam may reach 80°C and ethylene oxide may reach 55°C with considerable variations in pressure. Furthermore, not all endoscopes and accessories are totally submersible.

Two per cent activated alkaline glutaraldehyde has been the disinfectant of choice for flexible endoscopes for many years and is still widely used throughout the world. Although microbiologically effective, glutaraldehyde is an irritant to the skin, eyes and respiratory tract. Impermeable gloves (e.g. nitrile) and aprons should always be worn, as well as eye protection, if splashing is likely. Glutaraldehyde is also a fixative and its use has been discouraged owing to the potential for fixing prion protein (British Society of Gastroenterology, 2008; Advisory Committee on Dangerous Pathogens, 2003).

However, in the UK, its use has largely been replaced by alternative agents such as peracetic acid, chlorine dioxide and superoxidized/electrolysed water (see Chapter 5). These agents are often more rapidly effective than 2 per cent glutaraldehyde, particularly against mycobacteria (5 min) and spores (10 min). However, they may be more damaging to instruments and processing equipment, and their long-term toxicity is not known. Users are strongly advised to inform their Infection Control Team, to seek assurance on compatibility from the manufacturers of the instrument and processor (as use may invalidate guarantees and service-level agreements), to cost the change (bearing in mind the stability of the disinfectant and any personal protective equipment and environmental controls) and to keep those responsible for national guidelines informed of progress whether it is favourable or not (Babb and Bradley, 1995). In view of the toxic, irritant and sensitizing properties of aldehydes, it is necessary to find an effective, non-damaging and less irritant alternative to glutaraldehyde.

Selection of a disinfectant for flexible endoscopes

When selecting an instrument disinfectant, the following advice should be followed:

1 Inform your Infection Control Team; they should be familiar with national guidelines and current research.
2 Review manufacturers' efficacy and other claims. Seek confirmation from an independent peer-reviewed source wherever possible.
3 Consult the instrument and processor manufacturers about compatibility, as use may cause damage which could invalidate guarantees and service arrangements. Under the European Medical Devices Directive, the manufacturers of reusable medical devices are required to state process compatibility. This includes tolerance to heat, moisture, pressure and processing chemicals. Washer–disinfectors are also classed as medical devices.
4 Carefully cost the change, bearing in mind the use-life of the disinfectant and dilution rates.
5 Establish what is needed to meet local/national health and safety legislation

(Control of Substances Hazardous to Health in the UK; e.g. ventilation, personal protective equipment, processing equipment etc and the cost).
6 Re-validate processing equipment with the new chemicals. This applies to a change in detergent or disinfectant.
7 Ensure processed items are thoroughly cleaned before immersion and that the manufacturers' stated times are achieved..
8 Keep those irresponsible for local and national policy informed (e.g. national bodies, professional societies, opinion leaders, etc.)

Endoscope washer–disinfectors

These have become an essential part of endoscopy units, as they provide a controlled assurance of processing. The washer–disinfectors must be effective, safe, reliable and able to cope with endoscope design and throughput. They do not negate the need for manual cleaning (i.e. insertion tube, suction/biopsy channels, instrument tip, valve recesses). However, the washer–disinfectors themselves, if not disinfected at least on a daily basis, may become a source of recontamination.

In the UK, HTM 2030 'Washer disinfectors' (Department of Health, 1997) has had a major impact on the design of washer–disinfectors, in particular those used for heat-sensitive instruments (i.e. flexible endoscopes), which has led to numerous models now appearing on the market. EN 15883 Part 1 'General requirements for washer–disinfectors' was published in 2006, EN 15583 Part 4 'Washer–disinfectors for thermo-labile instruments' was published in 2008 (British Standards Institution, 2006). A model engineering specification MES C32 has been published by NHS Estates (2003), which, combined with HTM 2030 and the European Standard, can leave the User feeling slightly confused.

A typical cycle as described in HTM 2030 consists of the following stages.

1 A leak test to verify that the endoscope is undamaged.
2 Flushing with water not exceeding 35°C.
3 A flow test to verify that all channels are free of blockages for effective cleaning, disinfection and rinsing to take place.
4 Washing with detergent solution at an appropriate temperature not exceeding 60°C and an appropriate contact time.
5 Rinsing to remove detergent residues.
6 Drying to remove excess fluid, which may dilute the disinfectant.
7 Disinfection with a suitable agent that is microbiologically effective and compatible with endoscope and washer–disinfector. Contact time, temperature and concentration should be controlled by the washer–disinfector.
8 Rinsing to remove disinfectant residues.
9 Drying to remove excess fluid so the endoscope is available for immediate patient use.

It is important for the User to appreciate and understand the issues associated with the use of endoscope washer–disinfectors (EWD). These include the following.

Contamination of the washer–disinfector

The washer–disinfector should be designed in such a way as to discourage the proliferation of micro-organisms within the EWD. All pipework within and associated with the EWD should be free draining and there should be no water storage tanks. The MHRA (2002) recommend that the EWD should be subjected to a daily self-disinfect process, preferably at the start of the day. This may be carried out thermally or chemically. HTM 2030 states that the chemical used should be different to that used for disinfection of the endoscope. This is to avoid the selection of disinfectant-resistant strains, which has been reported when glutaraldehyde was used (Griffiths *et al.*, 1997). Ideally, the machine should have the facility to be programmed to perform the self-disinfect cycle at the start of the day so the machine is ready for use when the staff arrive for duty. Proof of the cycle having taken place should be available and retained.

Treatment of the incoming water supply

It is recommended that the final rinse water used for cystoscopes, bronchoscopes and ERCP procedures should be free of bacteria to reduce the risk of infection and/or misdiagnosis of infection. HTM 2030 recommends that 100 mL samples of rinse water taken on a weekly basis should contain no bacteria. Incoming water will contain bacteria and therefore have to be removed usually by using physical methods (e.g. filtration, reverse osmosis or the addition of biocides). The water treatment system itself may become a source of contamination and like the washer–disinfector should also be subjected to a regular disinfection regime.

Dilution of the disinfectant

Machines vary in the method in which the disinfectant is provided at use dilution. Some have a disinfectant storage tank, which is loaded with disinfectant at use dilution, and others use a concentrate disinfectant, which is diluted to use concentration within the machine. The User should be aware of the need to ensure that the use-life of the disinfectant, if reused, is not exceeded or, if single use, that there is adequate supply of concentrate in the machine to reproducibly supply the required concentration to perform a cycle. The washer–disinfector should have a system within the machine to alert the User of any problems.

Suitability of endoscope connection systems for the endoscopes being processed

Endoscopes vary in design and channel configuration. It is important that all channels of the endoscopes are connected correctly to ensure thorough irrigation. The EWD should be fitted with a mechanism to detect if a channel is blocked or not connected at all.

Traceability

It is advisable to have a system in place to provide evidence of decontamination and a unique identifier to link the process to the patient. Validation of the EWD should take place as described for sterilization processes (i.e. performance qualification and periodic testing; see Chapter 4). HTM 2030 (Department of Health, 1997) and EN 15883 Parts 1 and 4 (British Standards Institution, 2006) describe the tests to be carried out and the required frequency. It is essential to ensure that all channels of the endoscope are irrigated during all stages of the cycle, that the disinfectant is at an effective concentration and the water quality is suitable for the endoscopes processed.

Endoscope accessories

In the UK, single-use endoscopy accessories (e.g. biopsy forceps, brushes, snares) are now widely used owing to the risk of transmission or transfer of prion protein and the difficulties in cleaning these devices. However, if this is not an issue, it is advisable to purchase autoclavable accessories. These should be dismantled where possible, cleaned thoroughly, dried, reassembled and processed preferably in the SSD or in a dedicated area of the endoscopy suite. A porous load or vacuum bench-top sterilizer (Medical Devices Agency, 1996, 1998) should be used for packaged and lumened accessories. An alternative to non-autoclavable accessories should be sought, but if these alternatives are not available, accessories should be dismantled, cleaned and immersed in a high-level disinfectant.

Respiratory equipment

Ventilators

Many types of ventilator are available, most of which can be adequately protected by filters, thus minimizing the need to decontaminate the ventilator itself (Das and Fraise, 1997). Some ventilators have a removable internal circuit that can be autoclaved or disinfected using low-temperature steam. The circuits are now predominantly single use. In areas where single use is not used, chemical disinfection may sometimes be required. Most methods of chemical disinfection are not practicable and will not work efficiently in the presence of organic matter; none of the methods is entirely reliable. Two methods have been used, namely nebulization with hydrogen peroxide – a modification of the method described by Judd *et al.* (1968) – and the use of formaldehyde vapour. The hydrogen peroxide method is quick, and the peroxide readily breaks down and is not toxic to patients or staff. If the ventilator is visibly contaminated, it must be stripped down and cleaned prior to disinfection. An alternative method of disinfection is by the use of formaldehyde (Benn *et al.*, 1973). This method can be used only on machines with closed circuits, and great care is needed to remove residual formaldehyde and protect SSD staff from exposure to the irritant vapour. Formaldehyde cabinets are also effective provided that the ventilator is kept running during the cycle (Babb *et al.*, 1982). If the patient is known or suspected to be suffering from pulmonary tuberculosis, and the ventilator is not protected by filters, the use of the formaldehyde method is advisable. Nebulized hydrogen peroxide may be used on machines with single circuits, although these may often be dismantled more easily, washed and disinfected by heat. Small machines (e.g. infant ventilators) may sometimes be sterilized using ethylene oxide. If gaseous methods are used, care should be taken to ensure that all toxic residues are removed by flushing with air or oxygen before the ventilator is reused.

The preferred method of patient humidification is with either a water bath or a heat-moisture exchanger. Less condensation is produced in the tubing with the latter method, thereby reducing the risk of contamination with Gram-negative bacilli. The ventilator external circuitry and humidifier (if used) can be cleaned and thermally disinfected using a washing-machine or disinfected with low-temperature steam. Some circuits are autoclavable, although this may reduce the life of the equipment. If water humidification is used, it is recommended that the circuits are changed every 48 hours in adult patients (Craven *et al.*, 1982), and between patients or weekly in neonatal units. Although filters are hydrophobic, moisture traps may be incorporated to protect the filter. If heat-moisture exchangers are used, circuits may be changed between patients or weekly (Cadwallader *et al.*, 1990).

Humidifiers

Humidifiers in which water vapour (not an aerosol) is blown towards the patient are not a serious infection hazard. They should be changed, together with the ventilator circuit, every 48 hours. The condensate may contaminate the hands of staff, and humidifiers should be cleaned and disinfected, preferably by heat, before being refilled with sterile water. Alcohol (70 per cent) may be used to disinfect evaporator-type humidifiers in infant incubators. Antiseptics such as chlorhexidine added to the water are unlikely to be effective, and may select resistant organisms.

Contaminated nebulizers, which produce an aerosol, may be responsible for lung infections caused by Gram-negative bacilli, especially *Pseudomonas aeruginosa*. Their use should be avoided unless they can be disinfected by heat daily. Water should be replaced and not topped up. If the nebulizing part of the machine is liable to damage by heat, it should be flushed through with water and dried. If drying is not possible, it should be rinsed in 70 per cent alcohol and allowed to dry.

Oxygen tents

These should be washed and dried after each patient. Oxygen masks and tubing should be disposable. There is no evidence that piped medical gases become contaminated with bacteria, provided that the lines remain dry.

Anaesthetic equipment

The anaesthetic machines themselves are unlikely to become significantly contaminated during an operation, and routine decontamination is rarely possible or necessary, especially if a filter is fitted. However, if filters are not used, decontamination may be required after use on a patient with a known or suspected communicable disease (e.g. pulmonary tuberculosis), when formaldehyde gas may be required. In this case, the equipment should be returned to the SSD. The external surfaces of the machine should be kept clean and dry. Contamination is most likely to occur in the facemask and tubing nearest to the patient. This equipment (i.e. tubing, reservoir, ambu-bags, facemasks, endotracheal tubes and airways), if not single use, should be cleaned and thermally disinfected. The Medical Equipment Cleaning Unit of an SSD is most suitable for this. Items should preferably be disinfected in a washer–disinfector (>80°C) or using low-temperature steam (73°C) as frequent autoclaving at 121°C or 134°C may damage the equipment. It is desirable to provide every patient with a decontaminated set of equipment, but this is not usually possible. Sessional or daily treatment of tubing and the reservoir bag is reasonable unless the patient has a respiratory infection or pulmonary tuberculosis is known or suspected (Deverill and Dutt, 1980). However, all patients should have a decontaminated facemask, airway and endotracheal tube. Disposable facemasks, tubing and reservoir bags may be preferred on patients with known or suspected infections, such as tuberculosis. If not disposable, all items used on such patients should immediately be autoclaved or disinfected using hot water or sub-atmospheric steam.

Other medical equipment

Laryngoscope blades

Single-use blades are available, but cleaning and drying may be sufficient. If disinfection is required, immersion in 70 per cent alcohol for 10 min should be effective.

Scavenging equipment

The tubing close to the patient should be autoclaved or, if it is heat labile, disinfected using low-temperature steam or a washer–disinfector. It should be changed regularly (e.g. weekly) and after use on an infected patient.

Suction equipment

In the absence of piped suction, a separate machine should be available for each patient requiring suction. After use, the contents should be discarded, the bottle washed and dried, and fresh connection tubing attached. Bacterial multiplication may occur in the aspirate if it is allowed to stand for long periods. This can be emptied in the sluice and the bottle washed in detergent solution and dried. Alternatively, a washer–disinfector may be used. The bottle should be emptied at least daily irrespective of the amount of fluid aspirated. Non-sterile gloves should be worn and the hands must be washed after handling bottle contents. A fresh catheter should be used each time a patient undergoes suction (e.g. bronchial aspiration). An anti-foaming agent may be used to prevent excessive foaming of the bottle contents (which may wet the filter and enter the pump mechanism). The filter should be changed if it becomes moist or discoloured. The use of a detergent or disinfectant in the bottle may be responsible for excessive foaming. Some disinfectants are ineffective and may be toxic to the patient. Disinfectants are therefore avoided during suction, but if the contents are considered to be hazardous to the staff, or the suction equipment is used to irrigate instruments, sufficient disinfectant (e.g. a chlorine-releasing agent) to give a final concentration suitable for a 'dirty' situation may be drawn through the tubing and added to the bottle and left for at least 10 min. The tubing should then be flushed and the bottle washed and dried before reuse. The machine should periodically be returned to the SSD, where the pump can be checked, the filter changed and the tubing, lid, non-return valve and bottle autoclaved or processed in a washer–disinfector. If a patient requires suction for more than 24 hours, the bottle and tubing should be changed. When the machine is not in use, the bottle should be kept dry and the catheter should not be connected until it is required. Disposable suction bottles are now available but they may be expensive. The container itself is disposable, or a disposable liner is fitted within a container. If these are in use, the waste-disposal policy should take into account the difficulties of transport and incineration (i.e. bursting of the canisters or bags).

Infant incubators

It is preferable for these to be cleaned in a dedicated area. After discharge of a patient, the inner surface of the incubator should be thoroughly cleaned with a moist paper wipe and detergent and dried. Special attention should be paid to the humidifier, ports and the mattress. As cleaning and drying are usually effective, disinfection is rarely necessary, and it may fail without preliminary cleaning. However, if disinfection is required, the cleaned surface can be wiped with a freshly prepared chlorine-releasing solution (e.g. 125 ppm available chlorine), rinsed and dried. Alternatively, surfaces can be wiped with 70 per cent alcohol. However, care should be taken as alcohol is flammable, and the incubator must be aired thoroughly before reuse.

Formaldehyde cabinets are occasionally used, but these are expensive and involve the use of a hazardous chemical. As prior cleaning of the incubator is still necessary, the routine use of a cabinet is of rather doubtful value (Babb *et al.*, 1982).

Vaginal and other specula and rigid sigmoidoscopes

Single-use instruments may be preferred. If not, the instrument should be thoroughly cleaned and autoclaved (MHRA, 2003). Centralized processing in an SSD is preferred but, if local processing is preferred, small bench-top washer–disinfectors and autoclaves are suitable for use in clinics (Medical Devices Agency, 1996, 1998). Boiling water (for 5–10 min) is effective, but care is necessary to ensure that items are thoroughly cleaned and completely immersed, and that the instrument is exposed to boiling water for the required time (i.e. at least 5 min). The boiling-water bath should have a timing mechanism and a lockable lid. The use of chemical disinfectants should be avoided if possible, especially for vaginal specula (Royal College of Obstetricians and Gynaecologists, 1997).

Tonometers

Single-use tonometers are now widely used. If reusable, they should initially be rinsed and immersed in a disinfectant solution for at least 5 min. The use of chlorine-releasing agents for 10 min (500 ppm available chlorine) or 3–6 per cent stabilized hydrogen peroxide is recommended by the Centers for Disease Control and Prevention (CDC; 2008). However, recent evidence suggest that 3 per cent hydrogen peroxide and 70 per cent ethyl alcohol are not as effective against adenovirus (CDC, 2008). Tonometers should be rinsed thoroughly and dried before reuse. Hydrogen peroxide in particular is an irritant to the conjunctiva, and thorough rinsing or neutralization is important. Wiping with 70 per cent ethanol is probably effective, although the exposure time is short and alcohol can damage the conjunctiva if it is still present on the instrument when used. Immersion in 70 per cent alcohol for 5–10 min should be effective, but care is needed to ensure that this does not damage the instrument, and that the alcohol has completely evaporated before use.

Decontamination of equipment used on patients with Creutzfeldt–Jakob disease

The main risk of spread of Creutzfeldt–Jakob disease (CJD) is from the central nervous system (i.e. brain and spinal cord), although care in handling blood is also advised. The Advisory Committee on Dangerous Pathogens (ACDP) and Spongiform Encephalopathy Advisory Committee (SEAC) have jointly prepared guidelines (Advisory Committees on Dangerous Pathogens and Spongiform Encephalopathies, 2003) on safe working practices and the prevention of infection with transmissible spongiform encephalopathy agents (see also NHS

Executive, 1999). These unconventional agents are extremely resistant to physical and chemical agents (Taylor, 1992). They are not significantly susceptible to the disinfectants normally used to disinfect instruments, environmental surfaces and the skin. They are also resistant to gaseous sterilants (e.g. ethylene oxide, formaldehyde), ionizing radiation, ultraviolet light, microwaves and conventional steam-sterilization cycles (i.e. 121°C for 15 min and 134°C for 3 min). The advice given by ACDP and SEAC is that instruments used on patients with known or suspected CJD or related disorders and at-risk patients (i.e. those who are asymptomatic, but have a clinical or family history that places them in one of the risk groups), and which have been exposed to brain, spinal cord and eye tissue, must be destroyed by incineration. Instruments used on at-risk patients where there has been no involvement of brain, spinal cord or eye tissue should be thoroughly cleaned, preferably using a validated automated system, and sterilized or disinfected using an appropriate physical or chemical process. The few processes that are currently identified as suitable are porous-load steam sterilization at 134–137°C for a single cycle of 18 min, immersion in sodium hypochlorite (20 000 ppm available chlorine for 1 hour, immersion in 2 M sodium hydroxide for 1 hour and, for histological specimens, immersion in 96 per cent formic acid for 1 hour. These chemical agents, at the concentrations and contact times described here, are likely to damage most instruments. Wherever practicable, the use of single-use instruments is advised. If the use of expensive reusable items is unavoidable, it is essential to confirm the process compatibility of the device with the manufacturers, and to clean the item thoroughly first.

DECONTAMINATION OF NON-CLINICAL EQUIPMENT (see also Appendix, p. 142)

Plastic washing bowls

The bowls should be thoroughly washed with a detergent and hot water after each use and dried. It is important to remove residual fluid remaining in the bowl after cleaning and, if possible, the bowls should be stored separately and inverted. Each patient should preferably have their own washing bowl, particularly in intensive care or other high-risk units. The bowl should be terminally disinfected by heat or with a chlorine-releasing agent before it is issued to the next patient. Thorough cleaning and drying is probably sufficient in general wards. A rack is convenient for storage of washing bowls under the bed.

Nailbrushes

Nailbrushes frequently become contaminated with Gram-negative bacilli even when they are stored in a disinfectant solution, and their use should be avoided except for special procedures (e.g. first scrub of the day in an operating-theatre). Nylon brushes kept in a dry state are less often contaminated than bristle brushes, but brushes should be avoided if possible. If nailbrushes are required in patient treatment or food production areas, they should preferably be single use or supplied sterilized or heat-disinfected by the SSD.

Soap dishes and dispensers

Soap dishes are rarely necessary and may encourage bacterial growth. If used, they should be washed and dried daily. The nozzles of liquid soap dispensers should be cleaned daily to remove residues, and the outside should be cleaned and dried. Disposable cartridge-type refills with an integral nozzle are preferred, but they tend to be expensive. If non-disposable reservoirs are used, topping up should be avoided and the inside of containers should be cleaned and dried before refilling. In cartridge-type dispensers, the channel and reservoir between the refill and nozzle, if not disposable, require periodic cleaning. Liquid soaps used in hospitals should contain a preservative (e.g. 0.3 per cent chlorocresol), which should prevent bacterial growth during periods of use.

Razors

For pre-operative hair removal, clippers with a disposable head are preferred to reduce the risk of surgical site infection. If used for this purpose, razors should be disposable or autoclavable. Communal razors used by the hospital barber should be wiped clean and disinfected after each shave with 70 per cent alcohol. Electric razor-heads should also be immersed in 70 per cent alcohol for 5 min.

Beds and bedding

Bed frames

Bed frames are rarely an infection risk but should be cleaned after discharge of a patient. Bed frames should be included in cleaning schedules and should be wiped with detergent solution and dried. If disinfection is considered necessary, a chlorine-releasing agent (1000 ppm available chlorine) is usually suitable. Expensive antiseptics should not be used.

Mattresses and pillows

Mattresses and pillows cannot readily be disinfected if they become contaminated. They should be enclosed in a waterproof cover and additional waterproof draw sheets used if contamination with body fluids is likely. Wiping the cover with a detergent solution and thorough drying usually provides adequate decontamination. Avoid excessive wetting during cleaning. Disinfectants, particularly clear soluble phenolics, can make covers permeable and should be avoided. If disinfection is required, use a chlorine-releasing (1000 ppm available chlorine) solution and then rinse well (Department of Health, 1991). Silver nitrate used for topical treatment of burns will also damage mattress covers. Stained mattress covers are often permeable to fluids and should therefore be changed (Lilly *et al.*, 1982). All mattresses should be routinely inspected for damage.

It may be possible to disinfect some pillows, hoists and patients' supports using hot water laundering at 71°C for 3 min or 65°C for 10 min, or by low-temperature steam (73–80°C).

Duvets

Duvets with a waterproof outer surface and covered with a launderable outer fabric cover are now used in some hospitals, but some patients find them uncomfortable, particularly in hot weather. Provided that the duvet does not become soiled or wet, replacement of the outer fabric cover of the duvet between patients is usually adequate. The plastic surface will need to be cleaned if it becomes soiled or contaminated. Thoroughly wiping the outer surface of the duvet with a detergent solution and allowing it to dry completely will usually be sufficient. If disinfection is required after spillage or use by an infected patient, proceed as described for mattresses and pillows. Launderable duvets without a waterproof outer surface are available, but routine disinfection of the whole duvet in the laundry could be a problem. The possible implications of this should be carefully considered by the Infection Control Team after discussion with the laundry manager before they are introduced (e.g. an outbreak of MRSA may require laundering of all duvets in a ward at the same time). Duvets are not recommended for incontinent patients or if gross contamination with body fluids is likely.

Bedding

Bedding can rapidly become heavily contaminated with colonized skin scales. Frequent changing is therefore of limited value in controlling the spread of infection. Procedures for laundering are described in Chapter 7.

Cotton blankets should be used, and these should be changed on discharge of the patient or if they become soiled or contaminated with potentially infectious spillage. Sheets should be changed on discharge of the patient, also at least twice weekly and if soiled, wrinkled, stained or contaminated with potentially infectious material.

Curtains

The level of microbial contamination on curtains is related to the level of dispersal by patients in the immediate vicinity and, if changed, will rapidly regain that level. Curtains should therefore be washed when they are obviously soiled or else every 6 months. The curtains in the vicinity of a disperser of an epidemic strain of *Staphylococcus aureus* may remain heavily contaminated for some hours, and should be changed if the area is to be reoccupied by a susceptible patient within 24 hours. The degree of microbial contamination is not usually related to the type of material used or the time since the curtains were last changed.

Bed-cradles

These should be kept clean and maintained in good condition. They only need to be disinfected after use by an infected patient. The cradle may then be wiped with a chlorine-releasing solution or a clear soluble phenolic and rinsed. Bed-cradles should not be stored in patient treatment areas.

Toys

Disinfection of toys is rarely necessary. Contaminated solid toys may be wiped with a chlorine-releasing agent and rinsed, or wiped with 70 per cent alcohol. Soft toys may be disinfected using low-temperature steam or hot water. If they are grossly contaminated they should be destroyed.

Dressing-trolley tops

To clean dressing-trolley tops, use a detergent solution and a disposable paper wipe, and then dry. To disinfect them, wipe with 70 per cent alcohol after cleaning.

Thermometers

Oral thermometers

Oral thermometers should be stored clean and dry, as growth of Gram-negative bacilli is possible if they are kept in a disinfectant. If separate thermometers are used for each patient, they may be disinfected by wiping with an alcohol wipe before returning them to their respective holders. Thermometers should be disinfected by immersion in 70 per cent alcohol or 1–2 per cent clear soluble phenolic solution for 10 min when the patient is discharged. If not kept for individual patients, thermometers may be wiped clean and disinfected with alcohol at the end of the round, and then stored dry.

Rectal thermometers

Disposable sleeves will reduce the risk of contamination and, if used, the sleeve should be removed and the thermometer treated as for oral thermometers. If a sleeve is not used, remove all traces of lubricant by wiping the thermometer clean, and then disinfect as described above.

Bedpans

To prevent transfer of faecal contamination, the hands should always be washed after handling a used or reusable bedpan, even if it is apparently clean.

Reusable bedpans

Where possible, bedpans should be washed and disinfected in a bedpan-washing machine with a heat–disinfection cycle. Thermal disinfection should ensure that all surfaces reach 90°C or are raised to 80°C and maintained at that temperature for at least 1 min (EN 15883 Parts 1 and 3; British Standards Institution, 2006). The cycle should be checked regularly to ensure that the required temperature is reached. Washing-machines without a heat–disinfection cycle are acceptable in most situations, but not on urological wards, infectious diseases wards or where enteric infections are likely to occur. In such cases they should be replaced by machines with a heat–disinfection cycle when a new machine is required. If washers are not available, emptying the bedpan into the sluice, washing it and allowing it to dry thoroughly before reuse are also acceptable for non-infected patients.

Alternative methods of disinfection

Bedpans may be placed in boiling water for 5–10 min but this should rarely be necessary. Chemical disinfection is not usually practicable. Immersion tanks should preferably be avoided, as they may be ineffective if not well maintained, and they can encourage the growth of resistant strains of Gram-negative bacilli. Wiping the entire surface of a cleaned bedpan with a clear soluble phenolic or a chlorine-releasing solution, rinsing it and allowing it to dry is an alternative, but this is not as effective as heat disinfection, and should be used only in an emergency or in countries with limited facilities.

Disposable bedpans

Single-use paper-pulp bedpans that are disposed of in a purpose-built macerator are an alternative to washer–disinfectors. To minimize the risk of blockages, the horizontal course of the soil pipe above ground should not be greater than 7 m and should have an overall fall of 1 in 40. Paper-pulp bedpans require a reusable support. These supports become contaminated during use and may require washing after use. If heavily contaminated with faeces, they should be washed and wiped with a chlorine-releasing agent or a clear soluble phenolic. An individual support is recommended for each patient. This should be disinfected if soiled and also on discharge of the patient.

Commodes

The container used in the commode should be treated as a bedpan; containers that fit bedpan washers are preferred. After use, the seat and frame should be cleaned, with particular attention paid to under the arms. If the seat becomes soiled or is used by a patient with an enteric infection, it should be disinfected with a clear soluble phenolic or a chlorine-releasing agent, rinsed and dried before reuse. Disposable wipes should be used for cleaning and disposable gloves and a plastic apron should be worn. Hands must be washed at the end of the task even if gloves are worn.

Urine bottles

Bedpan washers will also accommodate urine bottles and recommendations are as for bedpans. Washers with a heat–disinfection cycle are strongly recommended for urology and infectious diseases wards. Urine bottles not disinfected by heat should always be regarded as contaminated and hands should be washed after contact with them. If heat disinfection is not available, a separate labelled urine bottle should be supplied to patients with urinary tract infections. This should be rinsed after each use and disinfected on discharge of the patient as described above for bedpans.

Other human waste containers (e.g. vomit bowls and suction bottles) may also be decontaminated in thermal washer–disinfectors provided suitable loading racks to ensure adequate processing are used.

Disposable paper-pulp urine bottles for disposal in bedpan macerators are available, but may not be suitable for urology wards if direct visual examination of the urine is required.

HOSPITAL ENVIRONMENT

The inanimate environment of the hospital (i.e. usually with minimal risk) is of little importance in the spread of endemic hospital infection (Ayliffe et al., 1967; Maki et al., 1982; Collins, 1988), as it is unlikely to make contact with a susceptible site, but it may occasionally have a role in outbreaks. Recommendations for decontamination are listed in the Appendix, p. **142**.

Ward

A ward surface (floor, furniture, equipment or wall) that is physically clean and dry is unlikely to represent an appreciable infection risk. A clean environment is necessary to provide the required background to good standards of hygiene and asepsis, and to maintain the confidence of patients and the morale of staff (Maurer, 1985). Wet surfaces and equipment are more likely to encourage the growth of micro-organisms and to spread potential pathogens. Cleaning equipment and used cleaning solutions may be heavily contaminated with bacteria; they should be removed from patient treatment or food-preparation areas as soon as cleaning is completed. Thorough cleaning will remove micro-organisms and the organic material on which they thrive. This will render most items relatively free of infection risk and safe to handle. Disinfectants are not usually required and should only be used as part of a properly controlled policy. Disinfectants should be accurately diluted, freshly prepared for each task and disposed of promptly after use.

During an outbreak, the use of a chemical disinfectant may be recommended (e.g. for *Clostridium difficile* or norovirus, where the likelihood of environmental contamination may be high). The use of a chlorine-releasing agent at 1000 ppm has been shown to reduce the incidence of C. *difficile* infection (Wilcox *et al.*, 2003).

Antimicrobial agents are sometimes included in cleaning solutions not described as disinfectants. These may be highly selective and adversely affect the microbial ecology, and their use should therefore be avoided whenever possible. If cleaning services are contracted to an industrial organization, the cleaning solutions and equipment should conform to hospital policy.

Disinfection of rooms with vaporized hydrogen peroxide

Commercial systems which utilize vaporized hydrogen peroxide or other chemicals to decontaminate the environment have recently become available. These systems may be logistically difficult to implement because the area has to be vacated and the doors and windows of the area need to be sealed. Cleaning with a detergent solution is often a prerequisite to vaporization. They have potential use in decontaminating the environment where there is likely to be a significant environmental level (e.g. as a means of ending outbreaks of infection because of norovirus and C. *difficile*). These systems have been used to decontaminate side rooms where MRSA-positive patients have been nursed (French *et al.*, 2004) and have been used to fumigate buildings that have been contaminated with anthrax spores – bioterrorist incidents.

These systems are preferred to formaldehyde gas as they are safer from a health and safety point of view.

Disinfection of rooms with formaldehyde gas

Formaldehyde disinfection may be required for rooms that have been occupied by patients with viral haemorrhagic fevers, although the necessity for this is doubtful (ACDP, 1993). Formaldehyde is also used for disinfecting laboratory safety cabinets and for fumigation of Category 3 and 4 handling facilities following spillage (Health and Safety Executive, 2003). The method is not required or recommended for terminal disinfection of rooms occupied by patients with the common range of infectious diseases or hospital-acquired infections. If required, expert supervision should be available, as formaldehyde is a toxic gas. The windows and other outlets should be sealed and formaldehyde generated from formalin or paraformaldehyde. The amount needed depends on the volume of the room. For formaldehyde fumigation, 100 mL of formalin plus 900 mL of water are required for each 30 m^3 of space. The mixture is boiled away in an electrically heated pan fitted with a timing device. If paraformaldehyde is used, 10.5 g/m^3 is heated in the same way. After starting the generation of formaldehyde vapour, the door should be sealed and the room left unopened for 48 hours. The atmospheric formaldehyde levels should be checked before the room is reoccupied. The maximum exposure limit for formaldehyde is 2 ppm (2.5 mg/m^3) over a 15-min reference period and 8-hour time-weighted average.

Duties and responsibilities of domestic services staff

The Domestic Services Manager is usually responsible for hospital domestic staff, and should ensure that they are properly trained and supervised. Routine cleaning of the environment, including floors, toilets, baths, wash-basins, beds, locker-tops and other furniture, should be the responsibility of the domestic service in all wards and departments. Domestic staff who are specially trained and aware of possible infection hazards should be available to clean and, if necessary, disinfect the rooms occupied or vacated by infected patients. In the UK, National Cleaning Standards have been produced (National Patient Safety Agency, 2007). The cleaning procedures in use should be agreed with the infection control staff, and should include a list of the contents of the room to be cleaned or disinfected, methods for disposal of waste material, and methods of disinfection of cleaning equipment. Nursing and other patient care staff should, wherever possible, be relieved of cleaning tasks. Surfaces or equipment contaminated with potentially infectious material require immediate attention. Nurses should continue to clean and disinfect these items unless specifically trained domestic staff are available. If there is an unusual infection risk associated with the presence of a particular patient (e.g. in cleaning blood spillage from an HBV- or HIV-infected patient, or in a high-risk department), the ward sister should ensure that the domestic staff are aware of that risk. It may be considered that the task could be performed more safely by a trained nurse. Cleaning should be carried out in a carefully planned manner, and cleaning schedules should be drawn up for each area to include all equipment, fixtures and fittings. New items should be added to schedules as they are commissioned. Cleaning schedules should be sufficiently detailed to specify the method, frequency and timing, where relevant, of equipment to be used, and where that equipment is to be stored and how it is to be cleaned and disinfected. The responsibility for each task should be indicated and should include the maintenance of paper-towel cabinets and soap or dispensers, and replacement of cleaning materials and linen. The schedules should be agreed with the individuals in charge of the area to be cleaned and, in high-risk areas, with the infection control staff.

Floors

The bacteriological advantages of using a disinfectant rather than a detergent solution, or a wet method rather than a dry one, are marginal in routine hospital cleaning. In a busy ward, recontamination from airborne settlement or transfer from shoes and trolley wheels is rapid. Levels of bacterial contamination on floors may be restored to their original values within 2 hours of cleaning, whether or not disinfectants are used (Ayliffe *et al.*, 1966). Infection rates are not influenced by the use of a disinfectant and a detergent alone will normally suffice (Danforth *et al.*, 1987). Disinfectants should be used only where there is a known or predictable risk (i.e. removal of potentially infectious spillage such as salmonella, tubercle bacilli, HBV or HIV, or decontamination of cleaning equipment before use elsewhere). Disinfection of floors and other environmental surfaces may also be included in cleaning policies for specific areas (e.g. clean rooms, isolation units, etc.) and where recommended by the microbiologist to deal with a particular risk. However, the risks of acquiring infection from floors and other environmental sites in these areas – including operating-theatres – are low, and cleaning alone is usually adequate.

Dry cleaning

Brooms re-disperse dust and bacteria into the air and should not be used in patient treatment areas or food-preparation and service areas. Suitable methods are a vacuum cleaner or dust-attracting mop. The inner paper bag of the vacuum cleaner should be checked before use and discarded if it is more than half full. Bags should be exchanged away from patient treatment areas with the minimum dispersal of dust. Filters should be inspected at regular scheduled intervals (e.g. monthly), and must be changed if they are dirty or blocked.

The dust-attracting mop, although less efficient, may be used either as a supplement or as an alternative to a vacuum cleaner. Dust-attracting mops may be either impregnated with or manufactured from a dust-attracting material, and may be disposable or reprocessable. If used for an excessive period without replacement, they will fail to retain the dust, and may indeed disperse it and adherent bacteria into the air. An acceptable period of use should be decided upon for each area. To avoid dispersal during use, the head should remain in contact with the floor during sweeping and should not be lifted at the end of each stroke. Dry cleaning removes soil, but will not remove stains or scuff marks.

Microfibre is a recently introduced method of cleaning and many trials have been carried out in clinical settings.

Wet cleaning

Wet cleaning is required at intervals to remove stains and scuff marks. Sluice rooms, toilets and other moist areas require wet cleaning at least once daily. A neutral detergent is usually adequate and should be freshly prepared for each task. Mops and other equipment should be cleaned, drained where appropriate and stored dry. Buckets should be rinsed and stored inverted to assist drying. Mops are difficult to dry completely and are frequently contaminated with Gram-negative bacilli. Although these may be transferred to the surface during cleaning, they will disappear rapidly as the surface dries. Floors transiently contaminated in this way do not appear to cause infections in general surgical and medical wards. Mops require disinfection after use in the rooms of infected patients and possibly before use in rooms occupied by immunosuppressed patients. Laundering in a machine with a heat–disinfection cycle is the preferred method, but rinsing followed by a soak in 1 per cent bleach or an alternative chlorine-releasing agent (1000 ppm available chlorine) for not more than 30 min, re-rinsing and allowing to dry is an acceptable alternative. If disinfection is not required, mops should be kept clean and laundering is the preferred method.

All cleaning equipment should be examined at regular scheduled intervals and cleaned if it is soiled. Worn or damaged equipment should be repaired or replaced. Cleaning solutions should be changed frequently to prevent the accumulation or multiplication of bacteria, and should be discarded or removed from the patient treatment area as soon as cleaning is completed. A two-compartment bucket or a wheeled stand containing two buckets (which allows the used water from the mop to be discarded into a separate bucket or compartment) is an advantage. Surfaces should be left as dry as possible after cleaning. Poorly designed or inadequately maintained mechanical cleaning equipment may increase the bacterial count of the cleaned surface or the surrounding air, and should not be introduced into high-risk areas without consultation with the microbiologist or infection control staff. The cleaning and maintenance of all new equipment should be agreed upon before putting it into use. Protocols should indicate the acceptable area of use for the equipment and any attachments. It may be permissible to use a scrubbing machine in more than one area, but separate pads should be used. It is preferable that scrubbing machines with integral tanks which cannot be totally drained should not be used in patient treatment areas. If a machine has a solution storage tank it should be drained as completely as possible at the end of the day's session and kept dry until it is required.

Spray cleaning

It is important to ensure that solutions sprayed in patient treatment areas are not heavily contaminated with Gram-negative bacilli. Solutions should be freshly prepared and spray bottles that are not in use should be stored clean/disinfected and dry.

Carpets (or other soft flooring materials) in hospital wards

Although bacteria are usually present in large numbers and survive longer on carpets than on hard floors, there is no evidence that carpets are associated with an increased infection risk (Ayliffe *et al.*, 1974). However, although conclusive proof does not exist for the transmission of norovirus via a carpet, evidence would suggest this may be a route of transmission (Cheesbrough *et al.*, 1997). It is, therefore, still reasonable to minimize potential infection hazards by selecting carpets with specifically desirable properties. If installed in wards or other clinical areas, the carpets should have a waterproof backing and joints should be sealed. Pile fibres should preferably be water repellent and non-absorbent. Ease of cleaning and rate of drying are both improved by having a pile of short upright fibres. The carpet should be washable and, if possible, not damaged by the application of commonly used disinfectants. Spillage of blood, particularly from patients at high risk of bloodborne infection, may require disinfection with chlorine-releasing agents, which damage most carpets. Alternatives to chlorine-releasing compounds (e.g. peroxygen powders), which are less damaging to carpets, are available. However, spillage can usually be safely removed by thorough washing with a detergent solution, provided that gloves are worn by the operator. Before buying a carpet, it is important to ensure that it is resistant to the agents that are likely to be applied in the healthcare setting, and that stains can be easily removed. Carpets should be vacuum-cleaned daily and periodically wet cleaned with specially designated equipment (e.g. steam cleaners with a vacuum extraction facility).

The decision as to whether or not to fit carpets in clinical areas is a difficult one and is not entirely based on infection risk, as other factors need to be considered (e.g. appearance, comfort, sound reduction, etc.). Carpets in wards with frequent or large-volume spillage (e.g. units for the mentally handicapped) are usually inadequately maintained, and are therefore not recommended in these areas (Collins, 1979). Other clinical areas, such as surgical and obstetric wards, may also be contaminated with blood and other body fluids frequently, and again routine cleaning may be inadequate. Problems of smell and staining have been responsible for the removal of carpets in many clinical areas. In general, it would seem preferable to avoid carpets in these areas as attractive alternative flooring is now available. Washable floors are advisable in isolation wards, as carpets may prolong the survival of certain organisms (e.g. multi-resistant strains of *Staphyloccus aureus*, such as MRSA). If it is still decided to fit carpets in clinical areas, it is of major importance to ensure that, in addition to buying suitable carpets and cleaning equipment, the cleaning schedules are agreed upon before the carpet is bought and that they are achievable. The cleaning guidelines provided by manufacturers are often impracticable as ward areas need to be evacuated during the procedure. Facilities should also be available for the prompt removal of spillage. Absorbent powders are particularly useful for this purpose, followed by either vacuum cleaning or the spot application of a suitable carpet-compatible detergent. As it is not usually possible to use a disinfectant because of possible damage to the carpet, protective clothing (i.e. gloves and a plastic apron) should be worn when removing spillage.

Spillage

Cleaning with a detergent and water may be adequate for most spillage (e.g. food, urine, etc.). A disinfectant should be used for spillage containing potentially hazardous organisms (Babb, 1996; Hoffman *et al.*, 2004). Disposable gloves should always be worn when cleaning known contaminated spillage. If there is a risk of contaminating clothing, a disposable plastic apron should also be worn. A sprinkler may be used to cover small amounts of the spillage with sufficient chlorine-releasing granules or powder to absorb any moisture. When the fluid is completely absorbed, a disposable paper wipe should then be immediately used to remove the residue and discarded into a plastic bag. Finally, the surface should be washed using a disposable paper wipe and dried. All waste, wipes, disposable gloves and apron (if worn), should be discarded, sealed and disposed of as clinical waste. Powders or granules should be used on wet spillage only. Liquid disinfectants (e.g. chlorine-releasing agents or clear soluble phenolics) can also be used and may be necessary for larger spillages (>30 mL). Chlorine-releasing powder, granules or fluids containing 10 000 ppm available chlorine should be used for blood or body fluid spillage that is known or suspected to be contaminated with HIV or HBV. If chlorine-releasing agents are added to hot water, anionic detergents or acidic body fluids (e.g. urine), this may result in a rapid release of toxic levels of chlorine. At these concentrations, chlorine-releasing agents are toxic and corrosive, and likely to damage or decolorize many surfaces; 1000 ppm can be used for other spillage or pre-cleaned surfaces. Paper towels are useful for absorbing spillage of blood and other body fluids. These should be disposed of as clinical waste and the area wiped or mopped with disinfectant. If the surface is likely to be damaged by chlorine-releasing agents, other agents with antiviral activity (e.g. peroxygen compounds) may be more appropriate. Universal precautions assume that all blood and certain body fluids are potentially infectious and routine disinfection before cleaning is often recommended. This would seem to be excessive (particularly in hospitals where the infection rate with HBV or HIV is low) and unnecessary, provided that gloves and a plastic apron are worn and hands are washed. Thorough cleaning alone is usually sufficient. Clear soluble phenolics (0.6–2 per cent) are less likely to damage surfaces and are suitable for bacterial contamination (e.g. with enteric organisms or mycobacteria), but they are poor virucidal agents.

Disinfectants should be freshly prepared and accurately diluted for each task. Chlorine-releasing powders, granules and tablets (i.e. sodium dichloroisocyanurate; NaDCC) are stable, but solutions are not, and so should be discarded on completion of the task or at the end of the day.

Walls and ceilings

Only very small numbers of bacteria adhere to clean, smooth, dry, intact walls (Ayliffe *et al.*, 1967). These surfaces are therefore unlikely to be a significant infection hazard. Ceilings have an even smaller number of bacteria. The cleaning of walls and ceilings should be carried out sufficiently often to prevent the accumulation of visible dirt. Intervals between cleaning should not usually exceed 12–24 months in patient treatment areas, or 6 months in operating-theatres.

Disinfection is not required unless known contamination has occurred. Splashes of blood or known contaminated material should be removed promptly. When walls are cleaned, the surface should be left as dry as possible. Damaged paintwork exposes plaster, which cannot be effectively cleaned or disinfected, and which may become heavily colonized with bacteria if it becomes moist (e.g. through condensation). Damaged wall surfaces should be promptly repaired and redecorated, particularly in operating-theatres. A moist surface may encourage growth of fungi, especially *Aspergillus*.

Other surfaces

Locker-tops and bed tables should be wiped daily with a freshly prepared detergent solution using disposable wipes. Other furniture should be similarly cleaned as required. Shelves and ledges should be damp-dusted weekly, or more often if dust accumulates. Disinfection is not required unless the surface is contaminated with body fluids and other potentially infectious material.

Baths, sinks and hand wash-basins

Baths and hand wash-basins should be cleaned at least daily by the domestic staff and, if practicable, patients should be encouraged to clean the bath after each use. Detergent is adequate for routine cleaning. A cream cleaner may occasionally be required to remove scum, but should not be used on fibreglass baths unless its use is approved by the manufacturer. It is necessary to disinfect baths after use by infected patients or those carrying multi-resistant or problematic strains (e.g. MRSA), or before use by patients with open wounds. A non-abrasive chlorine-releasing powder can be used for this purpose. Abrasive powders are effective, but they damage porcelain surfaces and must never be used on fibreglass.

Alternatively, solutions or cream cleaners containing chlorine-releasing agents may be used with a detergent, but only if the detergent is known to be compatible. Hand wash-basins should be used solely for this purpose. Compliance is more likely if plugs are removed and elbow/wrist-operated mixer taps are installed. Chlorine-releasing agents may also damage the recirculating pumps of some hydrotherapy baths and birthing tubs. Quaternary ammonium compounds are often used but are less effective. The suitability of all cleaning agents and disinfectants should be checked with the equipment manufacturers before use. No attempt should be made to disinfect sink traps or outlets, as disinfection of these sites is usually ineffective and treatment may disperse potential pathogens.

Toilets and drains

Toilet seats and handles should be cleaned at least once daily, and also when they are visibly soiled. A detergent solution should be used for routine cleaning. Disinfection with a chlorine-releasing agent or clear soluble phenolic may be required if the seat is obviously contaminated, or after use by patients with a gastrointestinal infection. If a disinfectant is used, the seat should be rinsed with water and dried before use. Pouring disinfectant into lavatory pans or drains is unlikely to reduce infection risks.

Crockery and cutlery

Centralized arrangements for machine washing and drying of all crockery and cutlery are preferable to washing on individual wards. A washing-machine with a final rinse temperature of 80°C for 1 min or other appropriate disinfection time/temperature combination (e.g. 71°C for 3 min) is a satisfactory alternative in ward kitchens (see the section on kitchen hygiene in Chapter 7), and is desirable in isolation wards.

Cleaning materials

Wherever possible, single-use wipes should be used for cleaning surfaces (e.g. baths, sinks, bowls, mattresses, beds, furniture, etc.). They should also be used for mopping up spillages from a known source of infection and for cleaning cubicles occupied by infected patients. If disposables are not available for use in other areas because of cost, the following alternatives can be used.

- A nylon brush, which can be dried quickly, may be used for cleaning baths. Absorbent cotton mops or bristle brushes become heavily contaminated, are difficult to disinfect and should not be used.
- If non-disposable cloths are used for cleaning, these should be washed after use, preferably in a washing-machine with a disinfection stage in the cycle, and then dried. Separate cloths should be used in the kitchen, sluice and other ward areas. A colour code may be used to distinguish the different areas of usage.
- Toilet brushes should be rinsed well in the flushing water of the lavatory pan. After the excess water has been shaken off, they should be stored dry.

Sponges dry slowly, are difficult to disinfect and should not be used.

CLEANING AND DISINFECTION OF THE SKIN AND MUCOUS MEMBRANES

Principles

There are three principal reasons for removing or reducing the number of micro-organisms present on the skin or mucous membranes:

- to reduce the number of micro-organisms present prior to an invasive procedure;
- to remove or destroy potentially pathogenic micro-organisms present on the hands of staff;
- to treat a carrier or disperser of a resistant, virulent or highly communicable strain of bacteria.

The bacteria present in healthy skin have been classified for practical purposes as follows:

- resident organisms that colonize the skin;
- transient organisms that are deposited on the skin, but do not usually multiply there.

The resident organisms consist mainly of coagulase-negative staphylococci, diphtheroids and occasionally *Staphylococcus aureus*. Gram-negative bacilli (e.g. *Klebsiella*) are usually transients, but may be temporary residents for periods ranging from several days to many weeks. *Acinetobacter baumanii* has many of the survival properties of staphylococci, and may be considered a true resident.

Most of the transient bacteria can be removed by a wash with soap and water, which may be almost as effective as disinfection. However, the resident bacteria are mostly left on the skin after washing with soap and water, but these can be reduced by disinfection. Some naturally acquired bacteria that do not multiply on the skin (e.g. *Clostridium perfringens*, present through faecal contamination) may be difficult to remove by washing with soap and water.

Large numbers of bacteria are found as residents of the mucous membrane in the mouth, nose and vagina, but different organisms predominate in different sites. Antiseptics that are neither irritant nor damaging to the tissues have a limited, although potentially useful, effect in reducing these micro-organisms. The urethra normally has few commensal bacteria, but is liable to become contaminated on passage of catheters or other instruments. Disinfection of the urethra before instrumentation is one of the important features of prophylaxis against infection of the urinary tract (see Chapter 7). The conjunctiva also has few bacteria, but these may include *Staphylococcus aureus*.

Cleaning and disinfection of the hands

The hands are considered to be one of the main routes of spread of infection. Social handwashing is the washing of hands with non-medicated soap or detergent and water. Hygienic hand disinfection entails the killing of transient organisms, and may be associated with removal of organisms if an antiseptic detergent is used. Surgical hand disinfection involves the killing of transient organisms and a substantial number of superficial resident organisms, and may also be associated with removal of organisms if an antiseptic detergent is used (Newsom, 1998).

Effective handwashing or disinfection (referred to here as hand hygiene) is therefore probably the most important infection-control measure. Unfortunately, healthcare workers have very poor compliance with good hand hygiene practices. Several studies have shown compliance to be between 20 per cent and 40 per cent (i.e. workers only decontaminated their hands on 20–40 per cent of the occasions when protocols dictated that they should). Even when intensive educational campaigns were introduced, hand hygiene compliance only increased to 66 per cent (Pittet *et al.*, 2000). Studies using electronic counting equipment have found hand hygiene frequency to be much lower than that claimed (Ayliffe *et al.*, 1988) and, when physicians are asked to self-estimate their hand hygiene compliance, they significantly overestimate it (Prichard and Raper, 1996).

To improve compliance, it is essential that the soaps, detergents and hand rubs used in clinical areas are acceptable to staff, or else they will not be used. A thorough wash at the right time with a cosmetically acceptable formulation is more important than the agent used. Dedicated wash-basins and soft paper towels should be readily available. Alcoholic hand rubs are ideal for disinfecting clean hands because an alcoholic hand rub is effective in a much shorter time than hand soap. Consequently these products are more likely to be used when workload is high and hand hygiene is frequently required; for example, it has been estimated that, on an average intensive care unit, nurses who washed their hands before and after every patient contact would need to spend more than half their shift on hand hygiene, whereas use of alcohol rubs will significantly reduce the time required for adequate hand hygiene.

Guidance should be given by the Infection Control Team on when to wash or disinfect the hands (e.g. before aseptic or invasive procedures or preparing food, and after contact with secretions and excretions, going to the lavatory, cleaning duties or bed-making) (Infection Control Nurses Association, 2001). Gloves should be worn when handling heavily contaminated materials and the hands should be washed on removal of the gloves.

Washing with soap (or detergent) is required where the hands are visibly soiled, as water removes dirt and dead skin squames. Washing also removes the bacteria present on the hands but does not kill them. Non-medicated soap without disinfectant is usually adequate for most ward procedures (see Chapter 7) but bar soap may become contaminated with bacteria, particularly if left in a dish of fluid. Liquid soap or detergent is preferable, but the dispensers must be regularly cleaned and maintained. Washing with an antiseptic–detergent preparation is usually more effective in reducing transients than washing with non-medicated soap, but the differences are often marginal. The agents commonly used are 4 per cent chlorhexidine detergent (e.g. Hibiscrub, Hydrex) or 7.5 per cent povidone-iodine (e.g. Betadine, Videne). Triclosan preparations (e.g. Aquasept) are also used and are increasingly popular with staff, but they tend to be less effective. Repeated applications skin disinfectants, particularly chlorhexidine, show a residual effect against transient organisms, but it remains uncertain whether this effect alone would influence the transmission of infection. Nevertheless, if hands are visibly clean, an alcohol-containing hand rub (or product with similar efficacy) is now regarded as the standard of care.

Hand hygiene products need to be effective in order to be marketed. In Europe, there are a set of standards (European Norms), which are laboratory tests that the product needs to pass before it can be marketed. EN 1499 (British Standards Institution, 1997a) is the standard for hygienic hand-wash formulations, EN 1500 (British Standards Institution, 1997b) is for hygienic hand-rub formulations and EN 12791 (British Standards Institution, 2005) is for products used for surgical hand disinfection. When choosing a product, it is important to ensure that it satisfies the standard appropriate to its proposed use. International standards for disinfectant products are being developed and will apply outside Europe.

A single application of 60–70 per cent ethanol or isopropanol with an emollient (e.g. 1 per cent glycerol) and with or without an antiseptic (e.g. chlorhexidine, povidone–iodine, triclosan) is significantly more effective against transients than a soap-and-water wash (Ayliffe et al., 1988; Rotter, 1996). A volume of 3 mL is poured on to cupped hands and rubbed to dryness. It is important that the formulation used is popular with staff and that all areas of the hands are covered with the agent, as certain areas (e.g. the tips of the fingers and thumbs) are easily missed (Taylor, 1978).

The following standard procedure is recommended (Ayliffe et al., 1978). The hands are rubbed, with five strokes for each movement, backwards and forwards, palm to palm, right palm over left dorsum, left palm over right dorsum, palm to palm with the fingers interlaced, backs of fingers to opposing palm with the fingers interlaced, rotational rubbing of right thumb clasped in left palm and left thumb in right palm, rotational rubbing with clasped fingers of the right hand in the palm of the left hand, and the left hand in the palm of the right hand, complete hands and wrists (see Figure 6.1).

If the hands are visibly soiled, a preliminary wash with soap or detergent and water is required before application of an alcoholic solution. The same

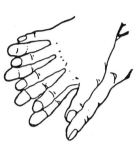

1 Palm to palm

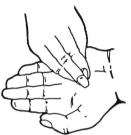

2 Right palm over left dorsum and left palm over right dorsum

3 Palm to palm finger interlaced

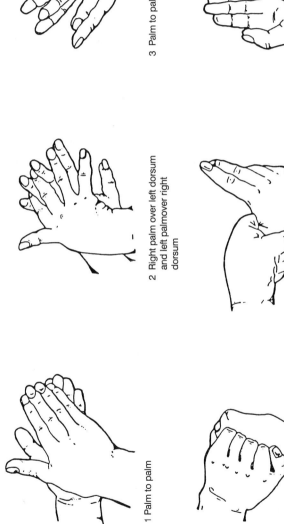

4 Backs of fingers to opposing palms with fingers interlaced

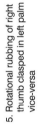

5 Rotational rubbing of right thumb clasped in left palm vice-versa

6 Rotational rubbing, backwards and forwards with clasped fingers of right hand in lef palm and vice versa.

Figure 6.1 Handwashing technique (Ayliffe et al., 1978). The hands are moistened and 3–5 mL of soap or detergent are applied to cupped hands. The hands are then rubbed together as shown. This technique, which normally takes 15–30 s, is suitable for handwashing and disinfection in all clinical areas and for surgical scrubs, provided that in the latter case the forearms are included. Additional aliquots of soap or detergent may be necessary for the more prolonged surgical scrub (2 min). The wrists are similarly rubbed. The same technique is used for alcohol hand rubs, but no water is used and the hands are rubbed together until dry.

technique may be used for a surgical scrub, but the application should be extended to cover the forearms.

Alcoholic solutions may not be effective against some viruses (e.g. enteroviruses), owing to the relatively short exposure time of the agent on the hands, and washing with soap and water prior to the use of alcohol is therefore preferable if contamination with these agents is likely (Davies *et al.*, 1993). However, 70 per cent alcohol is effective against rotaviruses on the hands (Bellamy *et al.*, 1993).

The same antiseptic–detergent or soap preparations (e.g. chlorhexidine and povidone–iodine) are commonly used for surgical hand disinfection as for hygienic hand disinfection (Lowbury and Lilly, 1973; Babb *et al.*, 1991). The main difference in the procedure is the longer application time (2 min instead of 10–30 s for hygienic disinfection). Triclosan or hexachlorophane preparations are less frequently used, but are still useful if hypersensitivity to other agents develops. Repeated applications of all of these agents reduce the superficial residents to low levels.

The antiseptic detergent should be thoroughly applied to the hands and wrists for 2 min and then rinsed off. A brush may be used for the first application of the day, but continual use is inadvisable, as damage to the skin increases the risk of colonization with *Staphylococcus aureus* or with an increase in the number of residents. An alternative and more effective method is the application of an alcoholic solution with or without an antiseptic (Lowbury *et al.*, 1974).

Two 5 mL amounts are applied, with the first allowed to dry before applying the second, to the hands, wrists and forearms using the standardized technique described above and rubbed to dryness. A single application as indicated for hygienic hand disinfection (3 mL applied for 30 s) may be adequate for invasive procedures where the resident flora of the hands is a less frequent cause of infection. Alcohol is also useful for the rapid disinfection of clean hands of surgeons following glove puncture during an operation. Alcohol without an added antiseptic surprisingly shows a persistent effect for several hours if gloves are worn. This is probably due to the delayed death of skin bacteria that are damaged but not immediately killed by alcohol (Lilly *et al.*, 1979). Where sensitization to commonly used aqueous formulations is a problem, soap and water followed by the application of an alcohol hand rub is a useful and effective alternative.

Cleaning and disinfection of the operation site

A rapid reduction of the skin flora is required in pre-operative preparation of operation sites. For this purpose, a quick-acting antiseptic is desirable. Alcoholic solutions containing chlorhexidine, povidone–iodine or triclosan are preferable to aqueous solutions for intact skin (Davies *et al.*, 1978).

The antiseptic should be applied with friction, on a sterile gauze swab, over and well beyond the operation site for 3–4 min. If a gloved hand is used to apply the antiseptic, a second glove should be worn by the surgeon over his or her operating glove, and removed when the preparation of the operation site is complete (Lowbury and Lilly, 1975). Alcoholic solutions must be allowed to dry. This is especially important if diathermy is to be used.

The effect of repeated washing or bathing with an antiseptic on infection rates remains controversial (see Chapter 7). A single antiseptic bath pre-operatively is unlikely to reduce the risk of infection. Repeated washing and bathing with chlorhexidine–detergent does reduce the level of the resident flora on the skin, and could be of value in cardiovascular or prosthetic surgery. However, a single application of alcoholic chlorhexidine rubbed on until the skin is dry, as described above, will reduce the number of resident bacteria to levels approaching the low equilibrium obtained on repeated applications of chlorhexidine detergent.

Before operations on hands with ingrained dirt (e.g. in gardeners) or on the legs of patients with a poor arterial supply (e.g. amputations for diabetic gangrene of the foot), the application of a compress soaked in povidone–iodine solution to the operation site for 30 min will greatly reduce the numbers of spores of gas-gangrene bacilli that present a special hazard in such patients. Ordinary methods of disinfection are ineffective against bacterial spores. However, some spores may remain and antibiotic prophylaxis is still required. Washing with detergents and grease-solvent jellies (e.g. Swarfega, Dirty Paws) helps to remove ingrained dirt and the dead skin scales on which organisms are carried.

Disinfection of the injection site

The necessity to disinfect the skin with 70 per cent ethanol or 60–70 per cent isopropanol before injection causes discussion. There is evidence that giving an injection without prior disinfection is not associated with an increased risk of infection in young, healthy individuals. Prior disinfection is not recommended for diabetic patients. Some hospitals have stopped using alcohol for disinfection of injection sites. However, alcohol is still used, usually with chlorhexidine, for cannulation procedures and taking blood cultures. However, disinfection of the injection site, particularly of the thigh, and in elderly and immunocompromised patients or if the site is close to infected or colonized lesions, is necessary. The area should be wiped thoroughly and allowed to dry before the injection is given. This will kill or remove most transient organisms.

Cleaning and disinfection of mucous membranes

Repeated applications (three or four times a day) of a cream containing 0.5 per cent neomycin and 0.1 per cent chlorhexidine (Naseptin) to the inside of the nostrils has been shown to remove *Staphylococcus aureus* from a fairly large proportion of nasal carriers. Possible alternatives include neomycin–bacitracin ointment or 1 per cent chlorhexidine cream (Williams *et al.*, 1967). Mupirocin cream (Bactroban) is more rapidly effective and more likely to eliminate the staphylococci than other preparations, and is particularly useful for treating carriers of MRSA (see Chapter 12).

Resistance to mupirocin has been described, and its widespread use should be avoided as it is useful for treating carriers of MRSA. *Streptococcus pyogenes* can usually be cleared from the throat by a course of penicillin (injected or given by mouth, but not by local application). Erythromycin is effective and should be used in patients who are sensitive to penicillin.

Applications of aqueous solutions of chlorhexidine or povidone–iodine are effective for disinfection of oral mucous membranes, but some dental surgeons consider disinfection to be of doubtful value. Treatment of the vaginal mucosa with obstetric creams containing chlorhexidine or chloroxylenol is considered to have little disinfectant action. An application of a povidone–iodine solution reduces the number of organisms, but the effect on clinical infection is uncertain.

APPENDIX

Table A6.1 Summary of methods for decontamination of equipment or environment

Equipment or site	Routine or preferred method	Acceptable alternative or additional recommendations
Airways and endotracheal tubes	Heat sterilize or heat disinfect	Chemical disinfection. For patients with tuberculosis, use disposables or heat
Ampoules	Wipe neck with 70% alcohol	Do not immerse
Baths and hoists	For non-infected patients: wipe with detergent solution or cream cleaner and rinse	For infected patients and patients with open wounds: chemical disinfection with a chlorine-releasing agent

Bedding	See Chapter 7
	
	Heat disinfection
	  65°C for 10 min
	  71°C for 3 min
		Heat-sensitive fabrics: low-temperature wash and chemical disinfection

Bed frames	Wash with detergent and dry	After infected patient/spillage disinfectant with chlorine-releasing agent
Bedpans	Washer–disinfector or use disposables. Wash carriers for disposable pans if soiled	Patients with enteric infections: if washer–disinfector or disposables are not possible, chemical disinfection or individual pan for infected patient

Equipment or site	Routine or preferred method	Acceptable alternative or additional recommendations
Bowls 　Surgical 　Washing	Autoclave Wash and dry	For infected patients, use individual bowls and disinfect. On discharge: heat disinfection or chemical disinfection
Carpets	Vacuum daily; clean periodically by hot-water extraction	For known contaminated spillage, clean, chemically disinfect with suitable agent if available, then rinse and dry
Crockery and cutlery	1 Machine wash, heat disinfect and dry 2 Hand wash by approved method	For patients with enteric infections or open pulmonary tuberculosis, heat disinfect, if possible, or use disposables
Duvets	Heat disinfect or wash with detergent solution and dry	Heat or chemically disinfect if contaminated. Do not soak or disinfect unnecessarily, as this may damage the fabric
Endoscopes	1 Clean and heat disinfect or sterilize 2 If heat sensitive, clean and chemically disinfect	See Chapter 5 for suitable disinfectants
Feeds bottles and teats	Pre-sterilized or heat-disinfected feeds	Use teats and bottles sterilized and packed by sterile services department. Disinfectant (i.e. chlorine-releasing agent) should be used only in small units where other methods are unavailable
Floors 　Dry cleaning 　Wet cleaning	Vacuum clean or dust-attracting dry mop Wash with detergent solution. Disinfection is not usually required	Do not use broom in patient areas For known contaminated spillage and terminal disinfection: chemically disinfect with a chlorine-releasing agent
Furniture and fittings	Damp dust with detergent solution	For known contaminated spillage and special areas, disinfect with a chlorine-releasing agent
Infant incubators	Wash with detergent and dry with disposable wipes	For infected patients: after cleaning, wipe with 70% alcohol or 125 ppm available chlorine
Instruments	Heat. If heat sensitive, chemically disinfect with a compatible agent	Contaminated surgical instruments should be cleaned before sterilization, preferably in a washer–disinfector
Locker-tops	See 'Furniture and fittings' above	

Table A6.1 Summary of methods for decontamination of equipment or environment – *contd*

Equipment or site	Routine or preferred method	Acceptable alternative or additional recommendations
Mattresses	Water impermeable cover: wash with detergent solution and dry	Chemically disinfect if contaminated; do not disinfect unnecessarily, as this may damage the mattress
Mops		
Dry, dust-attracting	Do not use if overloaded or for more than 2 days without reprocessing or washing	Vacuuming after each use may prolong effective life between processing
Wet	Rinse after each use, wring and store dry. Heat disinfect, rinse and store dry	Single-use mop heads. If chemical disinfection is required, rinse in water, soak (in 1000 ppm available chlorine) for 30 min
Nailbrushes	Use only if essential	A single-use, sterile or heat-decontaminated brush should be used for all clinical procedures
Pillows	Treat as mattresses	
Razors		
Safety and open	Disposable or autoclaved	Chemical disinfection with 70% alcohol
Electric	Chemical disinfection. Immerse head only	
Rooms (terminal cleaning or disinfection)	For non-infected patients, wash surfaces in detergent solution and allow to dry	For infected patients, wash with detergent solution and allow to dry. Use chlorine-releasing agent or alcohol if required. Fogging is not recommended
Shaving brushes	Do not use for clinical shaving	Autoclave. Use brushless cream or shaving foam
Sputum container	Use disposable	Non-disposable containers should be emptied with care and heat-disinfected or sterilized
Suction equipment	Clean and dry. Heat disinfection or sterilization	Single-use containers. If chemical disinfection is required, clean and then use a chlorine-releasing agent
Thermometers	Individual thermometers: wipe with alcohol, store dry or use single-use electronic probe	
Toilet seats	Wash with detergent and dry	After use by infected patients or if grossly contaminated, chemically disinfect with a chlorine-releasing agent, rinse and dry
Tooth mugs	Disposable	If non-disposable, heat disinfect
Toys	Clean first, but do not soak soft toys. If contaminated, disinfect with heat or chemical disinfectant	Expensive or treasured toys may withstand low-temperature steam or ethylene oxide; the latter needs a long aeration period. Heavily contaminated soft toys may have to be destroyed

Equipment or site	Routine or preferred method	Acceptable alternative or additional recommendations
Trolley-tops	Clean with detergent and wipe dry	Clean first, then chemically disinfect with alcohol
Tubing (anaesthetic or ventilator)	Heat disinfect in washer–disinfector	Disposable tubing
Urinals	Use washer–disinfector or use disposables	Chemical disinfection
Ventilator (mechanical)	Heat disinfection or disposable circuit. Protect machine with filters	
Wash-basins	Clean with detergent. Use cream cleaner for stains, scum, etc. Disinfection not normally required	Disinfection may be required if contaminated
X-ray/electrical equipment	Damp dust with detergent solution; switch off, do not over-wet, allow to dry before use	Wipe clean and disinfect with alcohol

REFERENCES

Advisory Committee on Dangerous Pathogens (1993). *Management and control of viral haemorrhagic fevers.* London: HMSO.

Advisory Committees on Dangerous Pathogens and Spongiform Encephalopathies (2003) *Transmissible encephalopathy agents: safe working and the prevention of infection.* Available online at: http://www.advisorybodies.doh.gov.uk/acdp/tseguidance/Index.htm (accessed 12 September 2008).

Alvarado CJ and Reichelderfer M (2000) APIC guideline for infection prevention and control in flexible endoscopy. *American Journal of Infection Control* 28, 138.

Ayliffe GAJ (1999) Nosocomial infections associated with endoscopy. In: Mayhall CG (ed.) *Hospital epidemiology and infection control,* 2nd edn. Baltimore, MD: Williams and Williams.

Ayliffe GAJ, Collins BJ and Lowbury EJL (1966) Cleaning and disinfection of hospital floors. *British Medical Journal* ii, 442.

Ayliffe GAJ, Collins BJ and Lowbury EJL (1967) Ward floors and other surfaces as reservoirs of hospital infection. *Journal of Hygiene (Lond)* 2, 181.

Ayliffe GAJ, Babb JR and Collins BJ (1974) Carpets in hospital wards. *Health and Social Services Journal* 84, 12.

Ayliffe GAJ, Babb JR and Quoraishi AH (1978) A test for hygienic hand disinfection. *Journal of Clinical Pathology* 31, 923.

Ayliffe GAJ, Babb JR., Davies JG and Lilly HA (1988) Hand disinfection: a comparison of various agents in laboratory and ward studies. *Journal of Hospital Infection* 11, 226.

Ayliffe GAJ, Babb JR and Bradley CR (1992) Sterilization of arthroscopes and laparoscopes. *Journal of Hospital Infection* 24, 265.

Babb JR (1996) Application of disinfectants in hospitals and other health care establishments. *Infection Control Journal of Southern Africa* 1, 4.

Babb JR and Bradley CR (1995) A review of glutaraldehyde alternatives. *British Journal of Theatre Nursing* 5, 22.

Babb JR, Bradley CR and Ayliffe GAJ (1982) A formaldehyde disinfection unit. *Journal of Hospital Infection* **3**, 193.

Babb JR, Davies JG and Ayliffe GAJ (1991) A test procedure for evaluating surgical hand disinfection. *Journal of Hospital Infection* **18**(Suppl B), 41.

Bellamy K, Alcock R, Babb JR, Davies JG and Ayliffe GAJ (1993) A test for the assessment of 'hygienic' hand disinfection using rotavirus. *Journal of Hospital Infection* **24**, 201.

Benn RAV, Dutton AAC and Tully M (1973) Disinfection of mechanical ventilators: an investigation using formaldehyde in a Cape ventilator. *Anaesthesiology* **27**, 265.

Best M, Sattar SA, Springthorpe VS *et al.* (1990) Efficacies of selected disinfectants against *Mycobacterium tuberculosis*. *Journal of Clinical Microbiology* **28**, 10.

British Society of Gastroenterology (2008) BSG guidelines for the decontamination of equipment for gastrointestinal endoscopy. Available online at: http://www.bsg.org.uk/bsgdisp1.php?id=c7c0b1cf82751ba94159&h=1&sh=1&i=1&b=1&m=00023 (last accessed 9 September 2008).

British Standards Institution (1997a) EN 1499:1997 *Chemical disinfectants and antiseptics. Hygienic handwash – test method and requirements (phase 2/step 2)*. Milton Keynes: British Standards Institution.

British Standards Institution (1997b) EN 1500:1997 *Chemical disinfectants and antiseptics. Hygienic handrub – test method and requirements (phase 2/step 2)*. Milton Keynes: British Standards Institution.

British Standards Institution (2005) EN 12791:2005 *Chemical disinfectants and antiseptics. Surgical hand disinfection – test method and requirements (phase 2/step 1)*. Milton Keynes: British Standards Institution.

British Standards Institution (2006) EN ISO 15883:2006 *Washer disinfectors (Parts 1–4)*. Milton Keynes: British Standards Institution.

British Thoracic Society (2001) British Thoracic Society guidelines on diagnostic flexible bronchoscopy. *Thorax* **56**(Suppl 1), i1. Available online at: http://www.brit-thoracic.org.uk/Portals/0/Clinical%20Information/Bronchoscopy/Guidelines/Bronchoscopy.pdf.

Cadwallader HL, Bradley CR and Ayliffe GAJ (1990) Bacterial contamination and frequency of changing ventilator circuitry. *Journal of Hospital Infection* **15**, 65.

Centers for Disease Control and Prevention (2008) *Guideline for disinfection and sterilization in healthcare facilities, 2008*. Available online at: http://www.cdc.gov/ncidod/dhqp/pdf/guidelines/Disinfection_Nov_2008.pdf (last accessed 15 December 2008).

Cheesbrough JS, Barkess-Jones L and Brown DW (1997) Possible prolonged environmental survival of small round structured viruses. *Journal of Hospital Infection* **35**, 325.

Collins BJ (1979) How to have carpeted luxury. *Health and Social Services Journal* **28**, September.

Collins BJ (1988) The hospital environment: how clean should a hospital be? *Journal of Hospital Infection* **11**(Suppl A), 53.

Cooke RPD, Feneley RCL, Ayliffe GAJ *et al.* (1993) Decontamination of urological equipment: interim report of a Working Group of the Standing Committee on Urological Instruments of the British Association of Urological Surgeons. *British Journal of Urology* **71**, 5.

Craven DI, Connolly MG, Lichtenberg DA *et al.* (1982) Contamination of mechanical ventilators with tubing change every 24 or 48 hours. *New England Journal of Medicine* **306,** 1505.

Danforth D, Nicolle LE, Hume K *et al.* (1987) Nosocomial infections on nursing units with floors cleaned with a disinfectant compared with detergent. *Journal of Hospital Infection* **10,** 229.

Das I and Fraise AP (1997) How useful are microbial filters in respiratory apparatus? *Journal of Hospital Infection* **37,** 263.

Davies JG, Babb JG and Ayliffe GAJ (1978) Disinfection of the skin of the abdomen. *British Journal of Surgery* **65,** 855.

Davies JG, Babb JR, Bradley CR and Ayliffe GAJ (1993) Preliminary study of test methods to assess the virucidal activity of skin disinfectants using poliovirus and bacteriophages. *Journal of Hospital Infection* **25,** 125.

Department of Health (1991) Hospital mattress assemblies: care and cleaning. *Safety Action Bulletin* **91,** 65.

Department of Health (1997) HTM 2030 *Washer disinfectors.* London: Department of Health.

Department of Health (2007) Health Technical Memorandum 01-01: *Decontamination of re-usable medical devices, Part A.* London: TSO.

Deverill CEA and Dutt KK (1980) Methods of decontamination of anaesthetic equipment: daily sessional exchange of circuits. *Journal of Hospital Infection* **1,** 165.

Dyas A and Das BC (1985) The activity of glutaraldehyde against *Clostridium difficile.* *Journal of Hospital Infection* **6,** 41.

European Union (1995) 93/42/EEC *Council Directive, Medical Devices Directive.* Brussels: European Union.

French GL, Otter JA, Shannon KP, Adams NMT, Watling D and Parks MJ (2004) Tackling contamination of the hospital environment by methicillin resistant *Staphylococcus aureus* (MRSA): a comparison between conventional terminal cleaning and hydrogen peroxide vapour decontamination. *Journal of Hospital Infection* **57,** 31.

Griffiths PA, Babb JR, Bradley CR and Fraise AP (1997) Glutaraldehyde resistant *Mycobacterium chelonae* from endoscope washer disinfectors. *Journal of Applied Microbiology* **82,** 519.

Griffiths PA, Babb JR and Fraise AP (1999) Mycobacterial activity of selected disinfectants using a quantitative suspension test. *Journal of Hospital Infection* **41,** 111.

Health and Safety Executive (2003) *Health Services Advisory Committee. Safe working and the prevention of infection in clinical laboratories and similar facilities.* London: HMSO.

Hoffman PN, Bradley CR and Ayliffe GAJ (2004) *Disinfection in healthcare,* 3rd edn.

Infection Control Nurses Association (2001) *Hand decontamination guidelines.* London: Infection Control Nurses Association.

Judd PA, Tomlin PJ, Whitby JL *et al.* (1968) Disinfection of ventilators by ultrasonic nebulisation. *Lancet* **2,** 1019.

Lilly HA, Lowbury EJL, Wilkins MD *et al.* (1979) Delayed antimicrobial effects of skin disinfection by alcohol. *Journal of Hygiene* **82,** 497.

Lilly HA, Kidson A and Fujita K (1982) Investigation of hospital infection from a damaged mattress. *Burns* **8,** 408.

Lowbury EJL and Lilly HA (1973) Use of 4% chlorhexidine detergent solution (Hibiscrub) and other methods of skin disinfection. *British Medical Journal* **1,** 510.

Lowbury EJL and Lilly HA (1975) Gloved hands as applicator of antiseptic to operation sites. *Lancet* **ii,** 153.

Lowbury EJL, Lilly HA and Ayliffe GAJ (1974) Preoperative disinfection of surgeons' hands: use of alcoholic solutions and effects of gloves on skin flora. *British Medical Journal* **iv,** 369.

Maki DG, Alvarado CJ, Hassemer CA *et al.* (1982) Relation of the inanimate environment to endemic nosocomial infections. *New England Journal of Medicine* **307,** 1562.

Maurer IM (1985) *Hospital hygiene,* 3rd edn. Bristol: Wright PSG.

Medical Devices Agency (1996) MDA DB 9605: *Device bulletin: the purchase, operation and maintenance of benchtop steam sterilizers.* London: Medical Devices Agency.

Medical Devices Agency (1998) MDA DB 9804: *Device bulletin: the validation and periodic testing of benchtop vacuum steam sterilizers.* London: Medical Devices Agency.

Medicines and Healthcare Products Regulatory Agency (2002) MDA DB 2002(05): *Device bulletin. Decontamination of endoscopes.* London: Medical Devices Agency. Available online at: http://www.mhra.gov.uk/PrintPreview/PublicationSP/CON007329 (last accessed 9 September 2008).

Medicines and Healthcare Products Regulatory Agency (2002/2005/2006) *Sterilization, Disinfection and Cleaning of medical equipment: Guidance on decontamination from the Microbiology Advisory Committee to the Department of Health. Part 1, Principles 2002; Part 2, Protocols 2005; Part 3, Procedures 2006.* Available online at: http://www.mhra.gov.uk/Publications/Safetyguidance/Otherdevicesafetyguidance/CON007438 (last accessed 9 September 2008).

Medicines and Healthcare Products Regulatory Agency (2003) MDA/2003/019: *Reusable stainless steel vaginal specula.* London: MHRA.

Medicines and Healthcare Products Regulatory Agency (2006a) DB 2006 (04): *Reuse of medical devices: implications and consequences of reuse.* Available online at: http://www.mhra.gov.uk/PrintPreview/PublicationSP/CON2024995 (last accessed 9 September 2008).

Medicines and Healthcare Products Regulatory Agency (2006b) DB 2006(05) *Management of medical devices.* Available online at: http://www.mhra.gov.uk/PrintPreview/PublicationSP/CON2025142 (last accessed 9 September 2008).

Morris J, Duckworth GJ and Ridgway GL (2006) Gastrointestinal endoscopy decontamination failure and the risk of transmission of blood borne viruses: a review. *Journal of Hospital Infection* **63,** 1.

National Patient Safety Agency (2007) *The national specifications for cleanliness in the NHS: a framework for setting and measuring performance outcomes.* Available online at: http://www.npsa.nhs.uk/nrls/improvingpatientsafety/cleaning-and-nutrition/national-specifications-of-cleanliness/ (last accessed 29 September 2008).

Newsom SWB (1998) Special problems in hospital antisepsis. In: Russell AD, Hugo WB and Ayliffe GAJ (eds) *Principles and practice of disinfection, preservation and sterilization,* 3rd edn. Oxford: Blackwell Science, 416.

NHS Estates (1997) Health Technical Memorandum 2030: *Washer disinfectors. Operational management, design considerations, validation and verification.* London: HMSO.

NHS Estates (2003) Model Engineering Specifications C32: *Automated endoscope reprocessors for flexible endoscopes*. London: HMSO.

NHS Executive (1999) *Variant Creutzfeldt–Jakob disease: minimising the risk of transmission. Controls assurance in infection control: decontamination of medical devices*. London: Department of Health.

Pittet D, Hugonnet S, Harbarth S, Mourouga P, Sauvan V, Touveneau S and Perneger TV (2000) Effectiveness of a hospital-wide programme to improve compliance with hand hygiene. *Lancet* **356,** 1307.

Prichard RC and Raper RF (1996) Doctors and handwashing: instilling Semmelweis' message. *Medical Journal of Australia* **164,** 395.

Rotter M (1996) Hand washing and hand disinfection. *Hospital Epidemiology and Infection Control* **79,** 1052.

Royal College of Obstetricians and Gynaecologists (1997) *HIV infection in maternity care and gynaecology*. Working Party Report. London: RCOG Press.

Rutala WA (1990) APIC guidelines for selection and use of disinfectants. *American Journal of Infection Control* **18,** 99.

Spach DH, Silverstein FE and Stamm WE (1993) Transmission of infection by gastrointestinal endoscopy and bronchoscopy. *Annals of Internal Medicine* **118,** 117.

Taylor DM (1992) Inactivation of unconventional agents of the transmissible degenerative encephalopathies. In: Russell AD, Hugo WG and Ayliffe GAJ (eds) *Disinfection, preservation and sterilization*, 3rd edn. Oxford: Blackwell Scientific Publications, 222.

Taylor LJ (1978) An evaluation of handwashing techniques. *Nursing Times* **74,** 108.

Wilcox MH, Fawley WN, Wigglesworth N, Parnell P, Verity P and Freeman J (2003) Comparison of the effect of detergent versus hypochlorite cleaning on environmental contamination and incidence of *Clostridium difficile* infection. *Journal of Hospital Infection* **54,** 109.

Williams JD, Waltho CA, Ayliffe GAJ and Lowbury EJL (1967) Trials of five antibacterial creams in the control of nasal carriage of *Staphylococcus aureus*. *Lancet* **2,** 390.

Peter Hoffman

LAUNDRY

Many reusable fabrics in healthcare have close, prolonged contact with patients. They become contaminated with pathogens and, unless thoroughly decontaminated before reuse, transmit them to susceptible patients subsequently in contact with those fabrics. The decontamination of fabrics is probably the largest-scale decontamination procedure in healthcare and one with which Infection Control Teams have little routine involvement. In the past, healthcare laundries used to be part of a hospital, though often at a remote location. Now, in the UK, the most common way for fabrics to be supplied to hospitals is by commercial organizations that own, supply and launder the linen, with each laundry serving many hospitals. This further distances any Infection Control Team involvement.

This chapter was written while the long-standing UK guidance (Department of Health, 1995) was in the process of being updated. It will eventually be replaced by a Health Technical Memorandum (HTM) in the decontamination series (HTM 01-04, in preparation), which will give more precise guidance. This section will cover more general aspects around issues of infection control.

The laundry contract

There should be infection control input when a contract for linen supply is set-up or renewed. This is likely to be the only time when important matters can be specified; after this, they are likely to be fixed by the contract.

The setting up of a hospital's laundry contract is reviewed by Barrie (1994). The Infection Control Team's involvement should be as part of the team evaluating tenders and they should have access to documentation on the laundries' quality assurance procedures, external quality evaluations and their health and safety policies. There should be infection control representation on the team sent to inspect each laundry as part of the tender assessment process.

Quality assurance systems

It is important to evaluate any quality assurance (QA) schemes critically. The main QA scheme is likely to be BS EN 14065: 2002 'Textiles – Laundry processed textiles – Biocontamination control system' British Standards Institution, 2002, also known as 'RABC' (risk analysis and biocontamination control). In this scheme, the processor lists what they consider to be the microbiological hazards to the clean linen they produce, the control points for laundry contamination, tolerances for those points, monitoring schemes, corrective actions and verification that the whole system is working adequately. This system is only as good as those drawing it up, who should have an understanding of microbiology and infection control. The focus should be on robust decontamination and subsequent prevention of recontamination from soiled linen, either directly or indirectly. The primary quality assurance should be by monitoring the laundering processes. Environmental monitoring, particularly in areas used prior to linen decontamination, is far less relevant. There should be an emphasis on prevention of recontamination of laundered linen with microbes from used linen rather than from other environmental sources. If product sampling is included as an occasional or exceptional additional monitoring measure, it should be remembered that non-destructive testing methods, such as contact plates, recover only about 0.2 per cent of contamination compared with more efficient but destructive methods, such as fabric excision and immersion (Barrie *et al.*, 1994).

The washing processes

Tunnel washers

The majority of fabrics will be washed in a highly efficient process known as a 'continuous tunnel washer' or 'tunnel washer'. This is a metal cylinder, usually about 2 m diameter and 10 m length, divided into different functional compartments by an internal Archimedean screw, where soiled linen is added at one end and clean water at the other. These flow in opposite directions, with wash chemicals and heat being added to various compartments. The Archimedean screw has, at various points along the length of the tunnel, small holes in it such that water can pass though it, but linen cannot. The cylinder rocks back and forth, agitating linen, and then, every 2 min, rotates through 360° and linen moves via the Archimedean screw into the next compartment. At this point, a new load of soiled linen is added to the first compartment and clean linen is ejected from the last compartment. The majority of water is then removed from the ejected linen in a piston press and the compacted linen usually then travels automatically on conveyer belts to a tumble drier set for the drying parameters for a particular type of linen. This is an economically necessary measure; for example, drying sheets will not require the same energy input as drying towels. Such pre-wash segregation of linen drying types necessitates pre-sorting of the linen, bringing laundry workers in contact with the soiled linen. Some tunnel washer setups do not pre-sort linen but sort it into different drying types after decontamination in the wash; however, there is still a stage of emptying soiled linen on to a conveyer belt that carries it into the tunnel washer. This brings workers into a lower level of contact than pre-sorting, but contact still occurs.

Tunnel washers are very water efficient and, as a consequence, use little energy in heating these small volumes of water and do not have to use large quantities of wash chemicals to get the correct dilutions. They are rapid, producing a load of clean linen (around 40 kg) every 2 min. Thus they are the laundry industry's preferred wash methods and the economics of a laundry contract depend on the vast majority of linen being processed in this way.

Washer–extractors

These are larger versions of conventional washing machines. They take about 40 min to wash a load (around 40 kg) and use comparatively large amounts of water, energy and wash chemicals. However, linen can be loaded into them by opening a plastic bag and emptying it straight in with no pre-sorting or contact with the linen occurring. These machines are slow and expensive, and are only used where tunnel washers are not suitable, such as for infectious or themolabile linen.

Dry cleaning

This is not generally used for healthcare linen. While there is some evidence, both experimental (Bates et al., 1993) and theoretical, that the main solvents used will have some limited antimicrobial effects on bacteria and enveloped viruses, it is not a well-controlled decontamination process and should be used only on rare occasions such as, for example, decontaminating a child's prized but contaminated soft toy.

Laundry should be segregated at the point of generation according to the following three categories.

- *Used linen:* this is the majority of laundry generated by healthcare. It can include both general used linen ('soiled') and linen contaminated by faeces and blood ('fouled'), unless they are known to be highly infectious.
- *Infectious linen:* this is linen that represents a substantial hazard to those workers in hospital or the laundry who may come into contact with it. There is some uncertainty about the infections that make linen 'infectious' but, in the absence of national guidance or where national guidance can be supplemented by local alterations, the list should comprise linen likely to be contaminated with those microbes that can be transmitted to healthy humans such as salmonella, *Shigella*, norovirus, verocytotoxin-producing *Escherichia coli*, etc. Linen contaminated with microbes that limit their infectivity largely to compromised hospital patients, such as methicillin-resistant *Staphylococcus aureus* (MRSA) or *Clostridium difficile*, should not

be included. Linen will usually have to be classified as 'infectious' on clinical suspicion, rather than confirmed infection, for example, faecally soiled linen from a patient suspected of having a highly transmissible infection.

- *Thermolabile linen:* this is linen that would be damaged by the heat disinfection applied to used and infectious linen, and has to be disinfected chemically, a less reliable process than thermal disinfection. This category of healthcare linen is difficult to process and should be kept to a minimum.

Used linen is processed in tunnel washers wherever possible; the economics of the laundry process relies on the vast majority of the linens being processed in this way. The laundry workers who unpack and sort the bags of used linen always should be trained in safety and take basic infection control precautions (gloves, aprons or gowns, handwashing, use safe methods of working, etc.).

Infectious linen should be processed by washer–extractors. With these, the laundry should be carefully emptied from the bag (if insoluble) by trained staff directly into the washing machine or loaded as an intact bag (if they are water soluble or have a water-soluble seam). There should be as little handling of infectious linen as possible; even emptying, without sorting, on to a conveyer belt should be avoided.

Some hospitals operate a version of universal precautions and will classify all theatre linen and all linen from isolation rooms as infectious. Laundries cannot cope, physically or economically, with a high proportion of linen that has to go through the substantially more expensive washer–extractor process. If they receive large volumes of linen packed as infectious, they will have to put most of it through their tunnel washers and expose their workers to it in unpacking and sorting it prior to the washing process. So, ironically, such a version of universal precautions is counterproductive in terms of worker safety. The difficult task is to persuade hospital staff to differentiate between all bloodstained linen, or all linen from infected patients and that subset which contains a substantial hazard to healthcare and laundry staff.

Decontamination parameters

The standard disinfection process is thermal disinfection at 65°C for at least 10 min or 71°C for at least 3 min (Department of Health, 1995). This applies equally to 'used' and 'infectious' linen; the difference in classification is to identify separate hazard groups for those who may handle it, not to indicate a requirement for a higher level of decontamination. The precise control of the temperature of a large mass of water and linen is difficult and the requirements are, in practice, less critical than those for other washer–disinfectors or for steam sterilizers, and tend to be exceeded without damage to the items processed.

Thermolabile linens cannot be heat disinfected and chemical disinfection has to be employed in washer–extractors, which will add to microbial removal by dilution. It is recommended (Department of Health, 1995) that a chlorine-releasing agent is added to the penultimate rinse to achieve a concentration of 150 parts per million available chlorine. It needs to be in a rinse part of the cycle as that low level of chlorine would be inactivated by the organic matter on soiled fabrics and it should not be the final rinse to avoid the processed linens smelling of chlorine.

There is some economic and environmental pressure to use either chemical or thermochemical disinfection instead of the high-temperature thermal processes. If such processes are to be employed, they must be rigorously validated in exact simulations of wash processes used rather than just simple laboratory suspension tests. Their routine use must also be continuously monitored to ensure that the correct disinfection parameters are always met.

Washing machines on hospital wards

These should be discouraged as they cannot hope to have the same levels of control as carefully monitored industrial processes. However, there may be areas where wards would not send items (such as woollen baby clothes) to an industrial laundry. Here, the choice is more likely to be between washing in a domestic machine on the ward or rinsing in a sink and air drying; microbial removal would be superior in a domestic washing machine. If a ward is to have a domestic washing machine, the need for this should be negotiated with the Infection Control Team who should explore whether alternatives, such as single-patient use items, could be used. If there is no alternative to a washing machine being used on a ward, it should receive regular maintenance, not just on breakdown. The Infection Control Team should advise further in outbreak situations.

Healthcare linen and *Bacillus cereus*

There has been a report of a small cluster of *Bacillus cereus* postoperative infection linked to high level of contamination of non-sterile theatre wear, and the rest of the hospital's freshly laundered linen (Barrie *et al.*, 1992). This was thought to be the result of a combination of a general increase in aerobic spore formers on used laundry awaiting processing and the low dilution of tunnel-washing processes (Barrie *et al.*, 1994). It appears to be associated with high ambient temperatures during summer allowing greater *Bacillus* spp. replication than would normally take place and than could be removed by low-dilution washing processes. A similar phenomenon has been observed anecdotally during other hot summers. Control is by increasing the rate of water supply to the tunnel washers used to process this linen. This measure affects the economics of the laundering process and can meet with resistance from processors.

Staff uniforms

The laundering of uniforms can be an emotive issue for healthcare staff, the public and the news media. However, it should be remembered that healthcare workers' uniforms have neither the properties or functions of personal protective equipment. (If they did, staff would have to change out of them to eat or drink). The main source of microbial contamination of clothing, whether it is a uniform or not, will be from the skin of the wearer. In all but a few critical situations, exemplified by surgical procedures, this is not relevant to infection. If workers are likely to become contaminated directly or indirectly from patients, they should wear personal protective clothing, such as aprons or gowns, which should be removed as soon as that task has been completed. Similarly aprons or gowns, as part of aseptic technique, should be used to prevent acquired contamination being spread to patients during susceptible procedures such as dressing changes. Any minor contamination that may occur can be removed in a domestic washing machine by dilution without the thermal disinfection of an industrial process. There is no evidence that home laundry provides inadequate decontamination for uniforms (Wilson *et al.*, 2007). Care should be taken not to overload the washing machine and the temperature chosen should be one compatible with that fabric type.

KITCHEN HYGIENE

Hospital kitchens have the, usually under-rated, task of producing safe inexpensive food to suit a variety of tastes and dietary requirements, to be served in locations remote from those in which it was prepared. Many of those to whom this food is served have a higher susceptibility to infection with more severe consequences should it occur. The disruption from a food-poisoning outbreak originating in a hospital kitchen can be magnified, as this facility usually prepares food for staff as well as patients. That hospital-associated food-poisoning outbreaks are rare is a sign that the production of safe food is the norm. This occurs without much intervention from Infection Control Teams, the major input being from the kitchens themselves and from environmental health practitioners. However, Infection Control Teams may need to become involved in this area should there be outbreaks or possible outbreaks. Should this happen, they will require familiarity with both the principles of food hygiene and their hospital kitchen. One of the best ways of doing this in advance of a crisis is to accompany environmental health practitioners on some of their routine inspections of the kitchens and it is recommended that all those who may get involved in such outbreak investigations do so.

Food, such as sandwiches, made and sold by volunteers, and consumed by visitors and outpatients, is also within the hospital's responsibility. It is no less important than food produced in the hospital's own kitchen, and should be produced and stored prior to purchase in equally hygienic conditions.

Principles of food hygiene

It is not intended for this section to be an exhaustive work on food hygiene and food poisoning. Other works should be referred to if that is required (e.g. McLauchlin and Little, 2007); however, it does cover the outline principles of food preparation in healthcare.

Food hygiene depends on the following.

- *Good-quality ingredients*: ingredients should come from sources known to supply good-quality produce. Goods should be inspected on delivery, including their temperature where appropriate, and rejected if not adequate.
- *Storage:* where appropriate (e.g. meats and dairy products), goods should be stored in controlled-temperature refrigerated environments to limit growth of both pathogens and spoilage microbes. This does not apply to 'dry goods', such as sugar, salt, dry spices, flour, sauce powders and tinned goods. Where products have a significant chance of being contaminated (e.g. raw meats), they should be stored separately from other products, particularly those that are to be consumed without cooking, such as cooked meats, salad vegetables and dairy products. The areas where foods are stored must be easily cleanable and clean at the time of inspection.
- *Separate preparation areas for different categories of food:* as with storage, there should be separate preparation areas, each with separate equipment, for products that are likely to be contaminated. Effective separation of equipment is more readily achieved using colour coding (e.g. knife handles and chopping boards for raw meats may be coloured red).
- *Controlled cooking:* cooking food is a thermal disinfection process. It is globally the most common example of thermal disinfection and is the most effective of all food-hygiene interventions. In kitchens, it cannot be as precisely controlled as, for example, in sterile supply departments but should be monitored in processes where it may be deficient. For example, if something is boiled, adequate disinfection is assured without temperature assessment; if thermally non-conductive items such as meat are processed by hot air (e.g. roasting chicken), temperature probes should be used to assess that disinfection temperatures, normally 75°C, have been achieved in all parts of the food, and similarly for reheating ('regenerating') cook–chill food.
- *Post-cooking temperature control:* if cooked food is intended for imminent consumption, it should be kept hot, usually at or above 63°C until it is served. Similarly cold foods should be kept cold, usually at or below 8°C until they are served. If cooked food is not intended for imminent consumption, such as in a cook–chill system, it should be rapidly cooled after cooking, to 3°C or less within 90 min, and can be held there for up to 5 days.

- *Staff training:* this is an essential component of the routine production of safe food. In all the criteria listed above, staff behaviour is an essential component of quality assurance. Without knowledgeable conscientious staff, it is possible to negate almost any safety process. Staff must also be motivated to apply their training, a process that includes good supervision.

Safety systems in food production

The standard safety system currently used in food production is called 'hazard analysis and critical control point', more usually known by its acronym 'HACCP'. It is a multi-applicable hazard control system that can be used in many non-food industries as well as food-production processes from the smallest to the largest. A team, with all the relevant disciplines represented, defines the steps in each process and decides which steps are critical to safety; such steps are termed 'critical control points' (CCPs). The HACCP analysis involves the following steps.

1 *Defining the process:* this produces a flow chart defining the steps from raw material to served product. The flow chart should be verified as accurate against the actual process.
2 *Identify the hazards:* all possible hazards should be identified. These are not just microbiological, but could include the presence of non-food materials, allergic reactions, etc.
3 *Assessment of hazards:* this combines the theoretical hazard with the likelihood of its occurrence and its consequences. These hazards should be ranked according to overall severity.
4 *Identify CCPs:* based on data from the previous step, the steps ('control points') that can control the hazard are identified. These can be a control point that can completely eliminate hazards, termed a CCP1 (such as thorough cooking of a chicken portion) or a control point that minimizes a hazard (such as chilling post-cooking) termed a CCP2.
5 *Specifying the monitoring and control procedures:* this will set out how the CCPs are monitored (e.g. how the cooking of a chicken portion is assessed) and what action to take when there is a failure to achieve that level of control.
6 *Implementation of controls:* this sets out how controls will be implemented, for example, checking that items are within their use-by date or checking for indicator enzyme levels in pasteurized milk. Microbiological checks are usually impractical as they take too long.
7 *Verification:* this uses additional tests to verify that the controls are in place and effective as part of an ongoing verification of the whole process. This stage could use microbiological checks but this is unlikely in hospital catering, where internal audit of process controls is likely to be more meaningful.

The HACCP principles are adaptable and theoretically applicable to most risk situations. There have been attempts to apply them to other aspects of safety in hospitals, including the control of healthcare-associated infection.

Legislation

Catering in healthcare has no legal privileges, and premises can be closed or prosecuted as any other food-producing organization. From the start of 2006, new European Union food legislation has applied throughout the UK. The main regulation affecting hospital kitchens is Regulation (EC) 852/2004 (European Parliament, 2004), which applies general hygiene requirements to all food business operators. This requires that food business operators put into place, implement and maintain a permanent procedure based on the principles of HACCP (i.e. even if not true HACCP, it must use the same principles). It also requires that food business operators ensure that food handlers are supervised and instructed and/or trained in food hygiene commensurate with their work activity, and that those responsible for the development and operation of the safety system are also suitably trained. In essence, all food business operators have to be able to show that they have an effective food safety management system in operation.

Dishwashing and cleaning

In general, vessels and items used to contain, process, serve or consume food are not at high risk of significant contamination. Where they are, for example, chopping boards used for raw meats, physical separation from contact with foods that will be consumed without further cooking should occur. Thus dishwashers in kitchens do not occupy the same strategic needs as, for example, surgical instrument washer–disinfectors, and so do not need the stringent controls and monitoring that is applied in these more critical areas. Mechanical dishwashers produce disinfection by dilution during the washing and rinsing parts of the cycle, and heat disinfection mainly during the late rinsing part of the cycle. The hot final rinse that should be used in healthcare dishwashers is part of the drying process; hot items will dry spontaneously after the process. Final rinse temperatures should normally be in the range 70–90°C. There may also be some disinfection from chemicals used in the highly alkaline detergents, particularly when used at elevated temperatures, but this is poorly quantifiable and is likely to be secondary to the dilution and thermal effects.

Larger items may have to be cleaned by hand, either in sinks or where they are permanently located ('cleaning in place'). Here disinfection is achieved by cleaning alone, and the quality of the process is as good as the skill and motivation of the individual doing that task, combined with the facilities they are given to do it. Cleaning cooking vessels is important from the views of product acceptability and aesthetic considerations, although these vessels will be thermally disinfected during the cooking process. Work surfaces will legitimately make contact with food but have to be cleaned in place. It is difficult to ensure high-quality decontamination of these surfaces, emphasizing the requirement for separation of areas for processing foods at high risk of contamination, such as uncooked meats.

More remote surfaces (e.g. floors and gullies) are even less directly related to food safety, and cleaning here is a matter of pest control (removing a food source) and safety (preventing the slippery build-up of grease on a floor).

The relevance of chemical disinfectants, usually called 'sanitizers' in this context, is marginal at best. The agents usable in food preparation areas are mostly easily inactivated and the processes have poor quality control. Food hygiene should be achieved primarily by procedural means and should not rely on the use of sanitizers.

Hand hygiene

The hands of staff in kitchens, just as on wards, can be an effective means of transferring micro-organisms from contaminated to susceptible sites and, again as on wards, handwashing and the correct use of gloves can be used to interrupt such transfer effectively. Each area in a hospital's kitchen should have at least one hand wash-basin, and more in larger, heavily staffed areas. Hands should be washed under running water, delivered at a comfortable temperature via a mixer tap. Taps should be capable of being operated without soiled hands touching them (e.g. elbow taps, infrared-operated taps or similar). Hands should be washed whenever they may have become contaminated, either as a consequence of a person's work (e.g. after handling raw meat or uncooked eggs in their shell, handling rubbish), or may otherwise have become contaminated (e.g. using the toilet, sneezing or blowing the nose), and before starting work.

Staff health

Kitchen staff, particularly when working with foods that will be consumed without further heating, can pose a risk of transmitting their gastrointestinal infections on a large scale. Such transmission can have particularly serious consequences where already-debilitated people, such as hospital patients, may acquire the infections. Potential staff should complete a pre-employment questionnaire taking the risks of transmissible infections into account, as should visitors to food-preparation areas. It must be made clear to staff that they have an obligation to report symptoms of possible gastrointestinal infection (diarrhoea and/or vomiting) and that they should remain off work until 48 hours after symptoms cease. However, if it is known or suspected that the pathogen is verocytotoxin-producing *E. coli*, typhoid, paratyphoid or *Shigella dysenteriae, S. boydii* or *S. flexneri* in a high-risk food handler, stool screening should be carried out (Little, 2005) and the food-handler may return to work only when they no longer present a risk. Details of the prevention of person-to-person spread of these and other relevant infections can be found in a Public Health Laboratory Service Working Group report (Health Protection Agency, 2004).

Ward food hygiene

The process of food safety that starts in the hospital kitchen needs to continue at ward level as the food is served. Staff who serve food usually do this in combination with several other duties, many of which could bring them into contact with contamination that could transmit foodborne infections. This is a substantially higher risk than serving food outside the context of a hospital ward. Such staff should receive training in the hygiene of serving food on wards and their food-serving duties should be separated from other activities. They should wear single-use plastic aprons and, if gloves are worn, they must be changed if they may have become contaminated. Supervision of these aspects of staff serving food should be by the same clinical staff who supervise other aspects of infection control processes, usually the ward manager or those delegated by them.

If cook–chill food is heated-up ('regenerated') on wards, staff must be trained in thermometric monitoring of the regenerated food and in other associated aspects of food hygiene (e.g. that sandwiches should not be kept on the regeneration trolley unless in insulated compartments).

Ward-kitchen refrigerators and food stored in them should be managed by ward staff with the combination of adherence to good hygiene, and the wishes of patients and their relatives. The policy usually consists of allowing food only if labelled with a patient's name and the date of bringing-in, with the understanding that they will be discarded after 24 hours if home produced or by the use-by date if commercially produced. These refrigerators should be used for this purpose only.

Pests

Food premises need constant and permanent safeguards against pests; waiting until there is an obvious problem before taking action is not a productive approach. There will be a constant challenge of introduction of pests to all food premises from both the local environment and from items, particularly foodstuffs, brought in from other locations. Pest control can be summarized into the following areas:

Exclusion

The more pests that can be prevented from entering food production premises, the easier the task of control will be.

- *Pests from foodstuffs brought in:* this is probably the most important route of introduction. The kitchen should use reliable suppliers and inspect all batches of food for signs of infestation (such as gnawed packaging or droppings).
- *Pests from the local environment:* windows should be protected by mesh screens to exclude flying insects and birds. Other routes into the building, such as disconnected pipes and drains, should be blocked or removed. Doors into the building should seal such that pests cannot get through them when they are closed and they should be kept closed as much as possible.

Monitoring

Most pests will not emerge when there is activity around or when premises are well lit, so there is a need to look for indicators of infestation rather than the pests themselves. There should be regular inspections by trained staff for such signs such as: rodent droppings, gnaw marks or footprints; entry holes, particularly with characteristic smears around them; spills around sacks/bags of stored foods; cockroach droppings or egg cases; bird droppings; and any smell characteristic of an infestation.

Control

Pests should be denied food and water. Food remains should be cleared promptly and efficiently (known as 'clean as you go'), waste food should be stored in pest-proof containers and removed as rapidly as possible, and all food should be stored at least 15 cm above floor level. All foodstuffs that may be contaminated by pests should be disposed of carefully and ultraviolet-light insect traps should be used.

Pest control is a specialism that requires training, experience and facilities. It is unlikely that a hospital kitchen would be able to achieve suitable control without using a specialist contractor. It is particularly important in food premises that any pesticide is used only by trained operators. The contractor should give written reports on their observations and actions to feed into the HACCP system. However, this does not relieve kitchen staff from any responsibility in this area, and they should be trained and vigilant to spot signs of pests and must report any such observation.

All components of pest control (inspections, findings and actions) should be recorded as part of the HACCP system.

HEALTHCARE WASTE

Healthcare waste is a problem spanning many hospital departments. While the prime responsibility for this does not belong to the Infection Control Team, their input can be required. This section will attempt to guide those whose primary interest is infection control through the general approach to healthcare waste and to highlight those areas where they may be required to have an input.

After a period of comparative stability in the UK guidelines concerning clinical waste, matters have changed following the introduction of the European Waste Catalogue (EWC). This classifies all waste, not just that from healthcare, and includes hazardous wastes. The waste from healthcare is no longer to be classified as group A to E clinical waste (i.e. the former classification of clinical waste, where Group A is ward-generated clinical waste; Group B, sharps; group C, laboratory waste; Group D, pharmaceutical waste; and Group E, ward-generated urine, faeces, etc. and their containers). Instead, it now has to be classified under the EWC codes, which are mandatory on waste-transfer documentation. While this impacts predominantly on waste between the stages of commercial collection from hospitals and final disposal, there will be some impact on collection and handling closer to the point of generation. Overall, the impact on the input of Infection Control Teams will be little changed but they should be aware of the framework within which they are operating. The key guidance document dealing with healthcare waste in the UK is Health Technical Memorandum (HTM) 07-01 'Safe management of healthcare waste' (Department of Health, 2006).

The current approach, which includes infectious waste as just one of many categories of hazardous waste, gives a unified approach to all the wastes produced in any healthcare situation. This enables wastes with different hazards, as well as wastes with more than one associated hazard (e.g. sharp, infectious and cytotoxic) to be dealt with in the same system. Thus healthcare wastes are no longer a special category of waste with respect to transport and disposal, but now have to fit in with the general scheme used for all other hazardous wastes. The spectrum of healthcare can produce many different hazardous wastes; this section will only deal with those where there are infection control implications.

The laws around healthcare waste are numerous and there are sometimes, usually minor, variations between England and Wales, Scotland, and Northern Ireland (e.g. what is 'hazardous waste' in England, Wales and Northern Ireland is 'special waste' in Scotland). All of the relevant legislation is outlined in HTM 07-01 (Department of Health, 2006). In all systems, the organization producing healthcare waste has the following main responsibilities in their duty of care:

- to describe the waste fully and accurately;
- to complete and sign a waste transfer note prior to transfer to another party (usually the waste contractor);

- to pack waste in accordance with the carriage regulations;
- to store waste safely on site;
- to make all reasonable checks on their waste carriers;
- to select an appropriate final disposal method;
- to ensure the waste falls within the terms of their contractor's waste management licence.

Healthcare waste is defined as 'the waste from the diagnosis, treatment or prevention of disease and of natal care' (Department of Health, 2006). Examples included within this definition are infectious waste, sharps waste, anatomical waste, medicinal waste, and laboratory cultures and chemicals.

Infectious waste

Infectious waste is currently defined in the Hazardous Waste (England and Wales) Regulations (2005) as 'substances containing viable micro-organisms or their toxins which are known or reliably believed to cause disease in man or other living organisms'. This is reflected in the EWC as 'waste whose collection and disposal is subject to special requirements in order to prevent infection'. The general approach should be that infectious waste is the waste generated by healthcare practices, or produced by healthcare workers in the community, unless an assessment has taken place to indicate a lack of infectious risk. Such an assessment should be on an item-specific and patient-specific clinical assessment by a healthcare practitioner. Healthcare waste must be of a type specifically associated with the activities of healthcare in order to differentiate it from the domestic waste, such as patients' leftover food, or other hazardous waste, such as ambulance waste engine oil, produced in those activities.

There are two categories within 'infectious waste' – A and B. *Category A* is an infectious substance that is transported in a form that, when exposure to it occurs, is capable of causing permanent disability, life-threatening or fatal disease to humans or animals. HTM 07-01 essentially defines this as patient-derived healthcare waste contaminated with haemorrhagic fever viruses, monkeypox or variola (as well as laboratory cultures of hazard group 3 or 4 pathogens).

Category B is any infectious substance that does not fall into category A. Thus all routine infectious waste will be Category B.

Other relevant categories of healthcare waste

These are as follows:

- medicines –
  - cytotoxic or cytostatic
  - controlled drugs (which have legal restrictions other than hazardous waste)

- all other medicines;
- sharps;
- anatomical waste(i.e. body parts and blood/blood products);
- chemicals
  - containing hazardous substances
  - other chemicals;
- waste mercury amalgam;
- recognizable medical waste in no other category.

Collection and disposal of healthcare waste

The collection of healthcare waste should be in containers coloured according to their final disposal method. This colour scheme (Figure 7.1, see endpaper at back of book for full colour version) is recommended rather than mandatory, but use of this scheme should be standard.

- Yellow – for incineration only.
- Orange – for either incineration or 'alternative treatments', such as heating or microwave-based treatments validated to render the waste safe. These alternatives are generally less expensive than incineration.
- Purple – for incineration at facilities suitable for cytotoxic and cytostatic drugs.
- Yellow and black ('tiger') stripes – for landfill at sites licensed for 'offensive' waste.
- Black – for landfill at sites licensed for domestic waste.
- White – for recovery of ingredients such as metals from dental amalgam, or photography and X-ray waste.

Category A infectious waste must be incinerated. Category B infectious waste can either be incinerated or rendered safe by one of the validated alternative treatments. These alternative treatments are generally preferable on the grounds of cost. However, if category B infectious waste also contains other hazards, the disposal method has to be suitable for those hazards as well (e.g. if the waste is infectious category B and cytotoxic, it must be incinerated).

If waste contains more than one type of hazard, the container must indicate those hazards as in the following examples.

- Infectious waste for incineration that also contains cytotoxics should go in yellow containers with a purple band.
- If sharps waste also contains cytotoxics, it should be collected in a sharps bin with a purple lid.
- If sharps waste also contain medicinal products, and so requires incineration, it should be collected in a sharps bin with a yellow lid. If a syringe is fully discharged and only the dead volume in a luer connection

contains non-cytotoxic medicine, it is considered empty and does not need to be disposed of by incineration. However, medicinal products cannot be deliberately emptied from syringes just for the purpose of easier disposal.

- If sharps waste just contains blood (i.e. just infectious – no extra hazard), it should be collected in a sharps bin with an orange lid.
- Infectious waste for incineration that may have radioactive contamination should be put in yellow containers overstamped with a radioactive symbol.

Handling of healthcare waste within the healthcare premises

It is a legal requirement that healthcare waste should always be stored such that it poses no risk to the public. Such storage should be secure and away from public areas. Failure to do so could result in prosecution.

At ward level, waste should be placed in the correct receptacles as close to the point of production as possible; plastic sacks should be held within rigid sack-holders. Sacks and sharps bins should be taken out of use when they are three-quarters full at most. They should be securely sealed (e.g. with a plastic tie for waste sacks), labelled with their point of origin and collected frequently. Local storage near the ward should be secure and allow the packed waste to be segregated into the different waste classifications. All ward staff who handle healthcare waste should be trained in waste categorization and safe handling. Waste should then be moved promptly to a cleanable, secure, totally enclosed, well-lit and ventilated central bulk storage area to await collection. This area should be dedicated to healthcare waste and not be shared with any other activity. The more hazardous wastes, sharps and medicines may require separate storage with more restricted access within this area. Bulk healthcare waste storage areas must be readily accessible to the contractor's collecting vehicle.

Issues of staff hygiene, such as the provision of appropriate personal protective equipment and handwashing facilities should be considered for routine handling as well as spills. The issue of immunization of groups of staff is primarily one for the Occupational Health Department (see Chapter 11).

Spills

There must be written procedures for dealing with spillages of healthcare waste. All staff who handle healthcare waste must be trained in the safe clearance of spilled waste. This will involve the use of safe methods of working, personal protective equipment, chemical disinfectants and receptacles in which to deposit the cleared spill. There should be input from the Infection Control Team on all these matters, particularly on safe and effective chemical disinfectants. Infection Control Teams may advise the use of a chlorine-releasing agent as the disinfectant of choice unless other factors make it unsuitable; an example of such a factor being the presence of strong acids (chlorine gas hazard). It should not be regarded that the use of a disinfectant will, of itself, reliably negate any infectious hazard, and safe methods of work and the correct use of personal protective equipment are vital to safety. Spill kits containing all relevant materials should be available at those points where spills are considered most likely. If a spill occurs, there should be a means of reporting it and a subsequent investigation procedure with the intention of preventing such future spills.

Training

All staff who deal with healthcare waste should be trained, both in how to classify and segregate it and how to deal with accidents including spills. The detail of such training will vary with the group of staff concerned and should reflect their specific roles (e.g. whether their involvement is that of management, generation, storage or transport of waste). The Infection Control Team should have input into such training where this would be relevant. All groups of staff handling waste should receive relevant training as part of their induction and this should be recorded in their training record.

Infectious waste in community healthcare

This is perhaps the most contentious area of healthcare waste. The same regulatory framework governing the large-scale handling of infectious waste also covers the same, much smaller scale, issue in community settings; however, there will probably be more scope for individual risk assessments here. In this context, 'community' covers community nursing, as well as healthcare workers (including emergency care practitioners) who provide care to patients in their own homes and care homes (i.e. those without nursing care).

Community items can include the following.

- *Dressings:* large contaminated dressings are likely to be disposed of as infectious healthcare waste; smaller dressings (the example given is 220 × 130 mm or smaller), sticking plasters and incontinence products that have not been assessed as infectious can be wrapped in a plastic sack and placed in the domestic waste.
- *Used single-use instruments:* these should be treated as infectious waste.
- *The sharps of self-medicating patients:* these should be disposed of in sharps boxes, taken to the general practitioner's surgery or a local pharmacy for disposal.
- *Catheter/stoma bags:* these can be disposed of by a community nurse in the domestic, black-bag waste stream unless produced in bulk, when they would considered as offensive waste.

• *Vacuum wound drains:* these should always be treated as infectious waste.

Transporting waste in the community

Healthcare workers are responsible for the waste they produce in the community and should be trained to deal with healthcare waste. If they transport the waste in their own vehicles, it must be in secure rigid packing (boxes or drums to packing standard P621). If they leave the waste in the home for later collection (e.g. by a local authority, waste contractor or healthcare provider, it should be stored such that pets, pests or children cannot access it). A consignment note, a legal requirement for the transfer of waste between producers and operators under other circumstances, is not required for the transfer of waste from domestic premises.

REFERENCES

Barrie D (1994) How hospital linen and laundry services are provided. *Journal of Hospital Infection* **27**, 219.

Barrie D, Wilson JA, Hoffman PN and Kramer JM (1992) *Bacillus cereus* meningitis in two neurosurgical patients: an investigation into the source of the organism. *Journal of Hospital Infection* **25**, 291.

Barrie D, Hoffman PN, Wilson JA and Kramer JM (1994) Contamination of hospital linen by *Bacillus cereus*. *Epidemiology and Infection* **113**, 297.

Bates CJ, Wilcox MH, Smith TL and Spencer RC (1993) The efficiency of a hospital dry cleaning cycle in disinfecting material contaminated with bacteria and viruses. *Journal of Hospital Infection* **23**, 255.

British Standards Institution (2002) EN 14065:2002 *Textiles – laundry processed textiles – biocontamination control system*. Milton Keynes: British Standards Institution.

Department of Health (1995) Health Service Guideline HSG(95)18: *Hospital laundry arrangements for used and infected linen*. London: Department of Health. [This is in the process of being updated at the time of writing as Health Technical Memorandum 01-04.]

Department of Health (2006) Health Technical Memorandum 07-01: *Safe management of healthcare waste*. London: Department of Health.

European Parliament, Council (2004) Regulation (EC) No. 852/2004 of the European Parliament and of the Council of 29 April on the hygiene of foodstuffs. OJL 139, 30.4.2004, 1–54.

Hazardous Waste (England and Wales) Regulations (2005) *Statutory Instrument 2005 No. 894*. Available online at: http://www.opsi.gov.uk/si/si2005/20050894.htm (last accessed 29 October 2008).

Health Protection Agency (2004) Working Group of the former PHLS Advisory Committee on Gastrointestinal Infections preventing person-to-person spread following gastrointestinal infections: guidelines for public health physicians and environmental health officers. *Communicable Disease and Public Health* **7**, 362. Available online at: www.hpa.org.uk.

Little C (2005) Food handlers and fitness to work. *Health and Hygiene* **26,** 12.

McLauchlin J and Little C (eds) (2007) *Hobbs' food poisoning and food hygiene,* 7th edn. Hodder Arnold, London.

Wilson JA, Loveday HP, Hoffman PN and Pratt RJ (2007) Uniform: an evidence review of the microbiological significance of uniforms and uniform policy in the prevention and control of healthcare-associated infections. Report to the Department of Health (England). *Journal of Hospital Infection* **66,** 301.

PART TWO

Prophylaxis and treatment
of infections

8 USE OF ANTIMICROBIAL AGENTS

Elizabeth SR Darley and Alasdair P MacGowan

INTRODUCTION

Since the discovery of penicillin in 1928 antimicrobial chemotherapy has evolved into a major area of chemotherapeutics with a huge impact on treatment of patients. In many cases, infections once feared and considered invariably fatal are now managed with minimal morbidity and, in developed countries where antimicrobials and healthcare facilities are easily accessed, with almost negligible mortality rates.

Antimicrobial agents are used both to treat bacterial infections in patients who already have symptoms or signs of infection, and also to prevent infection developing in patients who are either considered at high risk of acquiring infection or at risk of developing severe consequences of infection even if the risk of acquiring it is low. Antimicrobials used to treat bacterial infection are the most commonly used drugs. Antifungals, antiviral and antiprotozoan drugs are used, respectively, to treat fungal infection (e.g. candidiasis), for viral infection (e.g. herpes zoster) and for parasitic infection (e.g. malaria or giardiasis). The decision to treat a patient with evident infection may be straightforward, based on recognized clinical symptoms and signs, and isolation of a classical pathogen, such as a patient with productive cough and a chest X-ray consistent with a diagnosis of pneumonia, or a patient complaining of dysuria with a positive culture of *E. coli* from mid-stream urine. In other cases, the diagnosis of infection may be less self-evident, for example, a patient who is not systemically unwell but who has a non-healing leg ulcer, which has *Pseudomonas aeruginosa* cultured from a swab of the slough at its base. In these cases, the decision to treat must be made with both a clinical understanding of the expected outcome, whether cure, suppression or merely short-term improvement, and the benefits and risks of using antibiotics for this indication.

There is no place for an overly cautious approach towards antibiotic use as exemplified by 'if in doubt about the diagnosis of infection, treat', as the adverse effects on the patient and the local microbiological environment may be significant.

Prophylaxis is defined as the use of antimicrobials to prevent infection in patients with no existing active infection. The use of antibiotics as prophylaxis should be considered in the context of how likely infection is to occur without prophylaxis and what effect that infection would have on the patient.

In this chapter we cannot give an exhaustive summary of antimicrobial chemotherapy. However, we will give an overview of the principles of antibiotic use, the meaning of antibiotic resistance, the issues concerned with antibiotic stewardship in hospitals, the role of antibiotic pharmacists and infection specialists in managing antibiotic use, as well as the administrative and management structures required for success.

PRINCIPLES OF PRUDENT ANTIBIOTIC USE

Prudent antimicrobial use in man is a central part of any strategy to combat antibiotic resistance (UK Antimicrobial Resistance Strategy and Action Plan, 2000). There are many strands to achieving this objective, namely promotion of optimal prescribing in clinical practice, improved diagnostics and susceptibility testing methods, changes in the drug regulatory framework, and both professional and public education.

While not directly discussed in this chapter, the slowing of antibacterial drug development and failure of widespread uptake of rapid diagnostics is a considerable concern and will have major impacts on antimicrobial therapeutics in the next decade (Finch and Hunter, 2006). These developments underline the need for excellent antibiotic stewardship in the near and medium-term future.

The basic principles of antibiotic use are listed in Box 8.1 with some audit standards shown in Box 8.2 (Reese and Betts, 1986).

Over time, the evidence for certain antimicrobial prescribing has been challenged so that, in general, there is a trend towards the recognition that oral therapy may be as useful as intravenous, shorter durations of therapy are as effective as longer (el Moussaoui *et al.*, 2006) and use of monotherapy is as good as combination therapy (Paul *et al.*, 2004; Safdar *et al.*, 2004).

The harmful effects of antimicrobials are well recognized; hence, the decision to use antibiotics must be weighed in the light of the proven or theoretical benefits, and also the broader implications of potential antibiotic resistance for the patient and in the wider environment. Mandatory reporting of *Clostridium difficile*-associated diarrhoea (CDAD) rates in the UK since 2003 and, more recently, outbreaks of very severe *C. difficile* disease have highlighted the extent of hospital-acquired CDAD and colitis (Healthcare Commission, 2006). *C. difficile* predominantly affects patients who have received broad-spectrum antibiotics, usually while in a healthcare establishment, and affects a significant proportion of hospitalized patients with associated morbidity and mortality. Studies and anecdotal reports have implicated some antibiotics or antibiotic groups more than others in precipitating CDAD (e.g. an increased risk following broad-spectrum cephalosporins or more recently fluoroquinolones). In contrast, there is an apparently lower association with *C. difficile* infection after use of piperacillin/tazobactam.

Box 8.1 Principles of antibiotic use (reproduced from Reese and Betts, 1986)

INDICATIONS FOR ANTIBIOTICS

- Certain bacterial infections; probable bacterial infection; infection versus colonization; urgency; severity

SPECIMEN COLLECTION BEFORE STARTING THERAPY

- Gram stains; cultures, rapid diagnostics

RATIONAL SELECTION OF ANTIMICROBIALS

- Focal findings: test results, likely pathogens
- Age
- Severity
- Epidemiology, hospital acquired; previous antibiotic exposure and known restrictions
- Prior culture results
- Prior antibiotic allergies
- Antibiotic pharmacokinetics, tissue penetration, excretion mechanisms
- Potential side effects and adverse interactions
- Bacteriostatic or bactericidal
- Likely clinical outcomes
- Cost
- Host factors (i.e. pregnancy/lactation)
- Narrow or wide *in vitro* potency

DRUG COMBINATIONS

- Improve spectrum, increase bactericidal activity, reduce risk of resistance

ROUTE OF ADMINISTRATIONS

- Intravenous antibiotics/oral therapy/home intravenous antibiotics

DOSE AND DURATION

SPECIFIC THERAPY ONCE PATHOGEN IDENTIFICATION OR ANTIMICROBIAL SUSCEPTIBILITIES AVAILABLE

Antibiotics have a major impact on the outcome for patients with infections whether as the mainstay of treatment (e.g. in patients with acute pyelonephritis) or as an adjunct, such as in the treatment of osteomyelitis following excision and debridement of infected bone. Antibiotics can also have a significant positive impact in reducing the risk of cross-infection to contacts of a patient with active infection.

> ## Box 8.2 Audit checklist for individual patient antibiotic management
>
> - Is the indication for prescription of the antibiotic given in the notes?
> - Have appropriate specimens been taken, examined and cultured?
> - Have the most likely pathogens been evaluated?
> - Has the risk of antimicrobial resistance been assessed (patient age, previous healthcare exposure, previous antibiotics, known colonization/infection with a resistant organism)?
> - Is the route and dose duration specified for prescribed drugs?
> - Was therapy de-escalated once culture results were known?
> - Was the reason for combination therapy stated?

Judicious use of antimicrobial prophylaxis may prevent secondary cases of potentially severe infection in exposed contacts of the index case as in the administration of isoniazid to infants born to mothers with active tuberculosis, or rifampicin to a household contact of a patient with meningococcal meningitis. Secondary prophylaxis is commonly used in hospital to prevent active infection developing in patients already colonized with a recognized pathogen, for example, administration of vancomycin preceding a vascular procedure for patients colonized with methicillin-resistant *Staphylococcus aureus* (MRSA), or administration of fluconazole to immunocompromised or ventilated patients colonized with *Candida* spp at two or more body sites, to prevent systemic candidaemia. This approach is logical and widely employed, although the evidence in support of the use of prophylaxis is sometimes sparse and usually not based on the results of sufficiently large randomized-controlled trials. Specific details regarding the numbers needed to treat and, in the case of MRSA, the endemic proportion of MRSA to methicillin-susceptible *S. aureus* (MSSA) in colonized patients to warrant prophylaxis against MRSA are not clearly defined. Individual units and Infection Control Teams must review internal surveillance data and the available experience from other units to inform the decision of when to implement prophylaxis and which organisms must be targeted by the antibiotic. It may seem the obvious conclusion is to simply cover all potential pathogens with the broadest spectrum antibiotic available 'just in case'. This is an inappropriate use of antibiotics and may even be harmful to the patients if a more narrow-spectrum antibiotic, potentially more active against the organisms most likely to cause an infection, is available but not used in favour of the broader spectrum antibiotic.

ANTIBIOTIC RESISTANCE

Antibiotic resistance is defined in two main ways: first, by reference to what is the normal population of bacteria and, second, related to clinical outcomes.

The minimum inhibitory concentration (MIC) is taken as the gold-standard method of measuring an antimicrobial potency against a pathogen or range of pathogens. It is a phenotypic *in-vitro* measure of drug potency. Clinical resistance as defined by the European Committee on Antimicrobial Susceptibility Testing (EUCAST) is a level of antimicrobial activity associated with a high likelihood of therapeutic failure. A micro-organism is defined as resistant by applying the appropriate clinical breakpoint in a defined phenotypic test system. The clinical breakpoint may be altered with legitimate changes in circumstances (e.g. changes in drug dose). Microbiological resistance is defined for a species by the presence of an acquired or mutational resistance mechanism to the drug. Microbiologically resistant (non-wild type) micro-organisms may or may not respond clinically to antimicrobial treatment (see www.eccmid.org).

Some organisms are inherently resistant to specific antibiotics (e.g. *P. aeruginosa* is always resistant to flucloxacillin), other organisms may be sensitive or have acquired resistance to a particular antibiotic. Aside from organisms with inherent resistance, antibiotic resistance occurs as a direct consequence of antibiotic use (American Society for Microbiology, 1995; The Copenhagen Recommendations, 1998). Antibiotic resistance in a clinical area or in a specific patient may arise from different routes, which can be simply summarized as:

- selection of a resistant strain or sub-population by effectively eradicating all sensitive strains by antibiotic exposure;
- induced resistance in species with 'inducible resistance' mechanisms by exposure to the antibiotics which act as an inducers;
- transfer of genetic elements coding for resistance from other bacterial strains;
- introduction of an inherently resistant organism from another source;
- poor infection control measures permitting cross-infection from a resistant organism from any other of the above sources (Gould, 1998).

The extent of drug use in terms of duration and frequency of use, dosage and total drug exposure associated with development of resistance varies, but to a large extent may be predicted with microbiological understanding of the organisms, the chosen antibiotic and the local patient factors (Guillernot *et al.*, 1998; Lang *et al.*, 2001). Some organisms develop resistance relatively quickly on exposure to a specific antibiotic; for example, in the case of patient with an infective exacerbation of chronic respiratory diseases caused by *P. aeruginosa*, the bacterium may become resistant to ciprofloxacin within one or two weeks. This is demonstrated by repeat culture and sensitivity testing of sputum culture isolates after a treatment course. Similarly, rifampicin, for the treatment of *Staphylococcus aureus* must always be given in combination with other systemic antibiotics, as resistance develops quickly if it is used as monotherapy.

In contrast, there are other common pathogenic organisms that have been treated over many years with the same antibiotic in millions of patients worldwide with no evident development of resistance. *Streptococcus pyogenes* (Group A streptococcus) has been treated with penicillin antibiotics with no emergence of resistant strains.

The minimum inhibitory concentration of an antibiotic for an organism may gradually drift upwards over time, with increased exposure to the antibiotic, but still not exceed those concentrations which can be achieved by simply administering larger doses of the same antibiotic. An example is penicillin resistance in pneumococci (Yu *et al.*, 2003). In many, but not all strains of penicillin-resistant pneumococci, the relative increase in MIC and, therefore, resistance to penicillin antibiotics can be overcome by an increase in the dose of penicillin. The extent of resistance for a specific strain of pneumococcus can be determined easily in the microbiology laboratory by measuring the MIC. An informed decision can then be made about whether the most appropriate antibiotic treatment is still penicillin, but in a higher dose than usual, or whether a different antibiotic, to which the pneumococcus is fully sensitive, is required.

This is in contrast to methicillin resistance in *S. aureus*. A completely different mechanism of antibiotic resistance exists here, which does not allow for degrees of increase in MIC to occur. Instead, the mutation coded on the *MecA* gene, confers complete resistance to all achievable concentrations or isoxzyl penicillins. It may appear that emergence of MRSA occurs in a patient during a course of treatment for MSSA. This, however, is not due to gradual increments in MIC occurring as a result of exposure to flucloxacillin, but to the acquisition of another strain of *S. aureus*, which already contains the genetic coding for methicillin resistance. The MRSA has been introduced from another source and is able to colonize or infect the patient by surviving in the body sites where the original sensitive *S. aureus* has been eradicated. As no dose increase can overcome this increase in MIC, an alternative class of antibiotic is required for treatment of MRSA.

Antimicrobial resistance can adversely affect patient outcomes both in terms of survival and symptom resolution. This occurs in a wide range of situations; for example, in medical patients with community- or hospital-acquired infection, *P. aeruginosa* bacteraemia or uncomplicated urinary tract infections (Raz *et al.*, 2002; Micek *et al.*, 2005; Aloush *et al.*, 2006; Giamavellos-Bourboulis *et al.*, 2006).

Furthermore, inappropriate antimicrobial chemotherapy has an adverse impact on clinical outcomes in a wide range of clinical settings (Table 8.1). In most cases, inappropriate antibiotic therapy is defined as treatment of the patient with an antibiotic to which the pathogen is resistant, either by intrinsic mechanisms (flucloxacillin and *P. aeruginosa*) or acquired resistance (flucloxacillin and MRSA).

It is interesting to note that appropriate chemotherapy is not required initially in all patient groups: a period of about 48 h is critical, hence the need for

Table 8.1 Clinical situations where inappropriate antimicrobial chemotherapy has been associated with adverse outcomes

Situation	Reference
Bloodstream infections by antibiotic-resistant Gram-negative rods	Kang *et al.* (2005)
Bloodstream infection by *Stenotrophomonas maltophilia*	Metan and Ozun (2005)
Bloodstream infection with MRSA	Romero-Vivas *et al.* (1995)
Infection in critically ill patients	Kolleff *et al.* (1999)
Bloodstream infection in ICU	Ibrahim *et al.* (2000), Harbarth *et al.* (2002)
Pneumonia in ICU	Krobot *et al.* (2004)
Intra-abdominal infection	Mosdell *et al.* (1991)

ICU, intensive care unit; MRSA, methicillin-resistant *Staphylococcus aureus*

appropriate chemotherapy is not an argument for broad-spectrum empirical therapy in all patients. This has been shown to be the case for MRSA bacteraemia and bacteraemia due to ESBL-producing Enterobacteriaceae (Kim *et al.*, 2004; Fang *et al.*, 2006).

SIGNIFICANCE OF ANTIBIOTIC RESISTANCE IN PRACTICE

It is not necessary for the Infection Control Nurse or link practitioner to be familiar with all the different methods of resistance in micro-organisms or to know which antibiotics are likely to result in rapid development of resistance and which are not. However, it is important that there is an awareness of the local resistance problems in specific units of a healthcare establishment, in the wider community and globally, and what antibiotic measures need to be employed to manage and reduce selection for resistance or emergence of resistance. In the UK, intensive care units often have specific problems with MRSA, *P. aeruginosa* or other multi-resistant organisms. Multi-resistant *Klebsiella* outbreaks have been reported in neonatal intensive care units and infection caused by *Acinetobacter baumanii*, which has become resistant to almost all antibiotics, is an increasing problem for burns units. Close collaboration is needed between the Infection Control Team, medical microbiologists, biomedical scientists, pharmacists and the healthcare workers on each clinical unit to restrict use of antimicrobials, and detect and minimize emergence and spread of resistant organisms while not compromising the need for antibiotic treatment of those with genuine infection.

ANTIBIOTIC STEWARDSHIP

There has been considerable interest in implementing and monitoring interventions to optimize prescribing of antimicrobial drugs. This is usually taken to mean use of antimicrobials to ensure the best therapeutic outcomes while minimizing the risks of adverse events, secondary infections (e.g. *C. difficile* diarrhoea) and reducing the risks of emergence of resistance. Antibiotic stewardship is a term which encompasses all these interventions. There are now a large number of reviews and guidelines in this area (Gould, 1998; Davey *et al.*, 2005; Gross and Pujat, 2001; Paskovaty *et al.*, 2005; ; Dellit *et al.*, 2007).

While it is possible to list the elements that would go into a programme to improve antibiotic use in any hospital, there is no hard evidence as to whether single interventions or multi-faceted interventions are best and what kind of intervention is optimal (e.g. automatic stop orders or educational interventions). However, there is evidence that, in the short term, restrictive interventions may be superior to educational ones, but this is not clear in the long term. Changes in antimicrobial use can probably result in a reduction in CDAD, but it is less clear how much impact they have on the burden of infection owing to resistant Gram-negative bacteria. There is little evidence to support an impact on MRSA infection.

The recent North American Guidelines (Dellit *et al.*, 2007) provide a useful discussion of the key elements of an antibiotic stewardship programme for a hospital, in contrast to the British Cochrane review, which provides a more critical evaluation of the published literature, but has less clear recommendations for practitioners.

Interventions associated with antibiotic stewardship programmes are listed in Box 8.3. The following should be considered:

- education (e.g. meetings, outreach visits, local opinion leaders);
- guidelines/clinical pathways;
- antibiotic order forms;
- streamlining/de-escalation;
- dose optimization;
- intravenous (iv) oral switch;
- information technology (IT) support of therapeutic decisions;
- clinical laboratory support, especially restricted antibiotic reporting and rapid results availability;
- therapeutic substitution;
- automatic stop orders.

There is little evidence that antibiotic cycling is of benefit in reducing resistance (Brown and Nathwani, 2005) or that routine use of combination antibiotics will help. In addition, the potential measurable outcomes of a programme of antibiotic stewardship are variable and include:

- reduced financial spend on antimicrobials;
- reduced use of antimicrobials as measured by defined daily doses (DDD), perhaps corrected for hospital activity;
- reduced burden of hospital-acquired infection;
- reduced burden of sentinel infection owing to multi-resistant organisms, for

> **Box 8.3 Possible interventions to improve antibiotic use in hospital**
>
> - Establish a multi-disciplinary team to lead on antimicrobial use. This should include medical infection specialists, clinical pharmacists, an information technology specialist and infection control professional
> - The multi-disciplinary team should have links to the Drugs and Therapeutics Committee, quality assurance groups and patient safety groups (i.e. Clinical Governance)
> - The multi-disciplinary team should be supported by hospital management
> - The multi-disciplinary team should define the outcomes of its programmes of work (e.g. through an annual plan)
> - Formulary restriction and pre-authorization of use of anti-infectives
> - Prospective audit with intervention and feedback

example, MRSA or extended-spectrum beta-lactamase (ESBL) producing *E. coli* bacteraemia;
- reduced adverse events associated with antibiotic use, for example CDAD.

USE OF ANTIBIOTIC POLICIES

It has been estimated that up to 50 per cent of antimicrobial prescribing is inappropriate in terms of choice, duration and indication for treatment. The issue for the clinician and specifically the medical microbiologist is, therefore, to reduce, as far as possible, inappropriate antibiotic use to minimize the emergence of resistance in the organisms causing the patient's infection, the colonizing flora of the patients and the local hospital flora in the immediate environment. Implementation of antibiotic guidelines or policy, restriction of available antibiotics within the hospital and use of an antibiotic pharmacist to help monitor prescription charts and to advise prescribers can help to reduce inappropriate or excessive antibiotic usage.

The simplest effective way to control antibiotic prescribing in a hospital setting is to employ a restricted formulary, so prescribing is limited to only those selected antibiotics stocked by pharmacy (see, for example, Box 8.4). To encourage acceptance of the formulary, the decision of which antibiotics to include and which to leave out must involve not only the pharmacists and the medical microbiologist, but also representatives of all major prescribing groups including intensive care, infectious diseases, general medicine, paediatrics and surgical specialities. Inevitably it will be necessary to stock some antibiotics that are very rarely indicated for patients with allergy or susceptibility to adverse drug interactions, and these might be restricted on the formulary. There will be other antimicrobials, which might be used relatively frequently within one speciality for a small group of patients, but for which there are almost no

Box 8.4 An example of a hospital formulary. (reproduced with permission from Chapter 5 'Infections', in *Formulary*, North Bristol NHS Trust, 2006)

Antimicrobial prescribing is strictly regulated within North Bristol NHS Trust for three major reasons:

1 To ensure the use of effective antimicrobials
2 To prevent the development and spread of bacterial resistance
3 To contain cost

The antimicrobials stocked are split into three categories.

– *Unrestricted* – may be prescribed by any medical staff without the involvement of the department of medical microbiology
– *Restricted* – only available after discussion with, or if recommended by, a medical microbiologist, Infectious Disease Consultant or Consultant HIV Immunologist, unless used in accordance with North Bristol NHS Trust-wide antimicrobial guidelines
– *Restricted (Specialty)* – when a specialty (directorate/area) is listed, then the restriction does not apply to medical staff from that specialty

Antibacterial drugs

– Penicillins
– Phenoxymethyl penicillin (oral)
– Benzyl penicillin (parenteral)
– Amoxicillin (oral and parenteral)
– Co-amoxiclav (oral and parenteral)
– Flucloxacillin (oral and parenteral)
– Piperacillin/tazobactam (parenteral) – restricted
– Procaine benzyl (parenteral) – named patient

Cephalosporins

– Cefradine (oral and parenteral)
– Cefuroxime (parenteral)
– Ceftriaxone (parenteral)
– Cefixime (oral) – restricted
– Ceftazidime (parenteral) – restricted

Other beta-lactam antibiotics

– Meropenem (parenteral) – restricted
– Ertapenem (parenteral) – restricted

HIV, human immunodeficiency virus; NHS, National Health Service.

indications for use in other patients (e.g. cotrimoxazole to treat *Pneumocystis* pneumonia infection for patients with acquired immunodeficiency syndrome; AIDS). When a restricted antibiotic is intended for a patient, authorization from the medical microbiologist or the antibiotic pharmacist is required for the pharmacy to dispense selected antibiotics. Other antibiotics may be dispensed only after the required prior consultation with the consultant medical microbiologist. The limits on type of restriction (i.e. who can prescribe the restricted antibiotics and which level of authorization is required) can be agreed locally. It may be necessary to allow pharmacists to dispense a single dose of a restricted antibiotic out of hours prior to receiving authorization, and to determine how pharmacy seeks authorization for restricted antibiotics, whether directly from the medical microbiologist or indirectly contacting the prescriber. This approach of restriction and authorization can be time-consuming but can reduce the amount of unnecessarily broad-spectrum prescribing (e.g. the carbapenems), the use of intravenous agents when oral bioavailability is acceptable (e.g. use of iv fluroquinolones) the cost of antibiotic prescriptions (e.g. restricting the use of liposomal amphotericin) and restricting individual antibiotics, which are associated with selection for resistant organisms in particular patients.

In this formulary, a number of beta-lactam antibiotics are not available for use (e.g. co-fluampicil, mecillinam, ticarcillin, timentin, cefaclor, cefadroxil, cefalexin, cefoxitin, cefpirone, cefpodoxine, ceftozil, cefotaxime, azteonam and imipenem/cilastatin).

Antibiotic policies may be introduced primarily to reduce total antibiotic use, to reduce inappropriate prescribing (e.g. the tendency by some clinicians to use the most broad-spectrum antibiotics as a first-line therapy), to contain costs of antibiotic prescribing, or to target specific resistance problems related to specific antibiotic use. Prospective and retrospective comparative studies of various methods to restrict or reduce antibiotic prescribing in specific hospital areas have demonstrated reduced resistance rates, reduced rates of infection caused by specific organisms of concern and reduced numbers of cases of hospital-acquired pneumonia. However, in most cases, these restrictions or introduction of a new policy have been employed as part of a clinical response to address a particular problem (e.g. to halt an outbreak of CDAD or to counter an increase in prevalence of a multi-resistant organism on a unit). The antibiotic restrictions or policies used have almost invariably been accompanied by increased infection control measures, additional surveillance cultures or increased dialogue with the medical microbiologists. It is difficult to determine the extent of the contribution of antibiotic policy or the restriction measures to the outcome observed, but it is apparent that improvement in resistance rates, infection rates or cost containments can be achieved, without increase in cost or detriment to the patient's health or overall outcome. To date there have been no published randomized-controlled trials to demonstrate that strict adherence to antibiotic policy reduces resistance or infections with resistant organisms, and some studies show no significant benefit of restrictive prescribing. Furthermore, there are instances where strict adherence to a policy can be detrimental. Recommendation of a single antibiotic for a common diagnosis, for example, for hospital-acquired ventilator-associated pneumonia (VAP) in an ICU, can lead to overuse of that antibiotic. This may be inappropriate if given without considering the individual patient's colonizing flora, or recent antibiotic history (which may have recently included that antibiotic), or risk factors for side effects or for developing CDAD. A policy is likely to reduce the thought given to confirming a possible or doubtful diagnosis, and is very unlikely to state that antibiotics are not required or should be withheld pending further culture results in support of the diagnosis. Junior doctors are particularly keen to have clear policies for a wide array of clinical conclusions and owing to the constraints of time and inexperience, juniors are most likely to follow an antibiotic policy without considering whether that antibiotic might be the most suitable. In this respect, a valuable learning opportunity, to revise some basic medical microbiology, is missed. This is not to say that restrictive antibiotic policies cannot be very useful, but rather that introduction of the policy or launch of a revised version to each group of prescribers should involve appropriate teaching about the antibiotics chosen, including side effects, spectrum of activity, therapeutic drug monitoring and the target organisms both in the community and in the local hospital environment. It may be more helpful to use 'antibiotic guidelines' rather than an 'antibiotic policy', and to prompt users to discuss cases with the medical microbiologist where the signs and symptoms do not lead to a clear-cut diagnosis of infection.

ANTIBIOTIC PHARMACISTS

Antibiotic pharmacy has a relatively new role in Europe; it is much more highly developed in North America. However, it is now recognized that the antibiotic pharmacist is central to optimizing antibiotic use in hospital as part of a multi-disciplinary team with medical infection specialists as recommended by the EU Copenhagen Recommendations (1998).

Infection pharmacists have the basic pharmacy skills such as prescription monitoring, taking accurate medication histories, provision of medicines information, patient counselling, regular liaison with medical teams and reducing medication errors. In general, there has been increasing specialization within pharmacy with the result that pharmacists have gained more responsibility and expertise in some areas, such as haemato-oncology, intensive care or renal medicine. Infection pharmacy development is part of this wider process. Hence, as well as a primary undergraduate qualification in pharmacy, many infection pharmacists have post-graduate qualifications at MSc and increasingly PhD level.

The potential role in ensuring clinical and cost-effective antibiotic use within hospital is enormous. However, infection pharmacists should be involved in:

• monitoring antibiotic prescribing either financially, by DDDs, or qualitative measures through audit;
• identifying problem prescribing areas via a ward-based pharmacy network, pharmacy or microbiology IT;
• education of fellow pharmacists and other healthcare professionals;
• participating in infection control;
• formulary development;
• appraisal of new antimicrobials as part of the Drugs and Therapeutic Committee or Antibiotic Sub-group;
• identification of potential cost savings;
• ward stocking;
• guideline development and audit (e.g. iv/oral switch policies);
• clinical audit;
• infection consultation hospital rounds with medical infection specialists.

In the longer term, infection pharmacists may have roles as supplementary prescribers and in therapeutic drug monitoring. At present, there are no well-developed roles for most pharmacists in the UK (Weller and Jamieson, 2004).

CONCLUSION

Prudent antibiotic use in hospital is an essential part of patient management. Despite this recognition, many courses of antibiotics used in hospital are probably unnecessary and compromise patient safety. This needs to be balanced against the clear benefits of appropriate antimicrobial chemotherapy in infected patients.

There are many ways of improving the quality of antibiotic prescribing, but it is less clear which approach is most effective for a given amount of resource. It is clear that prudent antibiotic use can be promoted only as part of a long-term effort involving many disciplines, but especially medical infection specialists, infection pharmacists and infection control professionals.

REFERENCES

Aloush V, Navon-Venezia S, Seigmann-Igra Y, Cabil S, Carveli Y. (2006) Multidrug-resistant *Pseudomonas aeruginosa*: risk factors and clinical impact. *Antimicrobial Agents Chemotherapy* **50,** 43.
American Society for Microbiology (1995) Report of the American Society for Microbiology Task Force on antibiotic resistance. *Antimicrobial Agents and Chemotherapy* (Suppl), 1.

Brown EM, Nathwani D. (2005) Antibiotic cycling or rotation: a systematic review of the evidence of efficacy. *Journal of Antimicrobial Chemotherapy* **55**, 6.

Copenhagen Recommendations, The. Report from the Invitational EU Conference on The Microbial Threat (1998) Copenhagen: Ministry of Health, Ministry of Food, Agriculture and Fisheries, Denmark. Available online at: http://www.microbial.threat.dk.

Davey P, Brown E, Fenelon L *et al.* (2005) Interventions to improve antibiotic prescribing practices for hospital inpatients. *Cochrane Database of Systematic Reviews* Issue 4. Available online at: http://www.cochrane.org/reviews/en/ab003543.html (last accessed 26 February 2007).

Davey P, Brown E, Fenelon L *et al.* (2006) Systematic review of antimicrobial drug prescribing in hospitals. *Emerging Infectious Diseases* **12**, 211.

Dellit TH, Owens RC, MacGowan JE *et al.* (2007) Infectious Diseases Society of America and Society for Healthcare Epidemiology of America guidelines for developing an institutional program to enhance antibiotic stewardship. *Clinical Infectious Diseases* **44**, 159.

el Moussaoui R, de Borgie AJM, van den Broek P *et al.* (2006) Effectiveness of discontinuing antibiotic treatment after 3 days versus 8 days in mild to moderate–severe community acquired pneumonia: randomised double blind study. *BMJ* 332, 1355.

Fang CT, Shau WY, Hsueh RR *et al.* (2006) Early empirical glycopeptide therapy for patients with methicillin resistant *Staphylococcus aureus* bacteraemia: impact on the outcome. *Journal of Antimicrobial Chemotherapy* **57**, 511.

Finch RR, Hunter PA. (2006) Antibiotic resistance – action to promote new technologies: a report of an EU Intergovernmental Conference held in Birmingham, UK, 12–13 December 2005. *Journal of Antimicrobial Chemotherapy* **58**(Suppl), i3.

Giamavellos-Bourboulis EJ, Papadimitriou E, Galanakis N *et al.* (2006) Multi drug resistance to antimicrobials as a predominant factor influencing patient survival. *International Journal of Antimicrobial Agents* **27**, 476.

Gould IM (1998) A review of the role of antibiotic policies in the control of antibiotic resistance. *Journal of Antimicrobial Chemotherapy* **43**, 459.

Gross PA and Pujat D (2001) Implementing practice guidelines for appropriate antimicrobial usage. *Medical Care* **39**(Suppl 2), II55.

Guillernot D, Carbon C, Balkau B *et al.* (1998) Low dosage and long treatment duration of beta-lactam. Risk factors for carriage of penicillin resistant *Streptococcus pneumoniae. JAMA* **279**, 365.

Harbarth S, Ferrieve K, Hugonnett S, Ricou B, Suter P, Pittet D (2002) Epidemiology and prognostic determinants of bloodstream infections in the surgical intensive care. *Archives of Surgery* **137**, 1353.

Healthcare Commission (2006) *Investigation into outbreaks of Clostridium difficile at Stoke Mandeville Hospital, Buckinghamshire Hospitals NHS Trust.* London: Commission for Healthcare Audit and Inspection. Available at: http://www.healthcarecom mission.org.uk/_db/_documents/Stoke_Mandeville.pdf.

Ibrahim EH, Sherman G, Ward S, Frazer VJ, Kollef MH (2000) The influence of inadequate antimicrobial treatment of bloodstream infections on patient outcomes in the ICU setting. *Chest* **118**, 146.

Kang CI, Kim SH, Park WB *et al.* (2005) Bloodstream infections caused by antibiotic resistant gram-negative bacilli – risk factors for mortality and impact of inappropriate initial antimicrobial therapy on outcome. *Antimicrobial Agents and Chemotherapy* **49**, 760.

Kim SH, Park WB, Lee KD *et al.* (2004) Outcome of inappropriate initial antimicrobial treatment in patients with methicillin resistant *Staphylococcus aureus* bacteraemia. *Journal of Antimicrobial Chemotherapy* **54**, 489.

Kolleff MH, Sherman G, Ward S, Frazer VJ (1999) Inadequate antimicrobial treatment of infections. *Chest* **115**, 462.

Krobot K, Yin D, Zhang Q, Sen S *et al.* (2004) Effect of inappropriate initial empiric antibiotic therapy on outcome of patients with community acquired intra-abdominal infections requiring surgery. *European Journal of Clinical Microbiology and Infectious Diseases* **23**, 682.

Lang A, De Fina G, Meyer R *et al.* (2001) Comparison of antimicrobial use and resistance of bacterial isolates in a haematology ward and intensive care unit. *European Journal of Clinical Microbiology and Infectious Diseases* **20**, 657.

Metan G, Uzun O (2005) Impact of initial antimicrobial therapy in patients with bloodstream infections caused by *Stenotrophomonas maltophilia*. *Antimicrobial Agents and Chemotherapy* **49**, 3980.

Micek ST, Lloyd AE, Ritchie DJ *et al.* (2003) *Pseudomonas aeruginosa* bloodstream infection: importance of appropriate initial antimicrobial treatment. *Antimicrobial Agents and Chemotherapy* **49**, 1306.

Mosdell DM, Morris DM, Voltura A *et al.* (1991) Antibiotic treatment for surgical peritonitis. *Annals of Surgery* **214**, 543.

Paskovaty A, Pflomm JM, Myke M, Seo SK (2005) A multidisciplinary approach to antimicrobial stewardship: evolution into the 21st century. *International Journal of Antimicrobial Agents* **25**, 1.

Paul M, Benuvi-Silbiger B, Soares-Weiser K, Leibovici L (2004) Beta lactam monotherapy versus beta lactam aminoglycoside combination therapy for sepsis in immunocompetent patients: systematic review and meta-analysis of randomised trials. *BMJ* **328**, 668.

Raz R, Chazin B, Kennes Y *et al.* (2002) Empiric use of trimethoprim-sulfamethoxazole in treatment of women with uncomplicated urinary tract infections in a geographical area with a high prevalence of resistant uropathogens. *Clinical Infectious Diseases* **34**, 1165.

Reese RE and Betts RF (1986) Antibiotic use. In: Reese RE and Gordon Douglas R (eds) *A Practical approach to infectious diseases*. Boston and Toronto: Little/Brown and Company, p. 559.

Romero-Vivas J, Rubio M, Fernandez C, Picazo JJ (1995) Mortality associated with nosocomial bacteraemia due to methicillin-resistant *Staphylococcus aureus*. *Clinical Infectious Diseases* **21**, 1417.

Safdar N, Handelsman J, Maki DG (2004) Does combination antimicrobial therapy reduce mortality in Gram-negative bacteraemia? A meta analysis. *The Lancet Infectious Diseases* **4**, 519.

UK Antimicrobial Resistance Strategy and Action Plan (2000) London: Department of Health.

Weller TMA, Jamieson CE (2004) The expanding role of the antibiotic pharmacist. *Journal of Antimicrobial Chemotherapy* **54,** 295.

Yu VL, Chinu CC, Feldman C *et al.* (2003) An international prospective study of pneumococcal bacteraemia: correlation with in vitro resistance, antibiotics administered and clinical outcome. *Clinical Infection Diseases* **37,** 230.

9 CONTROL OF BLOODBORNE VIRAL INFECTIONS

Samir Dervisevic and Deenan Pillay

INTRODUCTION

Numerous healthcare workers who are occupationally exposed to bloodborne pathogens have contracted serious viral diseases from exposure to blood and other potentially infectious materials in their workplaces. Bloodborne viral infections such as hepatitis B virus (HBV), hepatitis C virus (HCV), and human immunodeficiency virus 1 and 2 (HIV-1 and HIV-2) continue to be a significant infection control problem in healthcare settings. Clinical and nursing staff, students and laboratory workers are primarily at risk of acquiring any of these viruses owing to daily contact with patients, blood or body fluids (i.e. occupational exposure). An occupational exposure includes percutaneous exposures, where the skin has been broken by a needle or other sharp object, human scratch or bite, and mucocutaneous exposures, where the mucous membranes (mouth, nose or eyes), or non-intact skin have been contaminated by the patient's blood or other body fluids. Avoiding occupational exposures to blood and body fluids is the primary way to prevent the transmission of HBV, HCV and HIV. Immunization and post-exposure management are crucial elements in preventing infection with these pathogens and are key components of maintaining workforce safety.

HEPATITIS B

Hepatitis B, owing to higher virus load, is the most infectious of all bloodborne viruses and is a well-recognized occupational risk for healthcare workers (HCWs) (Mast and Alter, 1993). Infection with HBV in those who are non-immune can result in acute hepatitis or chronic hepatitis. Chronic hepatitis is attributed to a prolonged infection of the hepatocytes, which results in the persistence of hepatitis B surface antigen (HBsAg) in the blood for more than 6 months. This often results in serious sequelae, such as liver cirrhosis and hepatocellular carcinoma. The World Health Organization (WHO) places hepatitis B infection among the top ten causes of death in the world (Hoofnagle, 1990). HBV is present in blood and body secretions including breast milk, bile, cerebrospinal fluid, faeces, nasopharyngeal washings, saliva, semen, synovial fluid and sweat of those individuals who are infected with the virus (Bond *et al.*, 1977). Blood is the most important vehicle of transmission in healthcare settings and contains the highest HBV concentrations of all body fluids. Percutaneous infections are one of the most efficient routes of HBV transmission and the risk to a healthcare worker is primarily related to the degree of contact with blood as well as the infectious status of the source. Other modes of transmission include direct or indirect exposure to blood and body fluids (blood in contact with mucosal surfaces or damaged skin; Francis *et al.*, 1981) or HBV-contaminated environmental surfaces (noted during outbreaks among patients in haemodialysis units) (Snydman *et al.*, 1976).

Acute infection is usually mild and anicteric and complete recovery occurs in more than 95 per cent of infected adults. The risk of developing chronic hepatitis B after acute exposure ranges from 1 to 5 per cent for non-immune adults to more than 90 per cent for infants born to infected mothers, owing to a different response from the immature immune system.

Chronic hepatitis B infection has two phases: immunotolerant and immunoactive, characterized by different serological and molecular profiles. Testing for HBV markers includes detection of different virus components and antibodies against the virus components (see Table 9.1). The principal screening assay for acute and chronic HBV infection is detection of HBsAg. In those individuals whose sera contain HBsAg, further markers are determined. HBeAg is a marker of higher levels of replication (high infectivity, high level of HBV deoxyribonucleic acid; DNA). The presence of antibody to e (anti-HBe) indicates either seroconversion and suppression of HBV DNA or emergence of the precore or basal core promoter mutant virus infection (HBV DNA positive $>10^4–10^5$) (Carman *et al.*, 1989). Antibodies to core antigen (anti-HBc) develop soon after infection and, in most cases, persist for life. Hepatitis B core-specific immunoglobulin M (IgM anti-HBc) indicates recent infection. Antibodies to HBsAg develop with clearance of surface antigen and indicate immunity. Since hepatitis B vaccine is composed of surface antigen only, response to vaccine is also assessed by the presence of the surface antibodies (anti-HBs).

Hepatitis B virus DNA in an infected patient is an essential indicator of disease activity and a predictor of liver disease progression. It may be detected

Table 9.1 Interpretation of serological markers for hepatitis B virus disease

Serological markers	Clinical significance
HBsAg	Acute or chronic infection
Anti-HBc IgM	Acute infection; flare-up in chronic disease
Anti-HBc	Previous or current exposure; chronic infection
Anti-HBs	Immunity (natural or vaccine)
HBeAg	Active replication; high infectivity
Anti-HBe	Moving to lower infectivity, but also possible viral escape

anti-HBc, antibody to hepatitis B virus core antigen; anti-HBe, antibody to hepatitis B virus e antigen; anti-HBs, antibody to hepatitis B surface antigen; HBeAg, hepatitis B e antigen; HBsAg, hepatitis B surface antigen; IgM, immunoglobulin M.

and measured by molecular techniques often before the patient's serum becomes HBsAg positive (Kaneko *et al.*, 1990). Relative levels of HBV DNA often correlate inversely with the degree of necroinflammatory activity in the liver, reflecting attempts by the host's immune system to control and eliminate virus. It is a practical tool for gaining insights into viral dynamics and essential for predicting progression to disease as well as monitoring the response to therapy.

The prevalence of chronic hepatitis B in the Western World ranges from 0.2 per cent to 5 per cent of the population. In Asia, Africa and the Middle East, prevalence ranges from 5 per cent to 20 per cent. Groups at particular risk of acquiring the infection include intravenous drug users, men who have sex with men and, where infection control procedures are sub-optimal, renal haemodialysis patients and healthcare workers. Owing to the high risk of HBV infection among HCWs, routine pre-employment immunization against hepatitis B infection and the use of universal precautions in order to prevent occupational exposure to blood and body fluid have been adopted.

Following a needlestick injury with blood from an HBsAg- and HBeAg-positive individual, the risk of becoming infected is in the order of 25 per cent. On the other hand, the risk of developing clinical hepatitis if the source of the needlestick injury was HBsAg positive and HBeAg negative is from 1 per cent to 6 per cent, probably reflecting low HBV viral load (Werner and Grady, 1982). HCWs most at risk from such infection are those involved in invasive procedures (surgeons, gynaecologists), using sharp instruments whilst performing deep abdominal or pelvic surgery in which small innocuous cuts on their hand with suture needles are common. As stated above, HBV can also be detected in other body fluids, although at 1000–10 000-fold lower concentrations than in serum.

Antiviral therapy for chronic hepatitis B has changed dramatically during the past decade with the advent of new nucleoside and nucleotide analogue drugs and improved immunomodulator preparations. Apart from currently approved preparations (lamivudine, adefovir, pegylated interferon alpha-2a, entecavir, tenofovir and telbivudine), several investigational drugs are entering phase three clinical trials (emtricitabine and clevudine). Despite these advances in therapy, immunization against HBV remains by far the safest and most effective tool for control of this virus.

HEPATITIS B VIRUS IMMUNIZATION OF HEALTHCARE WORKERS

Active immunization

A safe and effective vaccine for HBV has been available since the 1970s. Vaccines currently used (Engerix-B®, Fendrix® and HBvaxPRO®) are made biosynthetically using recombinant DNA technology. Apart from the single-component vaccines containing recombinant (DNA) HBsAg, a new combined vaccine containing inactivated hepatitis A virus in addition to HBsAg have been released (Twinrix®). Immunization against hepatitis B should be offered to all HCWs (medical, dental, nursing, ancillary and technical staff, independent contractors, students and volunteers) whose line of duty may involve contact with blood, body fluids or human tissues. Current UK Department of Health guidelines stipulate that any HCW involved in exposure-prone procedures must demonstrate evidence of an HBV vaccine response, or otherwise, that they are not infected with HBV, before starting work (Department of Health, 1993). This also aims to protect patients against infection from HCWs. Immunization and testing must be undertaken by an Occupational Health Department or a general practitioner in order to ensure that the correct sample is tested.

Routinely, three doses of recombinant HBV vaccine are given at 0, 1 and 6 months (see Figure 9.1). The immune response to vaccine (seroconversion rate) is reduced by several factors, including older age (>50 years), male gender, history of smoking, obesity and the immune deficiency (HIV, transplant recipients and haemodialysis). Rates range in excess of 95 per cent in young women to 80 per cent in older men. A level of anti-HBs >100 mIU/ml has been considered an indicator of protection. If the initial response to hepatitis B course is <100 mIU/ml, a booster dose is indicated. If a HCW's post-immunization anti-HBs level is negative 1–2 months after the last dose of vaccine, the three-dose series should be repeated and the anti-HBs level should be determined 1–2 months after the repeated course. If the HCW is still negative after a second immunization series, the HCW is considered a non-responder to hepatitis B immunization. Low or non-responders should be advised that they are not protected and that they must seek prophylaxis by passive immunization if they suffer accidental exposure. Existing chronic HBV infection and past infection are among the reasons for non-responding to immunization. Therefore, testing for anti-HBc and HBsAg in vaccine non-responders is mandatory. Alternative vaccines are under development to improve the seroconversion rate for those who do not respond to current preparations. One of the approaches includes incorporation of hepatitis B pre-S1 and pre-S2 protein in the vaccine preparation.

Passive immunization

Hyperimmune hepatitis B immunoglobulin (HBIG) is prepared from human plasma taken from donors with high titres of anti-HBs. During the process used to manufacture HBIG, HCV and HIV are inactivated and eliminated from the final product. Doses of 200–500 IU are given intramuscularly. HBIG is used in the following circumstances:

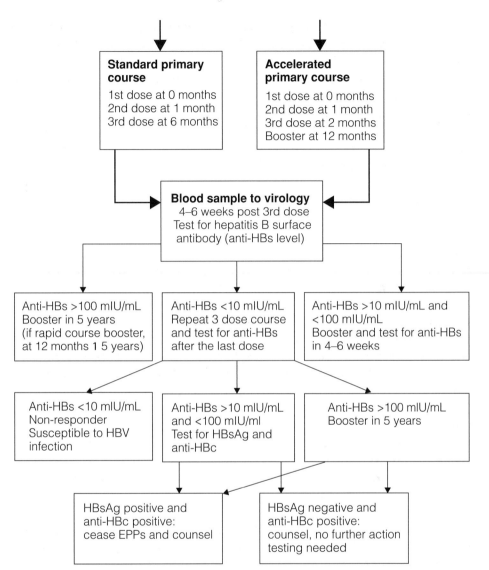

Figure 9.1 Hepatitis B immunization algorithm. anti-HBc, antibody to hepatitis B core antigen; anti-HBs, antibody to hepatitis B surface antigen; EPP, exposure-prone procedure; HBsAg, hepatitis B surface antigen; HBV, hepatitis B virus.

- after accidental exposure to high risk or known positive blood in those HCWs who are known non-responders or who never received hepatitis B vaccine;
- for neonates born to hepatitis B-infected mothers (in addition to vaccine);
- to prevent infection of a new liver transplanted for chronic HBV infection.

HEPATITIS D

Hepatitis D virus (HDV) is a sub-viral agent that can cause severe acute and chronic forms of liver disease in association with hepatitis B virus. HDV is highly endemic to several African countries, the Amazonian region, and the Middle East, while its prevalence is low in industrialized countries, except in the Mediterranean. It cannot replicate without assistance from HBV and, therefore, can only infect individuals simultaneously with HBV or as a super-infection of a chronic carrier of HBV. The mode of transmission is parenteral and the virus is particularly prevalent in intravenous drug users. The symptoms are similar to those of acute and chronic hepatitis B infection. However, the presence of HDV may exacerbate the severity of clinical picture compared with that seen with hepatitis B infection alone. Treatment of chronic hepatitis D infection, which relies on long-term administration of high doses of inter-feron-alpha, is not very effective (Niro *et al.*, 2005). Prevention of HDV trans-mission within a healthcare setting is the same as for control of hepatitis B.

HEPATITIS C

Hepatitis C virus, discovered in 1989, was the elusive pathogen that caused post-transfusion non-A non-B hepatitis. Its discovery led to molecular cloning of the complete viral genome (Choo *et al.*, 1991) and a rapid development of several antibody tests (1991) used to identify patients with HCV infection, and later on (1999) to introduction of nucleic acid testing (polymerase chain reaction; PCR) to improve the detection of HCV infection in blood donors, assess disease severity in those already infected and their response to treatment. In addition to these, new combination types of screening assay (antigen/antibody) with improved sensitivity and specificity have been developed and currently are being introduced into routine practice. The advent of a screening test for HCV infection helped virtually to eliminate the transmission of this virus by blood transfusion.

Acute infection is not usually associated with symptoms. Those who are symptomatic can experience malaise, nausea and right upper quadrant pain, followed by jaundice and dark urine. The incubation period is on average about 7 weeks; however, the patients become viraemic days after the exposure. A total of 15 per cent of those infected spontaneously resolve the infection and 85 per cent become persistently infected with long-term viraemia (Centers for Disease Control and Prevention, 2009). HCV is the leading cause of chronic liver disease, cirrhosis, liver carcinoma and liver transplantation.

Hepatitis C virus infection is mainly associated with exposure to blood. Among the specific risk groups are drug users who share needles, patients who have received transfusion of blood products before 1991, recipients of trans-planted organs or tissue grafts from an HCV-positive donor, individuals who have had body piercing, patients on haemodialysis and staff who have been occupationally exposed to blood products. HCV is transmitted less efficiently through occupational exposure to blood than HBV. The average incidence of seroconversion to anti-HCV following accidental percutaneous exposure from an HCV infected source is 1.8 per cent (range 0–7 per cent) (Lanphear *et al.*, 1994). Transmission rarely occurs from mucous membrane exposures to blood and no documented transmissions have been reported in HCWs from skin exposures to blood (Satori *et al.*, 1993).

If untreated, chronic HCV infection can lead to cirrhosis and liver failure in a large number of individuals. It is very important to recognize that chronic hepatitis C is a common driver of non-liver disorders and that effective treatment of chronic hepatitis C can prevent fibrosis and disease progression, and reduce complications of hepatitis C including cirrhosis and liver cancer. The standard of care for the treatment of chronic hepatitis C infection since early 2002 has been a combination of pegylated interferon-alpha and ribavirin. In 2004, the National Institute for Health and Clinical Excellence (NICE) recommended this form of treatment for patients with moderate to chronic hepatitis C, defined as histological evidence of significant fibrosis of the liver and/or significant necrotic inflammation of the liver. Combination therapy can lead to an overall viral eradication in more than 50 per cent of those treated (Flamm, 2003; Poynard *et al.*, 2003). However, sustained response to treatment differs between the HCV genotypes, and among persons infected with HCV genotype 1, particularly among those with high levels of baseline viraemia, it remains comparatively lower than for genotypes 2 and 3 (Zeuzem *et al.*, 2004). Furthermore, side effects associated with pegylated interferon plus ribavirin therapy preclude treatment of some patients and could substantially diminish the quality of life of some who start treatment for HCV (Hassanein *et al.*, 2004). In 2006, the search for less toxic and more efficacious therapies resulted in new molecular-based agents in development that specifically inhibit HCV replication and/or translation of viral RNA, progressing rapidly through clinical trials and testing. Among these are NS3 protease inhibitors, NS5 polymerase inhibitors and p7 inhibitors.

Many people with chronic hepatitis C are unaware of their infection. In order to increase awareness of hepatitis C, its risks and importance of reducing its associated morbidity and mortality, the UK Department of Health launched a hepatitis C awareness campaign: 'FaCe It', part of 'The Hepatitis C Action Plan', in 2004. The campaign targeted HCWs ahead of the general public with the aim to de-stigmatize the virus and empower HCWs with essential information on the risks, diagnosis, testing, referrals and treatment of HCV prior to the start of the public awareness campaign. A new NHS hepatitis C awareness website for HCWs and the public (www.hepc.nhs.uk) was launched and a national hepatitis C information line was introduced. The awareness campaign resulted in an increase of testing as well as of reports of confirmed infections and referrals to specialized hepatitis clinics.

Healthcare workers are at greater risk of HCV infection than the general population. There is at present no vaccine to prevent HCV infection owing to the fact that HCV is genetically highly diverse. Prevention of transmission of HCV infection in hospitals and healthcare settings relies on the employment of stringent infection control measures. Infection control policies include the safe handling and disposal of sharps, the avoidance of unnecessary exposure to blood and body fluids, and the decontamination and sterilization of instruments. In addition to these, in order to improve the safety of blood and blood products, special attention is given to selection and screening of blood donors. HCWs who are infected with active HCV infection are restricted from performing exposure-prone procedures (EPPs; see p. **201**) (Department of Health, 2002).

HUMAN IMMUNODEFICIENCY VIRUS

Human immunodeficiency virus evolved as a human pathogen very recently relative to most other known human pathogens and was identified in 1982. The global impact of HIV on healthcare resources and the degree of mortality and morbidity are enormous. Unlike hepatitis B and C viruses that primarily affect the liver (hepatotropic viruses), HIV infects a variety of cells of the immune system, including CD4-expressing helper T cells, macrophages and dendritic cells leading to their depletion and profound immunodeficiency. Two closely related types of HIV, designated HIV-1 and HIV-2, have been identified. Infection with the HIV-1, which is the most common cause of acquired immunodeficiency syndrome (AIDS), has become pandemic, spreading uncontrollably in Africa, China, India and the old Soviet Union. Infection with HIV-2, which shows less pathogenicity, is restricted mostly to West Africa and only a few cases have been diagnosed in the UK. HIV-2 infection also leads to AIDS, although the speed of progression may be slower.

Acute seroconversion illness (primary HIV) resembles glandular fever with flu-like symptoms and an enlargement of the lymph nodes. Following this stage, HIV establishes persistent infection which used to lead to AIDS prior to the advent of several antiretroviral drugs capable of reducing the risk of opportunistic infections. The development of AIDS is related to the ability of HIV to destroy the cells of the immune system and the inability of these to clear the infection. Antiretroviral therapy in the UK and the western world, continues to improve, leading to a suppression of the virus activity and immune reconstitution for years. The net effect of these interventions is that individuals infected with HIV are living longer with an improved quality of life.

The major routes of HIV transmission include sex, intravenous drug use/smoking crack cocaine, transfusion of blood product (a risk between 1978 and 1985) and perinatal infection. Widespread screening of blood donors has reduced the impact of transfusion-acquired infection, although such screening is by no means universal throughout the world. This leaves occupational per-cutaneous exposure to a patient's blood by 'needlestick' or 'sharps' injury the most common route of HIV transmission in the healthcare setting. Per-cutaneous deep injuries involving a hollowbore needle that has been in the vein or artery of an HIV-positive source patient, particularly those with late-stage disease and a high virus load, are associated with increased risk of HIV infection (Cardo et al., 1997). Data obtained from a number of prospective studies of occupational exposure events suggest that the risk of transmission to an HCW from an HIV-infected patient following such an injury to be around 1 in 300. Cases of occupationally acquired HIV infection are usually categorized as either 'documented' or 'possible', but the definitions used vary slightly from country to country. A 'documented case' is one for which there is documented evidence of HIV seroconversion (a recorded negative result of a test for anti-HIV followed by a subsequent positive result) associated in time with a specific occupational exposure to a source of HIV. The first documented case in the UK of an HCW becoming HIV positive following an occupational exposure was in 1984 (Anon., 1984). As a result of this incident, a system of passive sur-veillance of HCWs who have had significant occupational exposure to HIV in England, Wales and Northern Ireland was set up. Three more documented cases of occupationally acquired HIV infections in UK followed in 1992/1993 (Heptonstall et al., 1993) and a further one in 2000 (Hawkins et al., 2001). In 1997, an active surveillance scheme was implemented and expanded to include HBV and HCV exposures (Communicable Disease Surveillance Centre, 1998). Between July 1996 and June 2004, 122 reported HCWs exposed to an HIV-positive source were followed-up and tested for infection at 6 months post-exposure. Only one (0.8 per cent) seroconverted to HIV (Health Protec-tion Agency, 2005).

Laboratory diagnosis of infection with HIV-1 or HIV-2 relies on detection of HIV-specific antibodies or on detection of the virus itself, namely proviral DNA. HIV proviral DNA is integrated in the host cell genome and can be detected readily in peripheral blood mononuclear cells in those who are infected. Detection of proviral DNA is particularly appropriate in the diagnosis of an acute infection before seroconversion. The majority of those infected with HIV will seroconvert to HIV antibodies within 2–3 months, but some may take longer. Thus there is a 'window' period during which HIV-1 p24 antigen and HIV RNA will be detectable in blood. HIV RNA virus load is rou-tinely used for monitoring disease progression and response to treatment. Recently, a new generation of rapid detection methods/point of care tests have become available. Their potential use is in situations where a quick result on HIV status is important: in labour, for late antenatal clinic bookers, when no prenatal HIV test was performed, for sources of needlestick injuries to HCW, for the evaluation of acutely ill patients with possible *Pneumocystis jiroveci* pneumonia (PJP) or for patients who are unlikely to return for test results.

In order to prevent occupationally acquired HIV infections occurring, it is of paramount importance that HCWs receive adequate training and education on the management and prevention of occupational exposures. Universal precautions should be adhered to, where appropriate, and HCWs should experience the necessary training in their use, including the correct methods for disposing of sharps, routine use of gloves, double-gloving for invasive operations and wearing of masks, gowns and eye protection. The UK Department of Health published guidance for clinical HCWs on protection against infection with bloodborne viruses in 1998 (Department of Health, 1998). This guidance should be followed to minimize the risk of bloodborne virus transmission to HCWs from patients and to minimize the risk of transmission from infected workers to patients, and from patient to patient. HCWs who are infected with HIV, under these guidelines, must not perform EPPs (see p. **201**) and must seek further professional guidance regarding the limitations of their working practices.

At present, there is no vaccine against HIV, although several clinical trials are ongoing. However, therapy against HIV has been a tremendous success with the advent of highly active antiretroviral treatment (HAART). Four different classes of drugs are currently available:

1 nucleoside reverse transcriptase inhibitors (NRTI);
2 non-nucleoside reverse transcriptase inhibitors (NNRTI);
3 protease inhibitors (PI);
4 fusion inhibitors;
5 cellular chemokine (CCR5) co-receptor antagonists; and
6 integrase inhibitors.

MANAGEMENT OF NEEDLESTICK AND OTHER HIGH RISK INJURIES AMONG HEALTHCARE WORKERS

General

Each healthcare institution should have their own detailed and coherent local guidelines on prevention and spread of bloodborne viruses, including a written policy for prompt reporting, evaluation, counselling, treatment and follow-up of occupational exposures to pathogens. The guidelines should be implemented by an Infection Control Team whose primary responsibility would include all aspects of prevention, surveillance and control of infection in a hospital. The Infection Control Team should closely collaborate with the Occupational Health Service in order to provide advice to staff on measures to avoid the transmission of infection between patients and staff. For its part, the

Occupational Health Service needs to ensure that every HCW is immunized against hepatitis B as this is an integral component of complete policy to prevent infection with HBV following an exposure to blood or body fluids. There should be 24-hour access to clinical advice on management of occupational exposures, including weekends and ideally there should be an access to staff health records, including an immunization status whenever this is possible. Clinicians and other staff responsible for providing immediate post-exposure management should be familiar with the local guidelines on evaluation and prophylaxis, and have immediate access to hepatitis B vaccine, HBIG and HIV prophylaxis. Hospitals should ensure that all their staff are appropriately trained and proficient in the procedures necessary for working safely, and that both staff and patients are not placed at any avoidable risk, as far as this is reasonably practicable.

An exposure that might place a HCW at risk from bloodborne pathogens includes contact with blood and body fluids containing visible blood as described before in this chapter. Cerebrospinal fluid, synovial fluid, pleural fluid, peritoneal fluid, pericardial fluid, amniotic fluid, semen and vaginal secretions are also considered potentially infectious, although the risk for transmission of bloodborne pathogens from these fluids in healthcare settings is still unknown. Urine, saliva, sputum, faeces, vomitus, sweat and tears are not considered infectious unless they contain blood. In cases of human bites, there is a possibility that both the source of the bite and the recipient could be exposed to bloodborne pathogens and a thorough clinical evaluation is necessary. Documented evidence of transmission of HIV or HBV through bites is very rare (Vidmar *et al.*, 1996).

The source of occupational exposure to bloodborne pathogens should be evaluated for HBV, HCV and HIV infection. In addition to screening for bloodborne viruses, their medical records at the time of exposure should be reviewed, including results of blood tests, admitting diagnosis and past medical history. If the HBV, HCV and HIV status of the source is unknown, the source of the exposure should be approached by a senior member of staff informed about the incident, and informed consent should be obtained for testing for serological evidence of bloodborne viruses. Confidentiality should be maintained at all times. Testing for HBV, HCV and HIV should be done as soon as possible and the laboratories should regard the requests for testing as urgent and try to expedite the results.

Specific management of risk incidents

Hepatitis B virus

Percutaneous inoculations are the most efficient means of HBV transmission. In addition to these, broken skin in contact with environmental surfaces contaminated with blood poses a risk for transmission, as has been demonstrated in investigations of HBV outbreaks in haemodialysis units (Hennekens, 1973). HBV is capable of surviving in dried blood at room temperature for at least 1 week (Bond *et al.*, 1981).

Healthcare workers who contaminate their eyes or mouth, or fresh cuts or abrasions of the skin, with blood or body fluids from a known HBsAg-positive person should wash the affected area well with soap and warm water and seek medical advice immediately. The source of bloodborne exposure should be approached by the senior member of staff and consented for testing for bloodborne viruses. Advice about prophylaxis after such accidents should be obtained by telephone from the nearest virologist on call or the Health Protection Unit. If an accident occurred during working hours, advice can also be obtained from the Occupational Health Services, which should use the opportunity to check the HBV immunization history opportunistically. Prophylaxis with hepatitis B vaccine alone or in combination with HBIG, if the HCW was not previously immunized, is effective in preventing HBV infection after an occupational exposure. The decision to start prophylaxis is based on several factors, such as:

• whether the source is HBsAg positive;
• whether the HCW has been immunized;
• whether the HCW demonstrated immunity to HBV following the course of immunization.

The recommended protocol is shown in Table 9.2.

Table 9.2 Prophylaxis against hepatitis B virus infection following accidental exposure

Immune status of the recipient	Source known to be HBsAg positive	Unknown source
Completed course of hepatitis B immunization: anti-HBs >10 mIU/mL	Administer a booster dose of hepatitis B vaccine	Administer a booster dose of hepatitis B vaccine
Non-responder to hepatitis B vaccine: anti-HBs <10 mIU/mL	Administer single dose of HBIG and a booster dose of hepatitis B vaccine	Administer single dose of HBIG and a booster dose of hepatitis B vaccine
No previous hepatitis B immunization or only one dose received	Accelerated primary course of hepatitis B immunisation (0, 1 and 2 months) and single dose of HBIG	Accelerated primary course of hepatitis B immunization
Course of hepatitis B immunization not yet completed (last dose not yet received)	Complete the course by giving one dose of hepatitis B vaccine following exposure, and the second dose 1 month later	Complete the course (administer last dose of hepatitis B vaccine) at the time following exposure

anti-HBs, antibody to hepatitis B surface antigen; HBsAg, hepatitis B surface antigen; HBIG, hyperimmune hepatitis B immunoglobulin.

Hepatitis C virus

Hepatitis C virus is not transmitted efficiently following needlestick injuries. Transmission rarely occurs through blood contamination of mucous membranes, and no transmission has been recorded through intact or non-intact skin (Sartori *et al.*, 1993). Apart from haemodialysis units, environmental contamination with blood containing HCV does not pose a significant risk for transmission in the healthcare setting (Hardy *et al.*, 1992; Polish *et al.*, 1993). There is no vaccine against hepatitis C and no treatment following an exposure that will prevent infection. No clinical trials have been conducted to assess post-exposure use of antiviral agents (interferon with or without ribavirin) to prevent HCV infection. There have been nine reported HCWs who have seroconverted to HCV following significant occupational exposure between 1997 and 2004 in the UK (Health Protection Agency, 2005). In accordance with the Health Protection Agency's recommendations, HCWs exposed to an HCV-positive source should have blood samples taken at the time of the incident (baseline sample), and then at 6, 12 and 24 weeks post-exposure (Ramsay, 1999). An HCV ribonucleic acid (RNA) test should be performed on the 6- and 12-week samples and testing for HCV antibodies should be carried out on the 12- and 24-week samples. In the case of seroconversion, antibodies against HCV take between 50 and 70 days to develop, and should be detectable on testing the 12-week sample. As the risk of the infection is very small, there is no need for a limitation of clinical activity during this period. In the absence of post-exposure prophylaxis (PEP) for HCV, post-exposure management has the aim of an early identification of an acute infection and referral for evaluation of treatment strategies in order to prevent the progression to chronic hepatitis. Some studies have shown that the majority of patients who have recently seroconverted and commenced treatment within 6 months of the onset of infection successfully clear the virus and do not develop chronic hepatitis C (Jaeckel *et al.*, 2001; Rocca *et al.*, 2003). In these studies, the response to therapy was not influenced by the hepatitis C genotype, mode of transmission or the patient's sex.

Human immunodeficiency virus

Several factors might affect the risk of HIV transmission following an occupational exposure to bloodborne viruses. Studies have shown that the risk was found to be increased with:

- a large quantity of blood;
- procedures or cannulation involving a needle being placed directly in a vein or artery;
- deep injuries;
- visible blood on the device which caused the injury (Dienstag and Ryan, 1982).

If the source is known to be infected with HIV, the risk could also be increased in terminal HIV-related illness, reflecting the high HIV replication. The role of plasma HIV virus load from the source's blood for assessment of the risk for transmission has not yet been entirely clarified, as it reflects only the level of cell-free virus in blood (i.e. low virus load does not exclude the possibility of transmission).

There is now clear evidence that PEP following an occupational exposure to blood from an HIV-infected individual is beneficial. This is based on the role of the HIV pathogenesis, efficacy of PEP in animal studies, efficacy of antiretroviral drugs for PEP in human studies, and the risk and benefit of PEP to HCWs exposed to HIV.

Current practice is to use a PEP pack containing three antiretroviral drugs, as the combination therapy has been proved to be superior to monotherapy in reducing HIV virus load in HIV-infected individuals. In February 2006, The British Association for Sexual Health and HIV recommended the use of a PEP starter pack containing two NRTI drugs (recommended combinations include: azidothymidine (AZT) and lamivudine (3TC), stavudine (D4T) and 3TC, tenofovir and 3TC, or tenofovir and emtricitabine (FTC) plus one PI drug (lopinavir or fosamprenavir or saquinavir; Fisher *et al.*, 2006). The recommended duration of treatment remains 4 weeks in order to minimize the potential for HIV transmission.

Following the exposure to HIV, the procedure below should be adopted.

1 The site of exposure (e.g. the wound or non-intact skin) should be washed liberally with soap and water, but without scrubbing.
2 Assessment needs to be made urgently and the HCW evaluated within hours following their exposure about the appropriateness of starting PEP.
3 The HCW should be tested for HIV at baseline (to establish infection status at the time of exposure), and the blood sample should also be sent for baseline biochemistry.
4 PEP should be started as soon as possible (within the hour and not later than 72 hours). The exposed worker should take the first dose of PEP pending the more thorough assessment to inform a decision whether to continue with the rest of the PEP.
5 Following exposures for which PEP is considered appropriate, HCWs should be given time to discuss the balance of risks in their particular situation and they should be offered appropriate psychological support. They should be informed about the efficacy and toxicity of drugs used for PEP. It is important that their views about PEP are taken into account and that their preferences about what to discuss and with whom are respected. Although the risk for HIV transmission is low, HCWs who are exposed to HIV-contaminated blood and started on PEP are requested to practise safe sex (condom use or sexual abstinence) in order to prevent secondary transmission during the follow-up period.

If the exposed HCW is pregnant, the decision to start the PEP should be discussed with the pregnant woman and an experienced HIV clinician in order to discuss the potential benefits and risks for both the fetus and the mother. Some antiretroviral drugs should be avoided in pregnancy (e.g. efavirenz, stavudine and didanosine).

An HCW who was exposed to HIV-contaminated blood or body fluids, regardless of whether PEP was initiated or not, should have a regular follow-up with counselling and blood testing. HIV-antibody testing should be performed at 6, 12 and 24 weeks. HCWs who are commenced on PEP should be advised to complete the treatment and their blood checked for drug toxicity.

MANAGEMENT OF HEALTHCARE WORKERS INFECTED WITH BLOODBORNE VIRUSES

Hepatitis B

All blood and body fluids from HCWs as well as patients should be regarded as potentially infectious. Transfer of blood or other potentially infectious material from HCWs to patients must be avoided. In the past, several HCW-to-patient HBV transmissions have been documented in the UK (Heptonstall, 1991). Taken together, these outbreaks suggest a risk for HBV transmission from HCWs to patients, which is associated with certain types of surgical interventions called 'exposure-prone procedures'.

Exposure-prone procedures (EPPs) are those invasive procedures where there is a risk that an injury to the HCW may result in the exposure of the patient's open tissues to the blood of the worker (bleed-back). These include procedures where the worker's gloved hands may be in contact with sharp instruments, needle tips or sharp tissues (e.g. spicules of bone or teeth) inside a patient's open body cavity, wound or confined anatomical space where the hands or fingertips may not be completely visible at all times. Examples of EPP include: major pelvic surgery, vaginal hysterectomy, certain abdominal procedures (colectomy) and cardiac surgery.

Recommendations on restricting the practice of HBV-infected HCWs who perform EPPs were based on the presence or absence of serum HBeAg. HBeAg is considered to be a marker of high infectivity and associated with higher HBV DNA virus load and therefore high risk for transmission. This led to introduction of strict guidelines by the Department of Health in 1993 (National Health Service Management Executive, 1993), updated in 1998, restricting HBeAg-positive HCWs from practising EPPs. In 1997, the transmission of HBV to patients by surgeons who were HBV carriers without detectable serum HBeAg was reported (Anon., 1997). It is now clear that hepatitis B carriers who are HBe negative may also have high levels of HBV DNA, owing to changes in the HBV genome (Carman *et al.*, 1989; Pawlotsky,

2005). This led to restrictions in performing EPPs or clinical duties in renal units being extended to infected HCWs who are HBeAg negative and who have an HBV DNA (viral load) which exceeds 10^3 genome equivalents per millilitre (Department of Health, 2000). Subject to annual retesting, HCWs whose viral load does not exceed 10^3 copies/mL need not have their working practices restricted, but they should receive occupational health counselling. Hepatitis B-infected HCWs should not continue to perform EPPs while on interferon or oral antiviral therapy.

Human immunodeficiency virus

Transmission of HIV from an HCW to patients has been reported previously (Ou et al., 1992) and has been associated with performing the EPPs in which the injury to HCW might result in a worker's blood contaminating a patient's open tissues. However, the risk of such transmission is very small providing that general infection control measures are adhered to. Following identification of an HCW infected with HIV who is performing EPPs, it is recommended that, as far as is practicable, patients should only be notified if they have been at a distinct risk of bleed-back from the particular EPPs performed on them by HCW. Such patients should be contacted and encouraged to have pre-test discussion and HIV antibody testing. The decision on whether a patient notification exercise is undertaken should be made on a case-by-case basis using risk assessment. It is anticipated that, in most cases, this decision will be made locally by Directors of Public Health of Primary Care Trusts, supported as necessary by Regional Epidemiologists or Regional Directors of Public Health. Where there is still uncertainty, the UK Advisory Panel for Health Care Workers Infected with Blood-borne Viruses may also be approached for advice.

Any HCWs who believe that they might have been exposed to HIV in the past must seek confidential and professional advice on whether they should be tested for HIV infection. If found positive for HIV infection, an HCW must not perform EPPs and should obtain professional advice from the local Occupational Health Department about modification and limitation of their working practices. Those HIV-infected HCWs who do not perform EPPs, but continue to work with patients, should have regular medical and Occupational Health supervision (Department of Health, 2005).

All HCWs are under ethical and legal duties to protect the health and safety of their patients. Under the Health and Safety at Work Act 1974, and associated regulations, such as the Control of Substances Hazardous to Health (COSHH) Regulations 2002, HCWs who are employees have a legal duty to take reasonable care for the health and safety of themselves and of others, including colleagues and patients, and to cooperate with their employer in health and safety matters.

Hepatitis C virus

In the UK, there have been five recorded transmissions of HCV from HCWs to patients to date; similar accidents have occurred and have been documented worldwide Communicable Disease Surveillance Centre, 1995; Esteban *et al.*, 1996). The UK case involved a transmission during cardiothoracic surgery after which one patient developed acute hepatitis C (Communicable Disease Surveillance Centre, 1995). This incident generated a lookback investigation during which 277 patients were tested for HCV infection, but no other patients were identified (Duckworth *et al.*, 1999, suggesting that the risk of transmission of HCV is low.

In 2002, The Department of Health issued guidelines (HSC 2002/010) on HCV-infected HCWs, stating that those who perform EPPs and who believe they might have been exposed to HCV should promptly seek and follow advice from the Occupational Health Department on whether they should be tested for HCV antibodies. If HCV antibodies are detected, or if they already know that they are infected with HCV, they should be tested for HCV RNA in accredited laboratories and, if found positive, restricted from performing EPP (Department of Health, 2002). The effect of these guidelines is to reduce the inflow of HCV-infected HCWs into the pool of those performing EPPs and divert HCV-infected trainees away from EPP specialties at a time when they can retrain. If an HCW receives treatment for HCV infection and remains HCV RNA-negative 6 months after cessation of treatment, they should be allowed to perform EPP but should have a further check 12 months following the end of treatment and must remain HCV RNA negative.

Investigation of bloodborne infections possibly acquired in hospital

It is to be expected that awareness of the hazards of bloodborne viral infections by staff and patients has increased with the stringent infection control measures and regular training of the hospital employees. However, the evidence shows that lapses in good infection control occasionally occurs owing to the relative rarity of bloodborne infection outbreaks in healthcare settings. When a previously unidentified case of HBV, HIV or HCV is found, routine investigations may reveal a medical procedure as a possible risk factor (e.g. recent invasive pelvic surgery). There should always be a low threshold for conducting investigations in such circumstances, particularly in the absence of other risk activities. The investigation must include a hospital Infection Control Team, clinical virologists, public health specialists and the clinician involved in looking after the patient. If more individuals are identified as infected, molecular analysis of the isolates performed by the virology laboratory can help in establishing a common source of infection.

NON-BLOODBORNE HEPATITIS VIRUSES

Hepatitis A virus infection

Hepatitis A is an acute, self-limiting infection caused by enterically transmitted hepatitis A virus (HAV). This virus replicates in the liver, from where it is excreted in bile and found in high concentration in stool, making faecal excretion the primary source of the virus. The shedding of HAV in stool starts 2–3 weeks before and 1 week after the onset of jaundice. Young children and infants may continue shedding the virus for a longer periods than adults. The incubation period is 15–50 days (mean period 28 days) and the illness is often mild (the prodrome), including flu-like symptoms, fever, chills, malaise, fatigue and abdominal pain. This is followed by the onset of dark urine, pale-coloured stool and jaundice. The stool returns to its normal colour in 2–3 weeks, which coincides with the resolution of the illness, although some adults experience symptoms for several months. HAV does not result in chronic infection.

Transmission of the virus is by the faecal–oral route among close contacts, and by faecally contaminated food or water. Transfusion-related hepatitis A is now very rare and, in the past, used to be related to transfusion of blood product to patients suffering with haemophilia (Soucie *et al.*, 1998). Hospital outbreaks with HAV infection are rare because the majority of patients become admitted after they develop jaundice (i.e. when they are less infective). However, there are reports describing faecally incontinent in-patients transmitting HAV (Goodman, 1985); therefore, strict infection control measures are recommended in order to prevent nosocomial spread of the virus.

In the course of acute infection, liver enzymes, particularly alanine aminotransferase (ALT) and aspartate aminotransferase (AST), become raised but these are not specific for the diagnosis of HAV infection. Definitive diagnosis relies on the detection of HAV-specific IgM in an acute serum sample. Total antibody to the HAV is not helpful in the diagnosis. It can persist for many years, and most often reflects past infection or immunization against HAV.

The most effective way to control HAV infection in the hospital setting is adherence to good hygienic practices. HCWs employed in day or residential care centres for people with special needs may benefit from immunization owing to their higher risk for infection. On the other hand, there is no evidence that HCWs in hospitals are at increased risk of HAV infection; therefore, routine immunization in this group is not recommended. Active immunization with inactivated hepatitis A vaccine is recommended for prophylaxis in patients with haemophilia, HBV or HCV infection, liver cirrhosis of any cause and injecting drug users (Crowcroft, 2001). Further prophylactic use of HAV vaccine is for the protection from hepatitis A infection in close contacts (including HCWs in contact with incontinent patients) where the index case is identified promptly (i.e. within 1 week of the onset of symptoms). When the onset is more than 1 week, human normal immunoglobulin is recommended (Crowcroft, 2001) for prophylaxis.

Hepatitis E

Hepatitis E virus (HEV) was recognized as a cause of enterically transmitted non-A/non-B hepatitis occurring occasionally during large outbreaks of water-borne hepatitis in sanitation-poor regions in Asia, Africa and South America (Labrique, 1999). HEV is endemic in Southeast and Central Asia where it causes sporadic hepatitis in children and adults (Krawczynski, 1993).

Historically, HEV disease was associated with travel to areas of high prevalence. However, a recent study by the UK Health Protection Agency identified cases of non-travel-associated cases of HEV infection caused by the same virus as is carried by British pigs (Ijad *et al.*, 2005) indicating a possibility that pigs might act as a reservoir of HEV and that HEV is a zoonotic infection.

HEV is transmitted primarily by the faecal–oral route through faecally contaminated drinking water. Person-to-person contact does not appear to be an efficient mode of transmission. The incubation period ranges from 15 to 45 days (average 40 days). Clinical signs include fever, malaise, anorexia, nausea, vomiting, abdominal pain and jaundice. Overall, case fatality rate is between 1 and 3 per cent, increasing up to 25 per cent in pregnant women who are in the third trimester of pregnancy. There are no chronic sequelae associated with HEV infection.

Diagnosis of an acute HEV infection relies on detection of HEV-specific IgM, which subsequently disappears over the following 4–6 months. Finding of HEV IgG in the serum indicates a convalescent phase or previous infection.

Prevention of HEV infection for travellers to HEV-endemic regions includes avoidance of drinking water of unknown purity, uncooked shellfish and uncooked vegetables. Immunoglobulin prepared from donors in Western countries does not prevent HEV infection. Currently, a vaccine against HEV is in development, with preliminary results soon to be reported. There are no reports of nosocomially transmitted HEV.

REFERENCES

Anon. (1984) Needlestick transmission of HTLV-III from a patient infected in Africa. *Lancet* **ii,** 1376.

Anon. (1997) Transmission of hepatitis B to patients from four infected surgeons without hepatitis Be antigen. *New England Journal of Medicine* **336,** 178.

Bond WW, Favero MS, Petersen NJ et al. (1981) Survival of hepatitis B after drying and storage for one week [Letter]. *Lancet* **i,** 550.

Bond WW, Petersen NJ, Favero MS (1977) Viral hepatitis B: aspects of environmental control. *Health Laboratory Science* **14,** 235.

Cardo DM, Culver DH, Ciesilski CA *et al.* (1997) A case-control study of HIV sero-conversion in health care workers after percutaneous exposure. *New England Journal of Medicine* **337**, 1485.

Carman WF, Jacyna MR, Hadziyannis S *et al.* (1989) Mutation preventing formation of hepatitis Be antigen in patients with chronic hepatitis B infection. *Lancet* **ii**, 588.

Centers for Disease Control and Prevention (2009) *Hepatitis C Fact Sheet.* Available at: http://www.cdc.gov/hepatitis/HCV.htm (last accessed 3 January 2009).

Communicable Disease Surveillance Centre (1995) Hepatitis C virus transmission from health care worker to patient. *Communicable Disease Report. CDR Weekly* **5**, 121.

Communicable Disease Surveillance Centre (1998) Surveillance of health care workers with occupational exposure to bloodborne viruses. *Communicable Disease Report. CDR Weekly* **8**, 65, 68.

Choo QL, Richman KH, Han JH *et al.* (1991) Genetic organization and diversity of the hepatitis C virus. *Proceedings of the National Academy of Sciences USA* **88**, 2451.

Crowcroft NS, Walsh B, Davison KL, Gungabissoon U, on behalf of PHLS Advisory Committee on Vaccination and Immunisation (2001) Guidelines for the control of hepatitis A virus infection. *Communicable Disease and Public Health* **4**, 213.

Department of Health (1993) *Health Service Guidelines (93)40: Protecting Health Care Workers and Patients from Hepatitis B.* London: Department of Health.

Department of Health (1998) *Guidance for clinical health care workers: protection against blood-borne viruses.* London: Department of Health.

Department of Health (2000) *Health Service Circular 2000/020.* London: Department of Health.

Department of Health (2002) *Health Service Circular 2002/010.* London: Department of Health.

Department of Health (2004) *Hepatitis C action plan for England.* London: Department of Health.

Department of Health (2005) *HIV infected health care workers: guidance on management and patient notification.* London: Department of Health.

Dienstag JL, Ryan DM (1982) Occupational exposure to hepatitis B virus in hospital personnel: infection or immunisation? *American Journal of Epidemiology* **115**, 26.

Duckworth GJ, Heptonstall J, Aitken C for the Incident Control Team and others (1999) Transmission of hepatitis C from a surgeon to a patient. *Communicable Disease and Public Health* **2**, 188.

Esteban JI, Gomez J, Martell M *et al.* (1996) Transmission of hepatitis C virus by a cardiac surgeon. *New England Journal of Medicine* **334**, 555.

Fisher M, Benn P, Evans B *et al.* (2006) UK guidelines for the use of post-exposure prophylaxis for HIV following sexual exposure. *International Journal of STD and AIDS* **17**, 81.

Flamm SL (2003) Chronic hepatitis C virus infection. *JAMA* **289**, 2413.

Francis DP, Favero MS, Maynard JE (1981) Transmission of hepatitis B virus. *Seminars in Liver Disease* **1**, 27.

Goodman RA (1985) Nosocomial hepatitis A. *Annals of Internal Medicine* **103**, 452.

Hardy NM, Sandroni S, Danielson S, *et al.* (1992) Antibody to hepatitis C virus increases with time on hemodialysis. *Clinical Nephrology* **38**, 44.

Hassanein T, Cooksley G, Sulkowski M *et al.* (2004) The impact of peginterferon alfa-2a plus ribavirin combination therapy on health-related quality of life in chronic hepatitis C. *Journal of Hepatology* **40,** 675.

Hawkins DA, Asboe D, Barlow K *et al.* (2001) Seroconversion to HIV-1 following needlestick injury despite combination post-exposure prophylaxis. *Journal of Infection* **43,** 12.

Health Protection Agency (2005) *Eye of the needle. Surveillance of significant occupational exposure to bloodborne viruses in healthcare workers. Centre for Infections; England, Wales and Northern Ireland Seven-year Report: January 2005.* London: Health Protection Agency.

Hennekens CH (1973) Hemodialysis-associated hepatitis: an outbreak among hospital personnel. *JAMA* **225,** 407.

Heptonstall J, Gill ON, Porter K *et al.* (1993) Health care workers and HIV: surveillance of occupationally acquired infection in the United Kingdom. *Communicable Disease Report. CDR Review* **3,** R147.

Heptonstall J (1991) Outbreaks of hepatitis B virus infection associated with infected surgical staff. *Communicable Disease Report. CDR Review* **1,** R81.

Hoofnagle JH (1990) Chronic hepatitis B. *New England Journal of Medicine* **323,** 337.

Ijaz S, Arnold E, Banks M *et al.* (2005) Non-travel-associated hepatitis E in England and Wales: demographic, clinical, and molecular epidemiological characteristics. *Journal of Infectious Diseases* **192,** 1166.

Jaeckel E, Comberg M, Wedemeyer H *et al.* (2001) Treatment of acute hepatitis C with interferon alfa-2b. *New England Journal of Medicine* **345,** 1452.

Kaneko S, Kobayashi K, Miller RH *et al.* (1990) Detection of hepatitis B virus DNA using the polymerase chain reaction technique. *Journal of Clinical Laboratory Analysis* **4,** 479.

Krawczynski K (1993) Hepatitis E. *Hepatology* **17,** 932.

Labrique AB, Thomas DI, Soszek SK *et al.* (1999) Hepatitis E: an emerging infectious disease. *Epidemiologic Reviews* **21,** 162.

Lanphear BP, Linneman CC Jr, Cannon CG *et al.* (1994) Hepatitis C virus infection in healthcare workers: risk of exposure and infection. *Infection Control and Hospital Epidemiology* **15,** 745.

Mast EE and Alter MJ (1993) Prevention of hepatitis B virus infection among healthcare workers. In: Ellis RW (ed.) *Hepatitis B vaccines in clinical practice.* New York: Marcel Dekker, p. 295.

National Institute for Health and Clinical Excellence (2004*) Interferon alfa (pegylated and non-pegylated) and ribavirin for the treatment of chronic hepatitis* C. Technology appraisal 75. London: National Institute for Clinical Excellence.

Niro GA, Rosina F and Rizzeto M (2005) Treatment of hepatitis D. *Journal of Viral Hepatology* **12,** 2.

Ou C-Y, Ciesielski CA, Myers G *et al.* (1992) Molecular epidemiology of HIV transmission in a dental practice. *Science* **256,** 1165.

Pawlotsky J-M (2005) The concept of hepatitis B virus mutant escape. *Journal of Clinical Virology* **34,** S125.

Polish LB, Tong MJ, Co RL *et al.* (1993) Risk factors for hepatitis C virus infection among health care personnel in a community hospital. *American Journal of Infection Control* **21**, 196.

Poynard T, Yuen MF, Ratziu V and Lai CL (2003) Viral hepatitis C. *Lancet* **362**, 2095.

Ramsay ME (1999) Guidance on the investigation and management of occupational exposure to hepatitis C. *Communicable Disease and Public Health* **2**, 258.

Rocca P, Bailly F, Chevallier M *et al.* (2003) Early treatment of acute hepatitis C with interferon alpha-2b or interferon alpha-2b plus ribavirin: study of sixteen patients. *Gastroentérologie clinique et biologique* **27**, 294.

Sartori M, La Terra G, Aglietta M *et al.* Transmission of hepatitis C via blood splash into conjunctiva (Letter). *Scandinavian Journal of Infectious Diseases* **25**, 270.

Snydman DR, Bryan JA, Macon EJ, Gregg MB (1976) Hemodialysis-associated hepatitis: a report of an epidemic with further evidence on mechanism of transmission. *American Journal of Epidemiology* **104**, 563.

Soucie JM, Robertson BH, Bell BP *et al.* (1998) Hepatitis A virus infections associated with clotting factor concentrates in the United States. *Transfusion* **38**, 573.

Vidmar L, Poljak M, Tomazic J *et al.* (1996) Transmission of HIV-1 by human bite [Letter]. *Lancet* **347**, 1762.

Werner BG, Grady GF (1982) Accidental hepatitis-B-surface-antigen-positive inoculations: use of e antigen to estimate infectivity. *Annals of Internal Medicine* **97**, 367.

Zeuzem S, Hultcrantz R, Bourliere M *et al.* (2004) Peginterferon alfa-2b plus ribavirin for treatment of chronic hepatitis C in previously untreated patients infected with HCV genotypes 2 or 3. *Journal of Hepatology* **40**, 993.

10 IMMUNIZATION AND SPECIFIC PROPHYLAXIS

Jonathan North

INTRODUCTION

When basic infection control measures fail and an individual is exposed to a potentially infective inoculum of a pathogen, good immunity can reduce the chance of infection. Immunity to infection depends on the balance between several factors in the host and the infecting organism. A high-dose inoculum of virulent organisms in an un-immunized host is more likely to result in infection than lower doses of less virulent organisms in immune individuals. Healthcare workers (HCWs) are exposed to higher doses of potentially virulent organisms more frequently than the rest of the population and, therefore, specific measures to reduce the chances of infection are important. This chapter gives guidance on how to increase specific immunity where this is possible. The same measures can be undertaken to help protect patients whose immunity is impaired by their disease and/or its treatment, and also those in close contact with patients who have a communicable disease.

Healthcare workers should have their immunity against some specific infections assessed before commencing work in high-risk areas, but even optimal levels of antibody (e.g. against tetanus) may not provide protection against a large inoculum. All reasonable precautions to prevent exposure, therefore, must be undertaken even in the most 'immune' individual.

PRINCIPLES OF IMMUNITY AND IMMUNIZATION

Immunity can be gained by exposure to an infectious agent followed by recovery or by giving a non-infectious form of an infectious agent. An *active* process takes place wherein the various elements of the immune system produce protective antibody and specific T cells. An *antibody* has the ability to neutralize toxin (e.g. tetanus), prevent entry of the organism into the body or into host cells (e.g. polio) or aid killing of the organism by other components of the immune system, such as complement and neutrophils. For some antibodies, epidemiological studies of infected and non-infected individuals in an at-risk population give a good indication of a protective level, above which infection is rare. These are given below where appropriate. For others, however, a protective level has to be inferred from studies of normal populations and these levels (e.g. serotype-specific pneumococcal antibody levels) should be treated with more caution. Generally, antibody responses to typical antigens will be present for 5–10 years.

T cells are necessary for the production of antibody and also prevent viral spread by killing infected host cells, thus halting viral replication. They also play a major role in recruiting all components of the immune system to sites of infection and in stimulating an inflammatory response. Failure to produce an adequate antibody response can be due to impaired T cells; however, T-cell immunity is not routinely assessed directly. Immunization is not recommended during an acute infection as the majority of T cells will be engaged in the inflammatory and killing roles, and will not be capable of responding to a new antigen.

Natural protection arises to hundreds of organisms and their different strains throughout life. Infection is not necessary to produce natural immunity, as a small inoculum of a pathogen may survive locally in the host for a short time yet still stimulate a response that leads to long-term protection. Repeated inoculation will strengthen the protection, just as boosting with a vaccine does.

The young are more prone to infection for two reasons. The first is that full T-cell maturity occurs at around 2 years of age and antibody maturity can take up to 8 years to develop, especially for antibodies against bacteria that have a polysaccharide capsule, such as *Streptococcus pneumoniae*. The second reason is that new organisms or different strains are encountered as individuals meet more of the population who are carriers of, or infected with, previously unmet pathogens. This is typically seen when first-born children start attending play groups, nursery school, etc. A second phase of infections is seen in teenagers as organisms resident in the oropharynx are transferred directly.

Immunization involves presenting the immune system with a form of a pathogen that does not cause infection in normal individuals, but can elicit an immune response that recognizes the intended pathogen and prevent infection. Originally, killed pathogens were administered parenterally, but unwanted immune responses and consequent side effects were often encountered. Purified components of organisms are now used, where possible, but attenuated strains (i.e. non-virulent forms) of some are used when the immune response against an individual component of the organism is not protective.

Passive immunity occurs naturally when maternal antibodies are transported to the fetus towards the end of pregnancy. From birth, these antibodies last for about 3 months and this gives the neonate's own antibody responses time to develop. This can be mimicked later in life by giving exogenous antibodies with activity against specific pathogens. The antibodies are produced from the serum of individuals who have been infected or immunized, and given to a person who is particularly at risk in order to provide short-term protection. Active immunity to a pathogen can take several weeks to develop fully and passive immunization has the advantage of giving instant protection.

Cellular passive immunity by the transfer of specifically primed T cells can be undertaken only in very exceptional circumstances and is not routinely used to prevent infection, as primed T cells that are human leukocyte antigen (HLA) matched to the recipient are required.

INFORMATION ABOUT IMMUNIZATION

Immunization against Infectious Disease (the *Green Book*; Department of Health, 1996), is the standard Department of Health publication on immunization but chapter updates occur frequently making an up-to-date hard copy impractical. The new chapters can be found at http://www.dh.gov.uk/en/ Publichealth/Healthprotection/Immunisation/Greenbook/dh_4097254. The *Green Book* is a valuable source of information on the range of vaccines available, their uses and contraindications. The easiest method of keeping abreast of the current routine immunization schedules is at http://www.immunisation.nhs.uk, which provides the following.

- a guide to childhood immunizations for babies up to 13 months of age (ref. 275774);
- pre-school immunizations: a guide to vaccinations for 3–5-year olds (ref. 275776);
- teenage immunizations (ref. 275777);
- the influenza immunization programme 2006/2007 (PL/CMO/2006/3); the letter is issued annually;
- the pneumococcal immunization programme for older people and at-risk groups (PL/CMO/2005/2).

ROUTINE IMMUNIZATION FOR THE UK POPULATION

Patients (depending on their age) and staff will mostly have had their childhood immunizations, detailed in Table 10.1. All individuals raised in the UK should therefore have optimum immunity to tetanus, diphtheria, polio, pertussis, measles, mumps, rubella and meningitis C. Immunity to *Haemophilus influenzae* type b (Hib) and pneumococci develops naturally and immunization is intended to protect the infant for the first few years of life. This is not so important for adults who do not have an increased risk of infection. Boosting should occur for staff who have missed immunization doses and for selected

Table 10.1 Routine vaccination schedule for UK from September 2006

Age at vaccination	Vaccine(s)	Comment
2 months	DTaP/IPV/Hib + PCV	IPV is contraindicated in some immunosuppressed patients and killed vaccine should be used
3 months	DTaP/IPV/Hib + MenC	
4 months	DTaP/IPV/Hib + MenC + PCV	
12 months	Hib/MenC	
13 months	MMR + PCV	MMR is contraindicated in some immunosuppressed patients
3 years 4 months to 5 years	DTaP/IPV + MMR	
13–18 years	TD/IPV	Australia, Canada, France, Germany and USA administer an aP boost in adolescence
65 years and over	Pneumococcal vaccination	

aP, acellular pertussis; D, diphtheria; Hib, *Haemophilus influenzae* type b; IPV, injectable polio vaccine; MenC, conjugated meningococcal C vaccine; MMR, combined vaccine for measles, mumps and rubella; PCV, conjugated pneumococcal vaccine (seven serotypes); T, tetanus.

patient groups. Testing immunity to and immunization against tuberculosis (TB) was common practice in schoolchildren in the UK until the summer of 2005. Targeted testing and immunization of at-risk populations (Chief Medical Officer, 2005) has now replaced this policy. A vaccination history is, therefore, necessary in assessing immunity to TB (see Chapter 12). Targeted immunization of those at risk of influenza is also advised, as is pneumococcal immunization for at-risk groups.

IMMUNIZATION AND ASSESSMENT OF IMMUNITY FOR HEALTHCARE WORKERS

Under the Health and Safety at Work Act 1974, employers are required to assess the risk to health and safety of staff and others. The onus is not just on the employer but also on the employee, and both have a specific duty to take reasonably practical measures to protect workers and others who may be exposed to risks. The Control of Substances Hazardous to Health (COSHH) Regulations 2002 also call for employers to take reasonable measures to protect workers and others from the risks posed by pathogens. At the time of writing the Department of Health guidance, *Health Clearance for Serious Communicable Diseases: New Health Care Workers*, is in draft form but should be published and available on the Department of Health website shortly. The current draft guidelines explain how to test and immunize where necessary against hepatitis B, TB, hepatitis C and human immunodeficiency virus (HIV). There are different approaches for staff who will perform exposure-prone procedures and those who will not. Chapter 12 of the *Green Book* also details immunization and testing protocols for the above and other pathogens, which are summarized below (Department of Health, 1996).

Routine immunizations for healthcare workers

An immunization history should be taken from all HCWs and vaccination or boosting arranged if required. This is to help protect staff from infection and to prevent transmission of infection from staff to patients. For HCWs who have completed their full immunization schedule and have the appropriate documentation, no action is required. Immunity to tetanus, measles and rubella is especially important for all staff in direct contact with patients and, if the immunization history is unclear or recommended doses have been missed, antibody levels can be checked and boosting arranged where appropriate. Immunity to polio is important for staff who regularly handle faecal specimens (e.g. those working in a microbiology laboratory); therefore, regular boosting at 10-year intervals is recommended. Similarly, staff in laboratories or infectious disease units who are likely to be exposed to diphtheria should have antibody levels to this checked and boosting arranged where appropriate.

Antibody levels that are taken to be optimal or protective are given in Table 10.2.

Table 10.2 Antibody levels against pathogens and toxins used in determining the degree of protection

Pathogen/toxin	Antibody level	Significance
Diphtheria	<0.01 IU/mL	No protection
	>0.1 IU/mL	Protection for >10 years likely
Hepatitis B	<10 mIU/mL	No protection
	10–100 mIU/mL	Partial protection: boost
	>100 mIU/mL	Protection for >10 years likely
Hib	<0.15 µg/mL	No protection
	>1.0 µg/mL	Optimal protection
Measles	Negative	Presumed no protection
	Positive	Protective level presumed
Polio	Polio 1: >0.080 IU/mL	Protection.
	Polio 2: >0.180 IU/mL	Protection
	Polio 3: >0.075 IU/mL	Protection
Rubella	<10 IU/mL	No protection
Tetanus	<0.01 IU/mL	No protection
	>0.10 IU/mL	Protection for >10 years likely
Varicella	Negative	Presumed no protection
	Positive	Protective level presumed

Hepatitis B

New HCWs should be offered immunization against hepatitis B in accordance with the methods given in the *Green Book* (Department of Health, 1996). Those coming into direct contact with patient's blood, bloodstained body fluids or tissues (including staff who are at risk of being deliberately injured or bitten by patients) should also be tested for hepatitis B surface antigen (HBsAg). Those positive for HBsAg may be infected or be carriers of hepatitis B and further investigations should be arranged according to current Department of Health guidelines (see Chapter 9). Antibody levels against hepatitis B (anti-HBs) can be measured to assess the response to immunization. Levels >100 mIU/mL 1–2 months post-vaccination indicate a good response and protection does not need to be enhanced. The protection lasts at least 15 years for the majority of those vaccinated, but cases of breakthrough infection have been reported. An antibody response of 10–100 mIU/mL is classed as 'poor' and further boosting is advised. Non-responders have post-vaccination levels of <10 mIU/mL and a repeat course of immunization should be administered. The use of hepatitis B immunization in babies born to mothers with hepatitis B infection or carriage is given in Chapter 14 (Obstetrics and Gynaecology).

Tuberculosis

New staff with direct patient contact should be asked about the presence of symptoms suggestive of TB and have relevant investigations carried out if appropriate. Enquiry about past infection with TB or exposure to a family member with TB should be made. The presence of a BCG (bacille Calmette–Guérin) scar should be sought and unless there is clear evidence of such, or a formal record of TB immunity, a tuberculin skin test (Mantoux) should be administered. A Mantoux is recommended for all those who have spent time in areas of high TB prevalence, especially if HIV prevalence is also high. If the skin test is negative (grades 0–1), and the history or other investigations do not suggest immunodeficiency including HIV, BCG should be administered. It is important to be aware that BCG does not give complete protection against infection. If the skin test is positive, grades 2–4, the patient has immunity, but should be made aware of the symptoms of TB so that future active disease can be recognized at an early stage. If the skin test is strongly positive, grades 3–4, and there is a clinical suspicion of TB, a chest X-ray and formal investigation for TB should be arranged.

Immunity to TB is especially important for staff exposed to infectious patients and for those in paediatric, maternity, oncology and transplant departments. Non-clinical staff need not have routine testing or immunization.

Hepatitis C and human immunodeficiency virus

Immunization against hepatitis C and HIV is not available but antibody testing (and further investigation if positive) should be offered to new HCWs. It is recommended that this be done in the context of discussing their professional responsibilities and they are reminded of the ways in which they might have been exposed to these viruses. Testing should be undertaken for HCWs who will perform exposure-prone procedures and those who are positive should have further testing to assess infection and infectivity. HCWs who are HIV positive or hepatitis C ribonucleic acid (RNA) positive should not undertake exposure-prone procedures and should be managed according to current Department of Health guidelines.

Influenza

It is recommended that all staff in contact with patients should have the current annual influenza vaccination in order to help prevent infection of vulnerable patients and to help protect themselves.

Varicella

Staff who have a definite history of chickenpox and/or or shingles (herpes zoster) can be considered as being immune to varicella. If there is no history of such infection or the history is unclear, serological testing should be undertaken and staff who are antibody negative should be immunized.

IMMUNIZATION FOR STAFF AT SPECIAL RISK

For HCWs in infectious disease units or those handling particular organisms in reference or research units, immunization for the following organisms may be indicated. Immunization against some of these organisms carries a higher incidence of local or systemic reactions than the routine immunizations, so the risks of infection should be carefully evaluated for each member of staff:

- anthrax;
- cholera;
- hepatitis A;
- Japanese encephalitis;
- meningococcal disease (groups A, C, Y and W_{135});
- rabies;
- smallpox;
- tick-borne encephalitis;
- typhoid;
- yellow fever.

IMMUNIZATION FOR PATIENTS

Patients have many reasons to be more at risk of infection than the healthy population, not least of which is the effect of disease in general and of specific diseases and their treatment, on the immune system. Hospitalization *per se* is stressful and any form of stress (physical and/or mental) usually suppresses the ability to respond to infection or immunization by the action of endogenous glucocorticoids. Responses to immunization must, therefore, be assessed more carefully than in healthy individuals.

Patients with primary immunodeficiency or immunosuppression owing to treatment or HIV are likely to have impaired T-cell immunity and should not be given live vaccines, for example the combined vaccine for measles, mumps and rubella (MMR), Sabin polio and BCG, without specialist advice. Administration of these vaccines in such patients is likely to lead to infection with the immunizing organism. As neonates of Asian decent are often given BCG before discharge following birth, a family history of primary immunodeficiency should always be taken before administering BCG, and immunization withheld until specialist advice has been taken if there is such a history.

When immunosuppression is planned, inactivated vaccines should be given as far in advance of treatment as possible as all immunizations depend on T cells for an optimal response. Live vaccines can be used if there is sufficient time for the organism to be controlled by the immune system before immunosuppression but, again, specialist advice is required before administration. Bone marrow transplantation results in virtually absent immunity for several weeks (see Chapter 14) and the majority of patients will eventually require re-immunization with routine immunizations and possibly pneumococcal and Hib vaccines.

Table 10.3 is a summary of patient groups for whom protection additional to the UK routine schedule is recommended.

Table 10.3 Patient groups for whom additional immunization is recommended

Condition	Recommended immunizations
Asplenia or splenic dysfunction	Hib, influenza, meningococcal C and pneumococcal[a] vaccines (BCSH, 2002)
Chronic respiratory, cardiac, renal or liver disease and diabetes	Influenza and pneumococcal[a] vaccines
Cochlear implants	Pneumococcal[a] vaccine
Haemodialysis	Hepatitis B vaccine
Haemophilia	Hepatitis A and B vaccines

[a]Currently the 23 valent, unconjugated vaccine is recommended. Hib, *Haemophilus influenzae* type b.

PASSIVE IMMUNIZATION

The administration of antibodies collected from normal (immune) individuals gives instant but temporary protection against some infections. Preparations of human immunoglobulin enriched for immunoglobulin G (IgG) to particular pathogens are available. The donors and preparations of their immunoglobulin are screened for infectious agents (hepatitis B virus [HBV], hepatitis C virus [HCV] and HIV) and the serum used in UK preparations is sourced from non-UK (mainly USA) donors to decrease the potential risk of variant Creutzfeldt–Jakob disease transmission.

The half-life of IgG, the main immunoglobulin isotype that confers immunity, is 21 days. Although there is some variability between preparations, optimal protection beyond a month should not be assumed, although in practice some protection remains at 3 months. The variability in protection beyond a month is one of the factors that has led to the discontinuation of the use of passive immunization to cover staff who are temporarily assigned to high-risk areas and the use of passive immunization is no longer recommended for the protection of travellers.

Specific immunoglobulin is administered in order to give protection following exposure of non-immune HCWs, patients or close contacts to some pathogens. In a hospital or other healthcare setting, when a needlestick injury or contamination with a body fluid or tissue occurs, the source of the inoculum is usually identifiable and can be tested, with consent, for evidence of the major bloodborne viruses. When there is a risk that the source may be infective, passive immunization and/or antiviral agents can be administered to prevent the exposed individual becoming infected.

Information about the preparations available and their dosage and use is given in the *Green Book* (Department of Health, 1996) and also by the *Immunoglobulin Handbook* produced by the Health Protection Agency (HPA) (http://www.hpa.org.uk/infections/topics_az/immunoglobulin/menu.htm).

Generally, intravenous normal human immunoglobulin (NHIG) is used as replacement therapy and as an immunomodulatory agent in specific conditions, but not for prevention of specific infection. Intramuscular NHIG prepared by the Scottish National Blood Transfusion Service and issued by the Immunization Department of the HPA's Communicable Disease Surveillance Centre, certain Regional Health Protection Agencies and National Health Service laboratories, is licensed for use in preventing hepatitis A, measles and rubella. The same sources also issue specific immunoglobulin preparations for varicella-zoster (VZ), hepatitis B, rabies and diphtheria antitoxin. Human tetanus immunoglobulin and also human hepatitis B, anticytomegalovirus, VZ and rabies immunoglobulin preparations are available from Bio Products Laboratories.

The uses of intramuscular NHIG and specific immunoglobulin are given below. Passive or active immunization against mumps is not given post-exposure as there is no evidence that it prevents or attenuates the course of the disease.

Hepatitis A

Normal human immunoglobulin is recommended for use in household and other close contacts of an index case when the onset of hepatitis (indicated by jaundice) is over a week ago but, after 2 weeks, the use of NHIG is not likely to alter the onset of disease, although it may ameliorate the severity of the infection. If the index case is identified within a week of the onset of symptoms, hepatitis A immunization rather than NHIG is recommended. Hepatitis A virus (HAV) immunization has now replaced NHIG for the protection of travellers to high-risk areas. If an immunocompromised patient or patient with pre-existing liver disease is exposed to HAV, both NHIG and vaccine should be given. For well-defined communities, such as nursing homes or hospital units, NHIG should be used to prevent infection only if there is greater than a week's delay in identifying the index case *and* the exposure is clearly defined (e.g. contaminated food or drink), with HAV immunization being used in other circumstances.

Measles

Following exposure to measles, intramuscular NHIG should be considered in immunocompromised patients, pregnant women whose immunity to measles is unknown, and in infants under the age of 12 months. For immunodeficient patients receiving intravenous immunoglobulin at >100 mg/kg every 3 weeks, immunization with intramuscular NHIG is unnecessary, as they will have adequate antibody levels. If there is time, antibody levels to measles should be measured to determine whether or not NHIG is required. There is no evidence that NHIG prevents fetal loss in non-immune pregnant women exposed to measles, although it is likely to attenuate the disease. From the age of 6–9 months, infants in contact with confirmed cases of measles should have NHIG as soon as possible after exposure but, from the age of 9 months, they should receive MMR then continue with the routine national immunization schedule after an interval of 3 months. Up to the age of 6 months, infants should be protected by maternal antibody unless the mother did not receive measles or MMR immunizations, in which case NHIG should be considered.

Polio

There is no evidence that NHIG reduces the chance of paralysis if given to immunocompromised patients accidentally exposed to live polio vaccine or to close contacts who have had the live vaccine. It is recommended that exposed immunocompromised patients have antibodies levels checked immediately and be given NHIG. Weekly stool samples should be checked for poliovirus and NHIG given every 3 weeks until the stool is negative for virus for 2 consecutive weeks. If the exposed patient is antibody positive to all three virus types, or the recipient of the live vaccine is a school-age child, NHIG need not be given. If the patient is antibody negative or equivocal to one or more poliovirus types, a primary course of immunization with injectable polio vaccine should be given.

Rubella

The use of NHIG in non-immune pregnant women is recommended when termination of pregnancy for proven rubella infection is unacceptable. NHIG does not prevent infection in the pregnant woman but may reduce the risk to the fetus. The risk of intrauterine transmission from mother to fetus depends on the gestational age:

- <11 weeks – 90 per cent;
- 11–16 weeks – 20 per cent;
- 16–20 weeks – minimal risk of deafness only;
- >20 weeks – no increased risk.

Vaccines for MMR or rubella are ineffective for post-exposure prophylaxis.

Hepatitis B

The use of hepatitis B passive and active immunization in cases of exposure are summarized here with more details given in Chapter 9. Hepatitis B immunoglobulin (HBIG) is given with vaccination (at separate sites) and does not interfere with the formation of an active immune response. For those individuals already vaccinated against HBV and who have anti-HBsAg levels <100 mIU/mL 3 months after the third dose, a booster dose of vaccine without immunoglobulin should be given (unless the booster was given <12 months previously). For non-responders or those only recently immunized, HBIG should be given and repeated after 1 month unless the source is confirmed as HBsAg negative.

Specific human hepatitis B immunoglobulin (with vaccination) is indicated in:

- the newborn of mothers who are carriers of HBV, or who have had a recent acute infection with HBV and are consequently HBsAg positive;
- all individuals who are exposed to material containing HBsAg through percutaneous inoculation (e.g. needlestick, bite), mucous membranes (eyes or mouth) or non-intact skin (open wound, dermatitis);

• sexual contacts of individuals who have acute or newly diagnosed chronic HBV seen within 1 week of last unprotected sexual contact.

Immunization alone is undertaken for neonates whose mother is HBeAg negative and anti-HBe positive.

Varicella-zoster

Varicella-zoster specific human immunoglobulin (VZIG) is indicated for protection of non-immune individuals or those at risk of severe varicella infection who have been in close contact with an infective index case (CMO, 2003). Infective cases have one or more of the following features: acute chickenpox, disseminated zoster or exposed lesions (e.g. ophthalmic), immunosuppression with zoster (in which case there may be increased viral shedding). The index case with chickenpox is considered infective from 48 hours before the appearance of the rash until vesicles have stopped cropping and all lesions have crusted, whilst those with zoster are infective from the day of onset of the rash until crusting. Close contact is defined as being in the same room (includes classrooms and 2–4 bedded wards) for 15 minutes or more or having face-to-face contact with the index case. The administration of VZIG should also be considered for susceptible high-risk contacts in larger wards when the degree of contact may not be well defined.

Varicella infection poses a risk to immunosuppressed patients, neonates and pregnant women. After exposure to an index case, urgent VZ antibody testing should be arranged but if the results will not be available for 7 days or longer, VZIG should be given immediately if indicated rather than waiting for the result. Immunosuppressed patients include the following.

• those undergoing treatment with chemotherapy or generalized radiotherapy or immunosuppressed post organ or bone marrow transplantation;
• children who, in the previous 3 months, have received oral or rectal steroids at a daily dose of 2 mg/kg per day for at least 1 week or 1 mg/kg per day for 1 month (or equivalent doses);
• adults who have received approximately 40 mg of prednisolone per day for more than 1 week in the previous 3 months;
• patients with impaired T-cell immunity such as those with severe combined immunodeficiency, Di George syndrome or HIV infection with a low CD4 T-cell count (immunodeficient or suppressed patients already receiving NHIG do not require VZIG);
• neonates whose mothers develop chickenpox within 7 days before and 7 days after delivery (VZ status of the neonate is not required) or neonates who are VZ negative and exposed to chickenpox or zoster in the first 7 days, or any infant who is exposed while still requiring intensive or

prolonged special care nursing (infants born before 28 weeks' gestation or who have had extensive transfusion may lack maternal antibody and VZ antibody testing is recommended for these cases if they are exposed, irrespective of a history of maternal infection);

• pregnant women who have not had chickenpox and who are VZ antibody negative and exposed at any stage of pregnancy, provided the VZIG can be administered within 10 days of exposure.

Anti-viral treatment alone may be required for patients in whom an attenuation of the attack may be desirable (e.g. patients with cystic fibrosis). VZIG has not been shown to be effective for treatment of severe varicella infection.

Diphtheria

Diphtheria antitoxin is no longer used for diphtheria prophylaxis in the UK, only for the treatment of confirmed or suspected cases. The antitoxin is prepared from horse immunoglobulin so intradermal (0.02 mL of 1:10–1:100 dilution) testing or topical application to the eye (1 drop of 1:10 dilution) is required before administration to ensure the patient is not hypersensitive to horse serum. Contacts of cases are vaccinated and given antibiotic prophylaxis, not the antitoxin.

Rabies

Administration of human rabies immunoglobulin (HRIG) is used to treat individuals exposed to rabies virus. The risk of rabies depends on previous immunization and also varies from country to country, but only bat bites (and not bites or scratches from other indigenous animals in the UK) are potential exposures. The nature of the exposure, as well as the animal source, also determines whether or not HRIG is indicated.

• If the animal is rabid at the time of exposure, but there are no skin lesions or the contact is indirect, no treatment is indicated.
• If there is licking of the skin with scratches or abrasions or minor bites, and the animal is suspected of being rabid, vaccination should be started but stopped if the animal can be observed for 15 days and is found to be healthy. If rabies is confirmed in the animal, then vaccination should be completed and HRIG given. If the animal is unavailable for observation or rabid (risk varies with country where contact occurs), vaccination and HRIG should be given.
• If there is licking of mucosa, major or multiple bites on face, head, finger or neck, then vaccine and HRIG should be administered but stopped if the animal can be observed for 15 days and is found to be healthy (otherwise continue with vaccine and HRIG).

Tetanus

Two tetanus immunoglobulin (TIG) preparations are available. Intramuscular TIG is used for prophylaxis in cases where there is a risk of infection with tetanus and intravenous TIG is used for the treatment of tetanus.

A tetanus-prone wound (TPW) is any open wound or burn sustained more than 6 hours before its treatment or one that shows (irrespective of the duration of the wound) a significant degree of devitalized tissue, a puncture-type wound, one that has been in contact with soil or manure likely to harbour tetanus organisms, or a wound where there is clinical evidence of sepsis. The decision to administer TIG and/or a vaccine boost also depends on the patient's immunity to tetanus:

- For a fully immunized patient (Table 10.1) who has a clean wound or a TPW, no vaccine or TIG is required unless the patient is immunosuppressed or immunodeficient and may not have protective tetanus antibody, in which case, intramuscular TIG is administered.
- For a patient who has had the primary immunizations to tetanus but not yet reached the time when their boosters are due, no vaccine is required for a clean or TPW (but it may be expedient to immunize if close to the date when the routine boost is due) and TIG should only be given to an immunocompromised patient with a TPW.
- For a patient whose primary immunization is incomplete or whose boosters are not up to date, a complete course of tetanus boosters should be given for either a clean wound or a TPW, and a dose of TIG given in addition for a TPW.
- For a patient who has not been immunized or whose immunization status is unknown, immediate vaccination should be given for clean wounds and a full immunization schedule followed if it is confirmed that prior immunization has not occurred. For a TPW, the patient should receive immediate vaccination and full immunization (if required) as well as TIG.

Combined adsorbed tetanus/low-dose diphtheria vaccine should be used in the vaccination of adults and adolescents (>10 years of age) who require primary immunization or boosting.

SAFETY OF VACCINES

There are contraindications to specific vaccines that are detailed in the *Green Book* but this section deals with some of the more common queries that arise in practice (Department of Health, 1996).

Infection

Immunization should be delayed for febrile illness and/or systemic infection, but not for minor infections. This is not because of an increased risk of an adverse event but because responses to immunization are likely to be sub-optimal in severe infection.

Egg allergy

This is not a contraindication to MMR (or single component), there being very rare reactions to excipients such as gelatine only (Fox and Lack, 2003). Severe egg allergy is a contraindication to influenza and yellow fever vaccines.

MMR and autism

There is no evidence of a causal link between MMR vaccine and autism or bowel disease. Updates on any new data are posted on the MHRA website (http://www.mhra.gov.uk/Safetyinformation/Generalsafetyinformationandadvice/Product-specificinformationandadvice).

Impaired immunity

Live vaccines (MMR, live polio, BCG, yellow fever, live typhoid) are contra-indicated in those with impaired T-cell immunity, for example patients with severe combined immunodeficiency, acquired immunodeficiency syndrome (AIDS), immediately before and for several months after transplantation, patients on immunosuppressive treatment, etc. Precise definitions of impaired immunity are given in the chapter for each vaccine in the *Green Book* and on the relevant data sheets (Department of Health, 1996). For non-living vaccines, responses are likely to be reduced or absent in such patients and protection by NHIG or specific immunoglobulin may be required for protection to exposure.

Pregnancy

The use of some of the above live vaccines may be contraindicated at some stages of pregnancy, so always check before use. Non-living vaccines are safe in pregnancy.

Allergic reactions to vaccines

No vaccine should be administered if there is a prior documented severe allergic reaction to the vaccine or any of its components. In practice, local induration, sometimes with low-grade fever, is the commonest immune reaction to vaccination. This is most likely to be due to: (1) an arthus-type reaction that occurs several hours post-immunization and is caused by pre-existing antibodies (not IgE) that may have arisen by natural infection from previous immunization to that vaccine; or (2) a mild hypersensitivity reaction to one or more of the excipients. Acellular pertussis vaccine has been associated with an increase in local injection site reactions since its routine introduction but reactions usually resolve within 5 days. Repeated administration of foreign animal protein, such as horse antidiphtheria immunoglobulin, readily leads to sensitization and test doses to animal immunoglobulin must be given before administration.

Thiomersal in vaccines

Thiomersal contains ethylmercury and is used as a preservative in several vaccines: DTwP, diphtheria, tetanus, (now replaced by DTaP in routine use) and some hepatitis B and influenza vaccines. Concerns over the effect on brain development arose but a review of the evidence by the CSM has shown that there is no toxicity (Statement from the Committee on Safety of Medicines). Further data support safety of thiomersal in vaccines (CSM, 21/03/03).

Neurological conditions

Stable neurological conditions are not a contraindication to immunization. In all other cases, immunization should be delayed until expert advice has been obtained.

VACCINE FAILURE

In non-immunosuppressed individuals, the failure rate despite full immunization ranges from 1 to 15 per cent depending on the vaccine. The rate is higher for neonates and immunosuppressed patients in general. For HCW, hepatitis B antibody levels are measured routinely and, if protective levels are not achieved after two full immunization schedules, the worker's situation requires discussion with an occupational health physician and the HCW's local manager. A history and possibly investigation to exclude immunodeficiency or immunosuppression is required. A risk assessment needs to be undertaken and the HCW fully appraised of the implication of their lack of specific immunity. A protocol for dealing with exposure to high-risk fluids, etc. will be in place for all staff but, for an HCW already known to be non-immune, it would be prudent for passive immunization to be administered as soon as infectivity of the index case is confirmed.

IN CONCLUSION

Immunity to infection, whether conferred by active or passive immunization or by recovery from natural infection, never provides 100 per cent protection. It is therefore crucial that all HCWs, patients and visitors adhere to the guidelines on hygiene, sterilization, disinfection, isolation, etc. detailed throughout this book in order to reduce the risk of exposure to infectious agents.

REFERENCES

BCSH (2002) Guidelines for the prevention and treatment of infections in patients with an absent or dysfunctional spleen. *Clinical Medicine (Journal of the Royal College of Physicians of London)* **2**, 440.

Chief Medical Officer (2003) *Chickenpox (varicella) immunisation for healthcare workers* (PL/CMO/2003/8). London: Department of Health.

Chief Medical Officer (2005) *Changes to the BCG vaccination programme* (PL/CMO/2005/3). London: Department of Health.

Department of Health (1996) *Immunization against infectious disease; the Green Book.* London: Department of Health. Updated version is available online at: http://www.dh.gov.uk/en/Publichealth/Healthprotection/Immunisation/Greenbook/dh_4097254.

Fox A and Lack G (2003) Egg allergy and MMR vaccination. *British Journal of General Practice* **53**, 801.

11 THE ROLE OF OCCUPATIONAL HEALTH SERVICES IN THE CONTROL OF INFECTION

Tar-Ching Aw

INTRODUCTION

The different chapters in this book refer to infections associated with hospitals. The individuals at risk of acquiring these infections are patients and healthcare staff. Once a healthcare worker is infected, there are health implications for third parties, such as members of the family, co-workers and patients. When a patient becomes infected, there are similar implications for family members, visitors and their colleagues at the workplace.

Occupational health services for the healthcare industry play an important role in preventing such infections and managing infected staff. In the UK, occupational health departments for the National Health Service (NHS) are an integral part of hospital functions. Healthcare departments not based in hospitals, such as Primary Care Trusts (PCTs) and community health services, are also required to have access to occupational health provisions (Department of Health, 2001a). The providers of occupational healthcare may be in-house staff, or services supplied by out-sourced commercial occupational health organizations or independent occupational health consultants.

STAFFING OF OCCUPATIONAL HEALTH SERVICES

The occupational health team is multidisciplinary. For hospitals, the main professions represented are occupational health physicians and occupational health nurses.

Occupational health physicians are employed at different levels of experience and expertise. In the UK, the consultant occupational physician is on the specialist register as an accredited specialist in occupational medicine. They have usually completed a 4-year specialist registrar training programme leading to an examination and award of Membership of the Faculty of Occupational Medicine. There are also other non-specialists with experience in occupational health practice and/or with a Diploma in Occupational Medicine. The Department of Health has indicated that, where occupational health units are not led by a specialist occupational health physician, there is a requirement to ensure access to such specialist advice when required. The specialist occupational medicine contribution would be for strategic management and quality assurance, and for dealing with difficult and complex occupational health issues such as healthcare workers infected with human immunodeficiency virus (HIV) or hepatitis B (Department of Health, 2001b).

Occupational health nurses are registered by the Nursing and Midwifery Council (NMC) as specialist practitioners in occupational health nursing. A recent development is for nurses to be appointed within the NHS at a senior level as nurse consultants. There are currently only a handful of these posts for occupational health in the NHS. To be appointed as occupational health nurse consultants requires specialist occupational health nurses to have an academic qualification (at Masters or PhD level), or to be prepared to undertake training at that level.

Other hospital occupational health team members may include the following.

- *Safety practitioners*, who advise on hazards (usually with an emphasis on physical and chemical hazards), safety legislation and safe systems of work.
- *Manual handling trainers*, whose role is to provide training and advice on lifting and carrying of loads, posture and aspects of ergonomics. Their inclusion in the team is a recognition of low back pain and other musculoskeletal problems as one of the most common causes of morbidity and sickness absence in healthcare staff.
- *Physiotherapists*. With increasing evidence showing that prompt referral to a physiotherapist for patients with low back pain and other musculoskeletal symptoms facilitates recovery and return to work, NHS occupational health departments often have arrangements for affected staff to have rapid access to physiotherapy. This is done either through purchased sessions of physiotherapy time, or by special arrangement between occupational health and physiotherapy departments.
- *Counsellors*. Stress and mental health problems in the workplace rank alongside low back pain and musculoskeletal problems as the main causes of sickness absence in the NHS. Access to counselling support is therefore provided by many NHS occupational health departments. Some departments have in-house counsellors; others arrange for external counselling sessions.
- *Industrial hygienists*. These non-clinical specialists are not widely available as members of in-house occupational health departments. Their role is to recognize hazards, evaluate exposure and advise on control measures. This resource is often purchased externally, especially when a detailed assessment of exposure is required.
- *Risk assessment experts* who also advise on risks, legal requirements and cost–benefit considerations.

Some of the above professionals may be employed in an occupational health department or in several hospital departments. There is often some overlap in roles and functions.

HOSPITAL OCCUPATIONAL HEALTH SERVICES: LINKS WITH OTHER CLINICIANS

Occupational health staff in the NHS often have good ties with other clinical departments such as respiratory medicine, dermatology, rheumatology, psychiatry and mental health. The availability of these clinical specialists enables occupational health practitioners to consult them on cases seen, especially on treatment regimes, duration of treatment and side effects of treatment. Cooperation with departments of genitourinary medicine and sexually transmitted disease are valuable in dealing with issues related to HIV, hepatitis B and other sexually transmitted and/or occupationally acquired infections.

Just as for all UK residents, hospital staff are registered with general practice surgeries. Their general practitioners (family physicians) are important avenues for communication between the doctors who provide treatment and the occupational health departments who advise on prevention. This communication is particularly important for managing sickness absence, return to work, fitness for work and retirement on the grounds of ill-health. Several health issues related to the work of an infected healthcare worker have to be considered both by general practitioners and by occupational health practitioners. Some of these issues are:

- Does the infected worker pose a risk to patients, co-workers and others and, if so, should there be a restriction in work duties until the infection has cleared?
- Is the infected worker fit to remain at work, or should the individual be redeployed temporarily, or be given a period of 'sickness absence'?
- How long should the period of absence be, and what adjustments can be made at the workplace to facilitate an early return to work?

The general practitioner is likely to have full records of the history and current state of the patient's health, including previous and present treatment. The occupational health practitioner would be more familiar with the patient's work environment and job tasks. Coordinating their efforts and advice would be to the benefit of both the infected healthcare worker and the employer.

Another important link with regard to control of infection is that between occupational health, public health, communicable disease, infection control and microbiology. This is especially in the area of information and advice to groups such as staff (including clinical, managerial, administrative and support staff, and emergency response crew) and members of the public on outbreaks of infection, nosocomial infections, and development of contingency plans for possible epidemics such as pandemic flu.

OCCUPATIONAL HEALTH SERVICES: SCOPE AND FUNCTIONS

The primary focus of occupational health services is on prevention rather than treatment. The levels of prevention include health promotion, immunization, early detection of ill-health through health surveillance, limitation of illness or disability, facilitating early return to work, and reducing morbidity or mortality.

Occupational health departments provide a range of services, and the Department of Health (2001a) recommends that, for healthcare staff, the minimum requirements for the provision of occupational health are:

- general advice and guidance;
- health issues;
- safety issues;
- health promotion.

The occupational health services and functions that have a direct bearing on infection control include the following.

Development of policies and standards

Hospital policies and procedures dealing with infectious hazards are often produced jointly by occupational health and control of infection staff in collaboration with other stakeholders. Consultation with clinical colleagues will facilitate the development and promulgation of sound, consistent agreed policies on screening, surveillance, prevention and control of infection for hospitals.

In the UK, the writing of local policies on health matters should also take into account documents from the Chief Medical Officer and the Department of Health, advice from communicable disease and public health experts from the Health Protection Agency, and local considerations including financial commitment for purchase of items required to comply with the policies.

Vaccination of staff groups

Occupational health personnel are responsible for immunizing different categories of healthcare staff, and for determining and confirming the immune status for infections such as tuberculosis (TB), varicella, tetanus, mumps and hepatitis B. For bloodborne infections, where there is currently no available vaccine (e.g. hepatitis C and HIV), there is a UK requirement to determine the immune status of new starters in the health service, especially those intending to be involved in invasive procedures. The purpose is to confirm non-carrier status. Procedures and requirements for immunization are outlined in a Department of Health (Salisbury et al., 2006) publication on immunization against infectious disease. Occupational health practitioners also have to explain and clarify the purpose, value, and any contraindications and possible side effects of the vaccines to those presenting for immunization, and to obtain signed, informed consent as needed.

While annual influenza immunization for vulnerable groups is usually provided by general practitioners, it is deemed more cost effective in some hospitals for occupational health staff to administer the vaccine to their healthcare staff at work.

Occupational health departments can provide up-to-date advice to staff on requirements for immunization in regards to travel abroad. This covers information on the risks of acquiring different infections (e.g. yellow fever, malaria, cholera, typhoid and other foodborne infections, and HIV and other sexually transmitted diseases), and the relevant immunizations and prophylactic measures that are available and necessary.

Dealing with needlestick injuries

Needlestick injuries continue to occur within healthcare settings despite efforts to minimize such incidents (Health Protection Agency, 2006). They can result from the careless use and/or disposal of sharp devices. The consequences of needlestick injuries can be drastic, and this includes the risk of acquiring infections such as hepatitis B, hepatitis C and HIV, in addition to the psychological trauma experienced by the injured person.

Occupational health staff working with infection control personnel and infectious disease experts can provide advice and counselling to the healthcare worker concerned. The main role of the occupational health service is to assist with the investigation of the circumstances of the incident; provide occupational health information on the immune status of the individual; help in taking blood samples from the affected person and the source if indicated; advise on further preventive measures; deal with queries on restriction of work duties including exclusion from performance of exposure-prone procedures; and monitor the affected individual with regard to health status and ability to continue at work. Specific post-exposure prophylaxis and follow-up treatment for needlestick injuries are usually the remit of genitourinary medicine and/or infection control clinicians. The UK Department of Health has referred to the necessity for a specialist in occupational medicine to be available to hospitals for advice on infected healthcare workers, especially regarding matters arising from and related to work (Department of Health, 2005).

Occupational health and safety services are often involved in discussions with their clinical, infection control and managerial colleagues regarding preventive measures to reduce needlestick injuries. These include ensuring that the right containers are made available for the safe disposal of used hypodermic needles and other 'sharps' and clinical waste. There are also possibilities for introducing safer needles such as those with a retracting protective sleeve.

Through occupational health statistics on sickness absence and reasons for staff consultations, trends in the occurrence of needlestick injuries and infections as a cause of sickness absence can be tracked. This can provide an indication of the effectiveness of preventive measures and can be useful for a review of existing strategies.

HEALTH SURVEILLANCE AND MAINTENANCE OF IMMUNE STATUS

Occupational health surveillance applies to staff exposed to infectious hazards. Occupational health departments have a responsibility for maintaining full immunization records for members of staff and to provide the immunization history should the staff member have to relocate to work at a different hospital. They need to ensure that, where booster doses of vaccine are required, there is a recall system that will enable timely provision of booster doses. The use of individual credit-card-sized electronic data storage cards ('smart cards') for doctors has been trialled in the UK health service in an attempt to retain up-to-date information, including immunization records with the individual doctor. However, several problems have been experienced with the implementation of use of these cards, including availability of cards and card readers, training of staff who will be responsible for entering and retrieving data, security of the data and cards, and accuracy, updating and completeness of stored information.

Hazard identification, risk assessment, elimination and control of infection

Identification and reduction of infection risks to patients and to staff in health-care is an important target for hospitals. This applies to nosocomial infections as methicillin-resistant *Staphylococcus aureus* (MRSA) and *Clostridium difficile*, both of which can cause septicaemia and death in patients. Hospital staff may be carriers of MRSA, and measures to eliminate carrier status have involved occupational health departments in taking swabs from the skin of staff, and then treating them if they are found to be MRSA carriers. This process has practical difficulties in that re-colonization can occur and that the procedures alone do not necessarily prevent MRSA infection among patients.

Advice on hazards and risks

With their background training in toxicology and risk assessment, occupational health practitioners are well-placed to provide advice, not only on infection risks, but also on the choice of measures that can be used to reduce such risks. For example, the previous use of glutaraldehyde as a disinfectant for sterilizing endoscopes led to several documented cases of occupational asthma and dermatitis (Health and Safety Executive, 1997). The risks were reduced by reduction of exposure and use of other non-aldehyde alternatives. These replacement disinfectants have to be effective, non-damaging to instruments and not pose a risk to the health of users. Occupational health input contributed to recognition of the risks and preventive measures to reduce the risk from this hazard particularly in endoscopy units.

Pre-placement assessments

In the UK, all new starters in hospitals have a pre-employment assessment. This is performed by occupational health services, with the complexity of assessments varying from the use of a short self-completed paper health questionnaire to a nurse-administered interview. The value of such assessments has been debated, as <1 per cent of NHS job applicants are rejected as being 'unfit' (Whitaker and Aw, 1995). With the implementation of the Disability Discrimination Act, there is now a tendency for employers, including the NHS, to make greater efforts to consider suitable adjustments at the workplace for qualified job applicants, regardless of disease or disability.

A major consideration for hospital occupational health services is to ensure that new starters do not pose a risk to themselves and particularly to third parties such as patients, colleagues and visitors. Some examples are hepatitis B carriers proposing to perform invasive procedures; clinicians who have TB, especially those from highly endemic areas of the world; and HIV-infected immunocompromised staff intending to work in infectious disease wards.

Advice on choice and provision of personal protective equipment

There is UK health and safety legislation on the choice of appropriate personal protective equipment (PPE) for prevention of occupational injuries and diseases including infections. The Personal Protective Equipment at Work Regulations 1992 puts an onus on employers to provide protective devices and on employees to use them. PPE is usually regarded as the last option of choice for prevention, primarily because there are usually other more effective measures in the hierarchy of control of exposure to workplace hazards. Compliance with the use of PPE is often poor. There can be incorrect or improper use of PPE such that the extent of protection accorded is minimal or non-existent. Occupational health services have an important role in working with safety practitioners to provide information, instruction and training to users where PPE is indicated.

Respirators and masks

Respiratory protective devices have been used and provided for healthcare staff responsible for the care of patients with serious infectious diseases transmitted by close contact and/or droplet infection, for example, severe acute respiratory syndrome (SARS), avian flu and pandemic flu. There is a range of different types of respirators available: from surgical masks to fit-tested personal issue respirators, to self-contained breathing apparatus. The more efficient but also more costly devices have been used for nursing patients with highly infectious diseases such as Ebola infection. The choice of masks or respirators would depend on the level of risk and extent of protection required. Occupational health services can advise hospitals and NHS Trusts regarding choice and availability of suitable respiratory protection for biological (and chemical) hazards.

Gloves

Gloves are widely used in healthcare to:

- reduce the risk of acquiring infection through direct skin contact between clinicians and patients; for laboratory personnel who have to deal with biological samples and specimens; ancillary staff who have to dispose of clinical waste; and
- reduce the likelihood of contact dermatitis in staff exposed to chemical agents.

Occupational health considerations in the choice of gloves in addition to their effectiveness, strength and durability, include ensuring that gloves do not cause dermatitis through contact allergy. This is recognized especially for powdered latex gloves, where skin and respiratory health effects can occur in sensitized individuals, who therefore need to avoid contact with these gloves (Ahmed *et al.*, 2004). Cross-allergy also exists between latex allergy and certain fruits and vegetables such as avocados, bananas, tomatoes and eggplant (Lee *et al.*, 2004). However, familiarity, comfort and ease of use, retention of manual dexterity and tactile sensitivity, have been reasons given by users against the replacement of latex with nitrile and other types of non-powdered gloves. Occupational health departments in hospitals are involved in the pre-placement assessment of new staff, and the assessment and health surveillance of staff with suspected allergy to glove material.

Other PPE

This includes aprons, safety boots and eye protection. Aprons protect the body against spills and splashes of chemicals, or blood and body fluids. Safety boots are primarily for physical and mechanical hazards. Goggles and safety spectacles provide eye protection.

Administration of medication to staff

Although treatment is not the primary remit of occupational health departments, there are a few limited instances where they may be asked to prescribe and dispense medication for staff, especially when prompt use of medication is indicated for prophylaxis. Good communications between occupational health, general practice and the individual is important in these situations. Some examples are listed below.

- administering antibiotics such as rifampicin or ciprofloxacin to staff (usually ambulance crew or Accident and Emergency staff) who have had close contact with confirmed meningococcal meningitis patients (close contact refers to procedures such as mouth-to-mouth resuscitation);
- dispensing treatment to clear MRSA colonization from affected healthcare staff;
- possibly providing oseltamivir to staff during an outbreak of pandemic flu. (Contingency plans for dealing with a possible outbreak have considered the use of occupational health staff in hospitals to treat healthcare workers. Clear guidance has to be agreed with regard to the criteria for deciding on individuals who need medication (oseltamivir is currently the treatment of choice), and those who need vaccination, especially when there may a shortage of supply of both vaccines and medication.)

Health promotion

Occupational health departments contribute to health education and health promotion campaigns in hospitals. In addition to giving advice and information to staff on diet, smoking cessation, sensible alcohol consumption, exercise and healthy lifestyles, occupational health services also promote practices that help in the control of infection. Examples are reinforcing messages to staff about proper hand-washing, and the use of soap and water and alcohol gel preparations to reduce hospital-acquired infection.

LEGISLATION AND GUIDANCE

There are European and UK laws that apply to the control of infections in the workplace, and occupational health departments are familiar with the requirements of this legislation.

The Health and Safety at Work, etc. Act, 1974 places a general duty on employers and employees to take reasonable care to ensure the health and safety of employed persons and third parties. Hence measures to prevent infection in healthcare settings, insofar as they may affect staff and co-workers, and patients, would have this statutory backing.

The Control of Substances Hazardous to Health regulations (COSHH) has had several revisions since it was first promulgated in 1994. COSHH includes pathogenic micro-organisms within their definition of 'substances hazardous to health'. Several sections of the regulations apply to the control of infection in healthcare. These include a requirement to assess the risks to health from work involving micro-organisms; provision, use and maintenance of measures to control exposure; health surveillance where appropriate; and provision of sufficient information, instruction and training for healthcare staff with regular exposure to micro-organisms (e.g. laboratory workers).

In addition, the Department of Health in the UK issues notes of Guidance, for example on immunizations (Salisbury *et al.*, 2006); and recommendations on practice (e.g. through communications from the Chief Medical Officer). The Health and Safety Executive (part of the Department of Work and Pensions) is the government agency responsible for enforcing health and safety legislation in the UK. It also issues codes of practice and guidance notes (e.g. in their 'MS - medical series' documents) on aspects of workplace health and safety, and some of these will apply to biological hazards and risks of infection. Some of these documents are available on the internet.

The Reporting of Diseases, Injuries, and Dangerous Occurrences Regulations, 1995 (RIDDOR) require that NHS hospitals as employers report to the Health and Safety Executive the incidence of a range of listed occupational illnesses. This list includes infections such as hepatitis, tuberculosis, legionellosis and any infection resulting from work in the course of treatment or investigation of patients. Occupational health services provide the necessary information to hospitals to facilitate the reporting of such cases and, therefore, ensure compliance with this legislation. Affected individuals can also obtain information from occupational health in regards to their entitlement for prescribed diseases benefits.

CONCLUSIONS

Occupational health services play an important role in the control of infection in hospitals. The range of functions is wide, and multidisciplinary team work is essential. Good liaison and communications between occupational health services and other healthcare disciplines, such as infection control experts, general practitioners and other clinicians, are vital to the success of preventive measures to reduce the risk of infection in hospitals.

REFERENCES

Ahmed S, Aw TC and Adisesh A (2004) Toxicological and immunological aspects of occupational latex allergy. *Toxicological Reviews* **23,** 123.

Department of Health (2001a) *The provision of occupational health and safety services for general medical practitioners and their staff.* London: Department of Health.

Department of Health (2001b) *The effective management of occupational health and safety services in the NHS.* London: Department of Health.

Department of Health (2005) *HIV-infected health care workers: guidance on management and patient notification.* London: Department of Health.

Health and Safety at Work, etc. Act, 1974. London: The Stationery Office.

Health Protection Agency (2006) *Eye of the needle: United Kingdom surveillance of significant occupational exposure to blood-borne viruses in healthcare workers.* London: Health Protection Agency.

Health and Safety Executive (1997) *Glutaraldehyde: criteria document for an occupational exposure limit.* Sudbury: HSE Books.

Lee J, Cho YS, Park SY et al. (2004) Eggplant anaphylaxis in a patient with latex allergy. Journal of Allergy and Clinical Immunology 113, 995.

Salisbury D, Ramsay M and Noakes K (2006) Immunisation against infectious disease. Department of Health. London: The Stationery Office.

Statutory Instrument No. 720. The Disability Discrimination Code of Practice (Goods, Facilities, Services, and Premises) (Appointed Day) Order 2002. Available online at: http://www.opsi.gov.uk/si/si2002/20020720.htm. London: The Stationery Office.

Statutory Instrument No. 811. The Social Security (Industrial Injuries) (Prescribed Diseases) Amendment Regulations (2007). Available online at: http://www.opsi.gov.uk/si/si2007/uksi_20070811_en_1. London: The Stationery Office.

Statutory Instrument No. 2677. The Control of Substances Hazardous to Health Regulations (2002). Available online at: http://www.opsi.gov.uk/si/si2002/20022677.htm. London: The Stationery Office.

Statutory Instrument No. 2966. The Personal Protective Equipment at Work Regulations (1992). Available online at: http://www.opsi.gov.uk/si/si1992/Uksi_19922966_en_1.htm. London: The Stationery Office.

Statutory Instrument No. 3163. The Reporting of Injuries, Diseases and Dangerous Occurrences Regulations (1995). Available online at: http://www.opsi.gov.uk/si/si1995/Uksi_19953163_en_1.htm. London: The Stationery Office.

Whitaker S and Aw TC (1995) Audit of pre-employment assessments by occupational health departments in the National Health Service. Occupational Medicine 45, 75.

12 SPECIAL PROBLEMS OF INFECTION

Christina Bradley, Georgia Duckworth, Adam Fraise, Gary L French, Savita Gossain, Peter M Hawkey, Donald J Jeffries, E Grace Smith, Mark H Wilcox

MRSA

Georgia Duckworth

Staphyloccus aureus is a ubiquitous organism, which can be part of the normal flora, but is also one of the commonest pathogens, causing infections ranging from mild skin sepsis to devastating life-threatening infections. It can attack the human host in many ways, still incompletely understood, and is capable of meeting most challenges. Sequencing of its genome showed that around 20 per cent consists of very variable genetic elements that spread extensively between strains, which may indicate why it is so successful (Holden *et al.*, 2004).

The introduction of penicillin in the 1940s dramatically reduced mortality and morbidity associated with invasive infections. However, in a very short space of time, *S. aureus* evolved resistance to the early antibiotics. In the 1950s, outbreaks of resistant 'golden staph' infections were commonplace in hospitals, many strains becoming penicillin-resistant through the production of β-lactamase. Again, the introduction of a new antibiotic, this time the β-lactamase-stable methicillin (similar to flucloxacillin), had a major impact on infection, but methicillin resistance was described shortly afterwards (Jevons, 1961). Resistance is due to the production of a low-affinity penicillin-binding protein (PBP), PBP2a, to which β-lactams cannot attach, so cell-wall construction continues. This is coded by the *mec*A gene, part of a mobile genetic element, the staphylococcal cassette chromosome mec (SCC*mec*). Evolutionary studies suggest that major strains of methicillin-resistant *S. aureus* (MRSA) are derived from a small number of clones, arising separately by integration of the *mec*A gene into successful epidemic strains of methicillin-susceptible *S. aureus* (MSSA) (Enright *et al.*, 2002). This may explain why MRSA defied some early expectations that it would be less successful and virulent than MSSA. Other mechanisms of resistance have a role in some strains with reduced susceptibility to methicillin through hyperproduction of β-lactamase or the presence of normal PBPs with lower affinity for β-lactams. These are distinct from intrinsically resistant strains and their clinical and epidemiological significance is unclear. Resistance has now also been described to the 'last stand' antimicrobials, the glycopeptides, as well as to a novel agent, linezolid.

Hospital infections owing to MRSA became prevalent in many countries during the 1960s. Gentamicin resistance was added in the 1970s, a period when the focus was on developing resistance in Gram-negative organisms (Shanson, 1981). New types of MRSA became apparent in the 1980s, described as 'epidemic' strains, or EMRSA, in the UK. EMRSA-1 affected England in the early 1980s and was superseded by other strains. EMRSA-15 and -16 become dominant in the 1990s, when MRSA rose from less than 5 per cent of all *S. aureus* bacteraemias to over 40 per cent by the end of the decade (Figure 12.1). The factors influencing the changing prevalence of particular strains are poorly understood. The UK was not alone in experiencing these increases in MRSA prevalence; reports from other countries indicated that MRSA is the organism most commonly reported as causing outbreaks of hospital-acquired infection and becoming increasingly multi-resistant. The situation has been described as a global epidemic, although resistance rates may vary widely within and between countries. European surveillance data show low rates in some of the northern countries (Scandinavia, Netherlands) and much higher rates in the UK and southern countries like Italy and Spain (European Antimicrobial Resistance Surveillance System, 2005).

In most countries, MRSA colonization and infection are mainly a problem in hospitals, the prevalence in the community being low (much lower than for MSSA). However, 'spillover' of hospital strains of MRSA into community set-

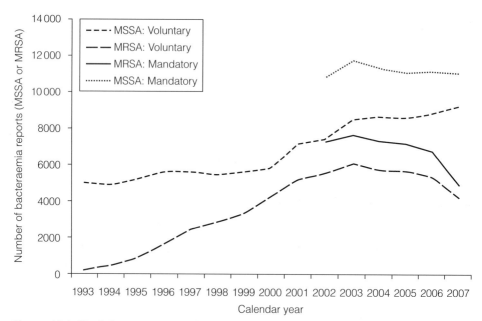

Figure 12.1 *Staphylococcus aureus* bacteraemias (methicillin-resistant *Staphylococcus aureus* [MRSA] and methicillin-susceptible *S. aureus* [MSSA]): voluntary and mandatory reporting systems, England 1993–2007. Source: Health Protection Agency.

tings, particularly care homes, has been recognized for a while (Cox *et al.*, 1995; Grundmann *et al.*, 2002). Long-term care settings now provide significant reservoirs for MRSA, the frequent transfer of elderly patients from care homes to hospitals 're-seeding' hospitals with MRSA. These patients often have chronic ulcers which, when colonized with MRSA, are very difficult to clear. In addition, more recent developments in healthcare are changing the interface between acute and community care: complex healthcare is increasingly undertaken outside hospitals, with home care for particular groups of patients, such as renal and oncology patients. These factors allow more transfer of strains between the two settings. In the past, control of MRSA has been less rigorous in the community setting, raising the issue of whether this should now change. Although residents of care homes may be colonized with MRSA, the evidence suggests that they are at less risk of becoming infected than their counterparts in acute hospitals. In this situation it is important to consider how to minimize the risk to acute hospitals without requiring excessive measures in residential care homes.

Further developments have been described recently, the appearance of distinctive strains of MRSA causing community-acquired infections. Some of these strains produced Panton–Valentine leucocidin, raising the spectre of severe skin infections and necrotizing pneumonia in the community (Dufour *et al.*, 2002). These tend to differ from the traditional hospital strains in having more diverse clonal lineages and being susceptible to more antimicrobials, although they are becoming increasingly resistant. They are causing significant problems in some countries, such as the USA, but are still relatively infrequent in the UK. They usually cause sporadic infections in previously healthy people, although some small clusters have been identified in groups (intravenous drug users, prisoners, sports teams and gay men). Younger people tend to be affected and infection is probably related to activities that damage the skin through cuts and abrasions. Transfer to the healthcare setting has also been described. MRSA has also been described in domestic animals, but it is not clear whether household pets have acquired the organism from their owners. The prevalence is considered to be low, although there is little information on this.

COLONIZATION AND INFECTION

Colonized or infected people are the main source of MRSA. Like MSSA, the anterior nares are the main ecological niche for *S. aureus*. It is likely that there is heterogeneity in terms of carriage in the human population: some people normally carrying *S. aureus*, others rarely and some intermittently. The extent to which this applies to MRSA is unknown. Rates of infection tend to be higher in carriers than non-carriers; infections are usually due to the colonizing strain. The role of nasal carriage is probably more important in terms of seeding other skin sites and causing infection elsewhere in that individual, rather than in causing direct transmission (other than in those with an upper respiratory tract infection). Eradication of carriage through decontamination regimens, such as nasal mupirocin, is associated with a reduction in infection rates in particular patient groups. Other carriage sites include the axillae, perineum, throat and areas of damaged skin. Carriage may be widespread; such carriers are more likely to be 'shedders' or 'dispersers' of skin squames containing staphylococci into the environment. Males are more likely to be carriers and shedders than females. Colonization may last a long time and rates may vary within different institutions. In addition, the ratio of infection to colonization may vary widely. This is likely to reflect differences in strains, risk factors and control measures. Colonization in healthcare workers is usually considered to be transient, unless other risk factors are present, such as dermatitis. However, transient carriage can also result in transmission from staff to patient. Colonization tends to be relatively uncommon in healthy contacts outside hospital, such as relatives. Most transmission is through contact spread (directly via hands or indirectly through fomites), but airborne transmission may occur. Airborne spread is more likely to occur from those who are heavily colonized, particularly if dermatitis is present. This poses a special hazard for control. Staphylococci may survive in dust and dry conditions for prolonged periods, and are often found in the environment of positive patients. However, there is a relative scarcity of literature suggesting that the environment is an important factor in transmission. This is likely to be more of a risk in units caring for especially vulnerable patients, such as burns units.

Broken skin is a particular risk factor for colonization and infection, whether the site of abrasions, cuts, chronic ulcers, injecting drug use, eczema or burns. Risk factors for MRSA colonization and infection are generally similar to those for MSSA, but ones which are more specific for MRSA include long length of stay in hospital, treatment in a high-risk unit (critical care, burns and certain surgical units), previous antimicrobials, severe underlying disease and exposure to MRSA. There are indications that exposure to certain antimicrobials, such as third-generation cephalosporins and fluoroquinolones, is more likely to be associated with MRSA colonization and infection. High bed occupancy, many inter-unit transfers and low staffing levels are likely to contribute to the difficulties controlling spread of infection.

WHY CONTROL MRSA?

The control of MRSA can be controversial, as there is a lack of robust evidence for some of the main interventions. Furthermore, containment strategies may be disruptive and expensive, and impact on other targets for the institution. Added to this, it is not always possible to predict the course of events after the introduction of a strain whether sporadic, endemic or epidemic infection will result. Initially, it was also believed that MRSA would be less transmissible and virulent than MSSA. In these circumstances it is perhaps not surprising that there has been much debate about whether it is worth controlling MRSA and the most (cost-) effective approach, particularly when MRSA has become endemic in an institution.

However, the following should enable reconsideration of the importance of MRSA control to protect the most vulnerable patients and to safeguard current therapeutic options.

- Experience has shown that strains of MRSA can cause largely the same spectrum of colonization and disease as MSSA, including many of the severe toxin-related infections. Mortality and morbidity is equivalent to that of MSSA or worse (Cosgrove *et al.*, 2003).
- Many strains are eminently transmissible, adding to the burden of S. *aureus* infections in hospitals, rather than replacing MSSA.
- Glycopeptides are not as effective as standard anti-staphylococcal β-lactams in MSSA infections, rendering MRSA patients more vulnerable to treatment failure than their counterparts with MSSA.
- The main therapeutic agents may be difficult to administer, with poor penetration of particular body compartments and significant side effects. They are more costly than agents to treat MSSA infection.
- Vancomycin-intermediate (VISA) and vancomycin-resistant S. *aureus* (VRSA) have arisen in patients with pre-existing MRSA.

Yet, on the positive side:

- there is evidence that interventions can control spread and reduce clinical impact, and also impact on other multi-resistant bacteria.

In addition, the cost of treatment and extended admissions result in sizeable extra costs to health services.

SURVEILLANCE, PREVENTION AND CONTROL

Surveillance

Surveillance is a key element of an infection control programme, defining base-line rates of infection and enabling the identification of changing trends and untoward events. The objectives of the surveillance need to be clear and appropriate to the needs of users. How surveillance is undertaken, the information collected, the level of accuracy and validation all need to be suitable for their purpose: methods that are appropriate for monitoring the situation in an individual hospital unit over time may not be sufficiently rigorous for national benchmarking purposes. Surveillance has many uses, such as convincing decision-makers of the need for action, justifying the need for further resources, defence against litigation, demonstrating that the service is satisfying national standards, and staff training. However, in recent years, surveillance has become the Government's tool to drive down MRSA rates in UK hospitals in the light of high rates of infection and growing public concern. Surveillance of S. *aureus* bacteraemia has become mandatory. This has been allied to the setting of targets and publication of hospital infection rates, coupled with action on hospitals with outstanding rates in England (Department of Health, 2004). This action ranges from local performance monitoring to visits by Department of Health review teams and the setting of action plans.

Prevention

Prevention of MRSA colonization and infection is based on robust infection control, allied with antibiotic stewardship and rapid identification of affected patients and their containment. The foundation for robust infection control is handwashing by healthcare staff. However, healthcare staff do not wash their hands as often as they should, despite the efforts of infection control teams over many years. Campaigns now focus on alcohol hand rubs to make this easier, but there is increasing advocacy of a disciplinary approach (Goldmann, 2006). Although handwashing is crucial to the control of MRSA, early research established that air contamination could also be important in transmission, which determines appropriate containment measures to prevent transmission. There has been much work on an antistaphylococcal vaccine, some trials showing partial immunity against S. *aureus* bacteraemia in selected groups of immunized patients, but protection wanes and this is not yet ready as a tool for prevention of infection.

Control

A systematic review of the effectiveness of isolation measures indicated that concerted efforts that include isolation could reduce MRSA, even in endemic settings (Cooper *et al.*, 2003). However, despite numerous publications describing outbreaks and interventions used, few well-designed studies have assessed the relative contribution of individual control measures. Four sets of guidelines have been published to cope with the growing problem of MRSA in UK hospitals since the 1980s. With each iteration of the guidelines, the literature has been searched more vigorously and graded according to the strength of the evidence, but most of the evidence is still not robust enough for the strongest category of recommendation. Practice is still largely based on medical and scientific rationale and suggestive evidence, rather than on well-designed experimental studies – a problem also faced by the developers of guidelines elsewhere (Muto *et al.*, 2003). Conversely there is little to suggest that traditional interventions are ineffective, leading to the conclusion that current recommendations should continue to be applied until the research indicates otherwise. The UK guidelines started off in the 1980s with a rigorous 'search and destroy' approach, based on screening of patients and staff, and isolation of affected patients (Spicer, 1984; Anon., 1986). Various pressures on Infection Control Teams (increasing incidence against a background of poor senior management support, lack of isolation facilities, high bed occupancy rates, high workload) resulted in a more targeted approach, focusing on controlling MRSA in high-risk areas (Duckworth et al., 1998).

More recently, the focus has shifted again (Coia et al., 2006): increasingly healthcare-associated infection is seen as an issue of the quality of patient care and patient safety. Control of infection is 'everybody's business' and should be embedded in all clinical directorates, featuring in staff job plans and performance reviews. There should be clear individual accountability within a performance management framework. The key elements of the UK guidelines are: surveillance, antibiotic stewardship, standard infection control principles, and an active screening programme with isolation and decolonization of affected patients. This should be underpinned by robust laboratory methods for detection and susceptibility testing (Brown et al., 2005). There is increasing recognition of the importance of surveillance in the hospital's clinical governance framework and infection control programme, with a clear responsibility structure in clinical units for investigation and action on the results. An active programme of antibiotic stewardship is also central to prevention, particularly of VISA/VRSA, where affected patients often have chronic underlying disease and receive multiple courses of glycopeptides. This focuses on appropriate use of glycopeptides at the correct dose and duration, reducing the use of broad-spectrum antimicrobials, monitoring antimicrobial use and resistance, and ensuring key staff have designated responsibilities for action and staff education.

There should be active screening for MRSA carriage, especially in patients at high risk of carriage (for instance, those with multiple admissions, transfers from other hospitals or previously known to be positive) and units where MRSA poses a particular risk of serious infection, such as critical care, burns and certain surgical units. Screening in these areas should be routine and the Infection Control Team should consider whether this should also encompass other areas of the hospital. There should be consideration of increased screening of a particular area on the basis of positive screening results. Screening sites include the anterior nares, groin/perineum and sites of lesions/wounds/indwelling devices/tracheostomy. Sputum should be included when available and the umbilicus in neonates. Throat sampling should also be considered. The results of the screening programme should be reviewed by the Infection Control Committee. Screening of staff is not routinely recommended, but this may need to be considered in staff with skin lesions and if there are indications that staff carriage may be playing a part in continuing transmission. Screening should be coupled with decolonization and isolation of affected patients in a designated closed area, plus treatment of infection, as necessary (Gemmell *et al.*, 2006).

Decolonization is based on mupirocin ointment to the nares, and antiseptic bathing and hair washing, using chlorhexidine, triclosan or povidone iodine. Clearing throat carriage is more problematic, reliance being placed on nasal and skin decolonization regimens plus, possibly, antiseptic gargles or sprays. Occasionally systemic treatment may be required, under close supervision. Decolonization may be difficult in the presence of dermatitis, when clinical management should be discussed with a dermatologist. Attempts should be made to clear positive patients prior to an invasive procedure. It is not usually necessary to continue with decolonization regimens after discharge, although this may be warranted in certain circumstances, such as when readmission is planned. Clearance is normally deemed successful after three clear sets of screening samples have been obtained.

Isolation will usually be in single rooms or through cohorting, while consideration should be given to the provision of isolation wards, as it may be difficult to contain a growing problem in single rooms. Movement of affected patients within a facility should be kept to a minimum to reduce opportunities for cross-infection. Special arrangements need to be made if they are required to attend another department for investigations or invasive procedures. Communication of the patient's status and any infection control or treatment requirements is paramount on their discharge from hospital, whether to their home, another hospital or residential care facility. Other institutions should not refuse to accept patients with MRSA, as adequate procedures and facilities should be in place.

Vancomycin-intermediate *S. aureus* and VRSA usually arise from pre-existing MRSA reservoirs. The approach to control is similar to that of MRSA in a high-risk unit, with stringent application of infection control procedures and the addition of screening of other patients in the unit and exposed staff. There needs to be a high index of suspicion, especially in patients receiving multiple or prolonged courses of glycopeptides or those colonized with both MRSA and vancomycin-resistant enterococci. Timely reporting of VISA/VRSA cases to the relevant national authorities is crucial.

While the approach to the control of MRSA has changed in the UK over the years in response to changing pressures, some countries with low rates ascribe their success to an aggressive approach (Verhoef *et al.*, 1999). This would not be realistic in hospitals with an endemic situation, although it might be possible to work towards this through a process of progressively widening 'MRSA free zones' in a hospital, starting with the high-risk units. However, it is important that control interventions are not abandoned in an endemic situation, as there is evidence that an impact can still be made.

Glycopeptide-resistant enterococci

Gary L French

ENTEROCOCCI AND ENTEROCOCCAL INFECTIONS

Enterococci are common bowel commensals and sometimes also colonize the throat, vagina and skin. There are several species, but *Enterococcus faecalis* is the one most commonly found in humans stools and is responsible for about 90 per cent of clinical infections. In recent years, infections with *Enterococcus faecium* have increased in frequency, probably because of inherent and increasing antimicrobial resistance in this species (Murray, 1990, 2000; Moellering, 1992).

Enterococcal infections are usually endogenous, patients being infected by their own commensal organisms. Enterococci most commonly cause urinary tract infections, both in the community and hospital. They are also involved in abdominal and pelvic sepsis, usually mixed with other gut flora and following inflammation or perforation of the bowel. In hospitals they may cause wound or vascular catheter-associated sepsis. Enterococci are generally of relatively low virulence but they are often multiply antibiotic resistant, so have an increasing tendency to cause opportunistic infections, especially after prior antimicrobial therapy. In compromised patients they may be involved in serious infections, such as cholangitis, liver, abdominal and pelvic abscesses, bacteraemia, endocarditis, osteomyelitis and meningitis. In many cases enterococci are part of polymicrobial infection, and may be of less importance in pathogenesis compared with other, more virulent, organisms in the mixture.

In some studies enterococci are now the third most common hospital isolate after *Staphylococcus aureus* and *Escherichia coli*. They are responsible for 10–12 per cent of all healthcare-associated infections (HCAIs), 10–20 per cent of healthcare-associated urinary tract infections and 5–10 per cent of healthcare-associated bacteraemia (Schaberg *et al.*, 1991). Although most enterococcal HCAIs are endogenous, they may spread from person to person, initially causing colonization, followed by subsequent clusters of infection with the outbreak strain. Such outbreaks are difficult to identify unless organisms with unusual antimicrobial resistance patterns are involved.

ANTIMICROBIAL RESISTANCE IN ENTEROCOCCI

Enterococci are inherently more antibiotic resistant than other clinically important Gram-positive bacteria and frequently acquire additional resistances (Murray, 1990). They are more resistant to penicillin than the streptococci, owing to the low affinity of their cell-wall penicillin-binding proteins. *E. faecium* has higher penicillin minimal inhibitory concentrations (MICs;

16–32 mg/L) than *E. faecalis* (2–8 mg/L). Ampicillin MICs are about one dilution lower; thus *E. faecalis* is nearly always ampicillin susceptible while *E. faecium* is usually ampicillin resistant. Enterococci are usually clinically resistant to cephalosporins, they are not killed by co-trimoxazole and show inherent low-level resistance to clindamycin, the aminoglycosides and the quinolones. *E. faecalis* is inherently resistant to quinopristin/dalfopristin, although *E. faecium* is naturally susceptible. Furthermore, the enterococci readily acquire high-level resistance to ampicillin, the aminoglycosides, chloramphenicol, tetracycline and erythromycin/clindamycin.

Owing to their broad spectrum of antimicrobial resistance, enterococci may emerge following treatment with a range of antibiotics. In particular, they tend to appear in patients treated for Gram negative infections with cephalosporins, quinolones or aminoglycosides. Because of its more extensive resistance pattern, including resistance to ampicillin, *E. faecium* is especially favoured by prior multiple-antibiotic therapy.

The glycopeptides, vancomycin and teicoplanin, are usually the agents of last resort for the treatment of resistant Gram-positive bacteria, but some strains of enterococci (especially *E. faecium*) have now acquired high level glycopeptide-resistance. Furthermore, the enterococci (again, especially *E. faecium*) tend to be the first group to develop resistance to new antimicrobials active against Gram-positive infections, such as quinopristin/dalfopristin (Oh *et al.*, 2005), linezolid (Gonzales *et al.*, 2001) and daptomycin (Munoz-Price *et al.*, 2005; Sabol *et al.*, 2005).

The gradual accumulation of multiple resistances to the whole range of agents normally active against Gram-positive bacteria has resulted in some clinical isolates of enterococci – especially *E. faecium* – becoming resistant to all currently available therapy. Such strains are rare, but it is essential to limit their further emergence and spread. This is particularly important because glycopeptide-resistant enterococci can transmit high-level resistance to the more virulent and clinically more important *Staphylococcus aureus*.

GLYCOPEPTIDE-RESISTANT ENTEROCOCCI

The glycopeptides have become the primary agents for the treatment of serious infections with multiply resistant Gram-positive bacteria, especially MRSA; Gemmel *et al.*, 2006). Glycopepeptides inhibit the formation of Gram-positive bacterial cell walls by binding to the terminal D-alanyl-D-alanine sequences of the developing peptidoglycan polymer, where their large size impedes the action of polymerases and peptidases involved in cell-wall synthesis (Barna and Williams, 1984; Reynolds, 1989; Courvalin, 2006).

Most Gram-positive bacteria are susceptible to the glycopeptides, and enterococci usually have vancomycin MICs of 0.5–4.0 mg/L and teicoplanin MICs one or two dilutions lower than this. Vancomycin was introduced in the

1950s and for many years little or no resistance was seen in clinical isolates until it was reported in enterococci in 1988 (LeClerc *et al.*, 1988; Uttley *et al.*, 1988). The emergence of resistance at that time was probably related to the increasing use of vancomycin for the treatment of MRSA, methicillin-resistant coagulase-negative staphylococci and for gut clearance of *Clostridium difficile* (Kirst *et al.*, 1998).

Vancomycin resistance can be divided into 'low-level' (MICs 8–32 mg/L) and 'high-level' (MICs ≥64 mg/L). There are several resistance phenotypes, the most common of which are high-level, inducible transferable resistance to both vancomycin and teicoplanin (VanA), and low-level inducible resistance to vancomycin alone (VanB) (Woodford *et al.*, 1995; Courvalin, 2006). Enterococci resistant to one or both of the glycopeptides should properly be called glycopeptide-resistant enterococci (GRE), but they are often referred to as vancomycin-resistant enterococci (VRE).

VanA and VanB resistance is encoded by transposons that contain the *vanA* or *vanB* genes, respectively. The *vanA* transposon is usually plasmid-borne but may become incorporated into the chromosome; the *vanB* conjugative transposon is usually chromosomal but may transfer to other enterococci directly or by a plasmid. VanA and VanB resistance phenotypes are most commonly seen in *E. faecium* and, rather less frequently, *E. faecalis*. The constitutive low-level vancomycin resistance seen in *E. gallinarum, E. casseliflavus and E. flavescens* is called VanC. There are other less common phenotypic variants.

The vancomycin resistance transposons contain a series of genes that encode the production of altered bacterial ligases and facilitate their action. These enzymes replace the normal peptidoglycan D-alanyl-D-alanine terminal sequences with D-alanyl-D-lactate (VanA and VanB) or D-alanyl-D-serine (VanC), which have reduced binding affinity for glycopeptides. VanA high-level resistance has been seen in enterococci since the late 1980s but has remained rare in other Gram-positive species. The resistance was transferred to *S. aureus* in the laboratory in 1992 (Noble *et al.*, 1992), but no naturally occurring high-level glycopeptide-resistant isolates of *S. aureus* were seen until 2002, and only four such strains have been reported up to mid-2006 (Appelbaum, 2006). These were MRSA that are presumed to have acquired *vanA* transposons from GRE (Appelbaum, 2006; Courvalin, 2006). The control of GRE is important in itself but is also essential for preventing transmission of glycopeptide resistance to MRSA and other Gram-positive pathogens.

EPIDEMIOLOGY AND RISK FACTORS OF GLYCOPEPTIDE-RESISTANT ENTEROCOCCI INFECTIONS

The acquisition and spread of GRE are favoured by glycopeptide usage. GRE infections are therefore most frequent in hospital units where glycopeptide therapy is concentrated, such as renal, liver, haematology, oncology, transplant and intensive care wards (Cookson et al., 2006). Vancomycin, cephalosporin and quinolone therapy have all been associated with GRE colonization and infection, and the risk increases with the length of hospital stay and the length of therapy (Montecalvo et al., 1995; Tornieporth et al., 1996; Tokars et al., 1999). Other risk factors include hospital size and sophistication (Centers for Disease Control and Prevention, 1993). These risk factors of prolonged hospital stay, prolonged antimicrobial therapy, especially with glycopeptides, severe underlying disease and treatment in specialist high-dependency units and larger hospitals are interrelated.

Renal and haematology patients often have repeated admissions (both as inpatients and as day cases) over long periods, often associated with repeated courses of glycopeptide therapy. These patients often become chronically colonized with GRE and are sources of outbreaks on these units.

Outbreaks with GRE can be polyclonal or have one or a few predominant types; they can be restricted to a single unit or can be more widespread throughout a hospital or a city (Frieden et al., 1993; French, 1998). Polyclonal outbreaks with multiple strains are caused mainly by sporadic endogenous infections in groups of patients with common risk factors; single or dominant strain outbreaks are usually the result of cross-infection. Outbreaks most commonly involve E. faecium but some outbreaks involving E. faecalis and, rarely, other enterococcal species have been reported.

Significant differences have been reported between the epidemiology of GRE in the USA and Europe. In the USA, hospital infections are common: the proportion of GRE among all enterococcal bloodstream infections in the USA rose from 0 per cent in 1989 to 25.9 per cent in 1999 (Centers for Disease Control and Prevention, 1999). GRE are generally less frequent in European hospitals where glycopeptide resistance usually occurs in <3 per cent of enterococcal blood isolates (Schouten et al., 2000), although in England and Wales, vancomycin resistance in blood isolates of E. faecalis increased from about 3 per cent in 1996 to 5 per cent in 1998, and in E. faecium it increased from 6.3 per cent in 1993 to 24 per cent in 1998 (Reacher et al., 2000). In the USA, outbreaks are mainly due to hospital cross-infection with epidemic strains; in Europe there is more strain diversity, suggesting polyclonal endogenous infection arising from the community.

Although there is some debate and the evidence is sometimes inconsistent (Acar et al., 2000), the use of the glycopeptide avoparcin in animal husbandry appears to have contributed to the emergence of GRE in Europe. Until it was banned in the 1990s, in the Netherlands about 50 times, and in Denmark, about 1000 times more avoparcin was used for growth promotion in animals than vancomycin for treatment in humans (Wegener, 1998; van den Bogaard et al., 2000). Use in animal feeds favours the proliferation of GRE in animal bowels, resulting in contamination of carcasses, usually with E. faecium of the VanA phenotype. These organisms enter the food chain and some may colonize the bowels of normal Europeans. For example, between 5 and 19 per cent of healthy Dutch people have stool colonization with GRE (Endtz *et al.*, 1997; van den Bogaard *et al*, 1997). When asymptomatic Europeans enter hospitals and are treated with glycopeptides, GRE may be selected out and cause overt colonization and infection. This results in outbreaks with multiple strains, sometimes associated with clusters of cross-infection with the more epidemic clones involved. In the USA, avoparcin has not been used in farming, and meat products and the non-hospital population tend not to be contaminated or colonized with GRE; this may explain why polyclonal outbreaks appear to be less common there than in Europe (Goosens, 1998).

OUTCOMES OF GLYCOPEPTIDE-RESISTANT ENTEROCOCCI INFECTION

Serious infections with multi-drug resistant bacteria generally have worse outcomes than those caused by sensitive strains (French, 2005). Although infection with GRE tends to occur in patients with poor prognostic risk factors, a recent meta-analysis has shown that in enterococcal bacteraemia vancomycin resistance is independently associated with increased mortality, presumably because of the reduced treatment options available in these cases (DiazGranados *et al.*, 2005).

EPIDEMIOLOGY OF HOSPITAL TRANSMISSION OF GLYCOPEPTIDE-RESISTANT ENTEROCOCCI

Colonization with GRE can persist asymptomatically for months and sometimes years (Roghmann *et al.*, 1997). Transmission between patients is often via the hands of healthcare workers that have been contaminated by contact with patient urine, faeces, skin or mucous membranes (Bonten *et al.*, 1996). Enterococci may also contaminate the environment around affected patients, especially those with diarrhoea (Boyce *et al.*, 1994), and may survive for several days. Surfaces and items that come into contact with staff hands may also become contaminated and may be sources for secondary transmission.

SCREENING FOR GLYCOPEPTIDE-RESISTANT ENTEROCOCCI CARRIAGE

During outbreaks, previously unaffected patients may need to be screened for asymptomatic carriage of GRE to help decide on patient isolation for outbreak control. Some high-risk units, such as intensive care units, transplantation and haematology/oncology units may screen patients on admission in order to direct later therapy of suspected Gram-positive bacterial sepsis, but this is a local decision. Attempts have been made to clear GRE stool carriage with oral antibiotics, but none has been successful and this is not recommended. Staff have not been reported to be sources of GRE outbreaks and should not normally be screened for stool carriage.

The screening specimen most often positive for GRE is the stool; rectal swabs have a lower yield. Other sites may yield GRE, including throat, skin, vagina, perineum, wounds, urine and vascular access sites. The more sites that are screened, the more likely it is a colonized patient will be detected.

The use of a selective medium containing vancomycin is recommended for screening (Hospital Infection Control Practices Advisory Committee. 1995; Cookson et al., 2006) but there is no agreement on which is best. A UK Working Party (Cookson et al., 2006) suggested Enterococcosell agar with vancomycin 6 mg/L, but warned that surviving colonies should be confirmed as GRE by other methods. Enrichment culture increases laboratory time and cost but there are conflicting reports on whether it increases sensitivity (Ieven et al., 1999; Brown and Walpole, 2003). Molecular techniques have also been used, but their value in outbreak management is unclear.

PRINCIPLES OF PREVENTION AND CONTROL OF GLYCOPEPTIDE-RESISTANT ENTEROCOCCI

The recent UK Working Party Report gives comprehensive recommendations on the control of GRE and should be referred to for details (Cookson et al., 2006). Guidance on general issues of infection control, including hand hygiene, environmental cleaning, waste disposal, laundry, patient isolation and outbreak control are described in other chapters of this book. The principles of GRE prevention and control are as follows.

1 Produce a written policy for the prevention and control of GRE.
   • This should be tailored to local situations and will have guidance on the following issues.
   • The policy must include a programme for dissemination and education.
2 Maintain high standards of hospital hygiene, including the following:
   • hand decontamination, when hands are soiled and between each patient contact;
   • standard aseptic techniques, including wound dressings and urinary catheterization;
   • standard procedures for the insertion and care of intravascular catheters and other devices and avoiding unnecessary intravascular access, since this is a common source of bacteraemia;
   • environmental cleaning, both as a regular process and 'terminal cleaning' of isolation rooms and bays after patient discharge;

- safe handling and disposal of patient faeces and urine, and other excretions and secretions;
- proper management and disposal of waste;
- appropriate handling and laundering of linen.

3 Encourage and maintain prudent antimicrobial prescribing.
- This is part of the normal hospital system of governance.
- In particular, the use of glycopeptides should be monitored and controlled. Details are given by the Hospital Infection Control Practices Advisory Committee. (1995) and the UK Working Party Reports (Cookson *et al.*, 2006).
- Governments should monitor and control the use of glycopeptides in farm animals.

4 Maintain active hospital surveillance of GRE.
- Use an appropriate 'alert organisms' system and investigate cases as they arise.
- Isolates can be grouped by species and antibiogram; if necessary, molecular typing can be performed by reference laboratories. For details on typing, see the UK Working Party Report (Cookson *et al.*, 2006).
- In England, hospitals are required to submit monthly data on GRE bacteraemia to the Department of Health, expressed as episodes per 1000 occupied bed days, and this is published nationally. Hospitals can compare their rates with those of their peers. Detailed discussion of the use of GRE bacteraemia as a surveillance tool is given in Brown *et al.* (2006).
- Increased numbers of GRE cases should prompt an outbreak investigation.

5 Perform a risk assessment when a case of GRE infection or colonization is identified.
- Action will depend on the settings and risks involved. Since enterococci are of low virulence, the cost and risks of control should be assessed against the probable benefits. Mathematical models suggest that greatly enhanced hand decontamination and the cohorting of nursing staff may be needed to prevent cross-infection of GRE in wards affected by endemic infection (Austin *et al.*, 1999).
- In general, single cases should be isolated with standard precautions, ideally in single rooms.
- Staff and patient leaflets should be produced and used to explain the details and reasons for patient isolation in appropriate language.
- Appropriate hand hygiene and environmental cleaning should be implemented.

6 Perform a risk assessment when more than one case of GRE infection or colonization is identified.
- The significance of more than one case will depend on the setting and risks.

- If appropriate, screen other patients on the same ward or unit and isolate asymptomatic carriers.
- Assess the likely origin of each case and whether cross-infection is occurring, using an organism typing method, if necessary.
- Limit the movement of affected patients between wards and units as far as possible.
- If an outbreak is identified or suspected, convene an incident/outbreak meeting to determine the facts of the outbreak and implement appropriate control action.
- Review the use of glycopeptides and other antimicrobials in the units concerned, and reduce or restrict usage, where appropriate.
- Agree on treatment protocols for serious GRE infections (see Cookson *et al.*, 2006).

7 Arrange to inform others of GRE status when a patient is discharged or transferred.

- Once patients are GRE positive, they may remain carriers for prolonged periods. Their notes should be flagged so that appropriate action is taken at the time of the next admission.
- If the patient is transferred to another ward of healthcare facility, the receiving unit should be informed so they can take the appropriate control measures.
- The patients and their general practitioners should be informed, and it should be explained that GRE carriage is not normally a problem in non-compromised patients, and is of no danger to family and other healthy contacts.

HIGH-LEVEL GLYCOPEPTIDE-RESISTANT *STAPHYLOCOCCUS AUREUS*

High-level glycopeptide- or vancomycin-resistant *S. aureus* (VRSA) is so far extremely rare, and the strict control of GRE will reduce the likelihood of further strains emerging as the result of interspecies resistance transfer. However, because of the potential seriousness of VRSA, if a patient is identified as having such an organism, very strict isolation should be immediately implemented.

If a case of VRSA infection or colonization is encountered, specialist advice should be sought. However, in principle, extensive screening of patient contacts (including staff, other patients and family and community contacts) should be performed and carriers isolated and treated for clearance. Because of the public health risk of such cases, even one case should be regarded as a major incident and immediately reported to appropriate senior management and local health authorities. Advice should be urgently sought from public health reference laboratories, who in the first instance should confirm that the isolate is indeed VRSA.

Clostridium difficile

Mark H Wilcox

INTRODUCTION

Since its identification in the late 1970s as the major infective cause of diar-rhoea associated with antibiotic use, *Clostridium difficile* has emerged as a sig-nificant healthcare-associated pathogen. Laboratory reports of C. *difficile* have increased markedly, partly through increased detection methods, but also asso-ciated with the widespread use of antibiotics such as aminopenicillins, second- and third-generation cephalosporins and (less so) clindamycin. It is now clear that many if not all antibiotics can induce *Clostridium difficile* infection (CDI). This should not deflect from the recognition that clusters of cases of health-care-associated CDI occur because of cross-infection. Its profile has increased further following multiple outbreaks of CDI, notably characterized by severe disease associated with poor outcome, starting in Canada in 2002. Similar out-breaks have occurred in the USA, UK and mainland Europe, resulting in heightened medical, public and political awareness. Community-associated cases have certainly been underdiagnosed because laboratories did not rou-tinely examine faecal samples for C. *difficile* toxins. The aetiology and epidemi-ology of community-associated CDI remains unclear, not least because of the relative infrequency with which symptomatic individuals attend their general practitioner and/or are tested. However, it is becoming clear that a significant proportion of community-associated CDI cases are not associated with recent antibiotic prescriptions or hospitalization (Wilcox *et al.*, 2008). The number of death certificates in England and Wales that mentioned C. *difficile* increased from 1214 in 2001 to 6480 in 2006. Between 2004 and 2005, and again between 2005 and 2006, the number of deaths involving C. *difficile* increased by approximately 70 per cent, although these data are likely to be affected by ascertainment bias (Office for National Statistics, 2008). CDI is clearly associ-ated with an increased risk of death in the elderly, in whom 80 per cent cases are seen, but a causal relationship is often very difficult to prove in frail patients with multiple co-morbidities. Patients with CDI have considerably longer hos-pital stays, resulting in significant excess cost and resource utilization.

Some C. *difficile* strains have epidemic potential that may be potentiated by greater capacity to cause clinical disease and/or to spread. C. *difficile* ribotype 027 (also known as NAP1) has spread throughout Europe (Kuiper *et al.*, 2007), and has emerged as the predominant strain in the UK, and currently appears to be responsible for many of the additional cases being seen in hospi-tals during the last two years (Health Protection Agency, 2008). Other recog-nized epidemic C. *difficile* strains include ribotypes 001, 047 and 106. Evidence suggests that cases of CDI caused by C. *difficile* ribotype 027 are more likely to be severe with increased complications such as renal impairment, severe colonic dilatation and sepsis. These features may relate to increased (duration of) toxin expression by C. *difficile* ribotype 027 owing to a mutational frame shift in the gene that controls the cessation of toxin production (Freeman *et al.*, 2007). The contribution of the binary toxin that is produced by this strain remains unclear. C. *difficile* PCR ribotypes 027 and 001 sporulate more frequently than other strains which may contribute to survival and spread (Freeman *et al.*, 2007). Thus, the mainstay of controlling C. *difficile* in the healthcare setting is to reduce environmental contamination and transmission (Chapter 6), particularly of strains that have epidemic potential. Other ways of reducing CDI risk are discussed in the next section (Fawley *et al.*, 2007).

PREVENTION OF *C. DIFFICILE* INFECTION

Antimicrobial exposure

Antibiotics are the most important predisposing factor for CDI. Diarrhoea typically starts within a few days of commencing antibiotics, although antimicrobials taken 1–2 months ago can still predispose to CDI, and very occasional cases occur where no recent antibiotic consumption can be identified. In such cases it is possible that antimicrobial substances in food could have impaired the colonization resistance that is normally imparted by gut flora. There is considerable controversy about the role of proton-pump inhibitors with studies showing apparently directly contradictory evidence for these drugs as a potential risk factor for CDI (Leonard *et al.*, 2007). Until this issue is clarified, it is reasonable for patients with recurrent CDI who are receiving proton-pump inhibitors to have this therapy reviewed to determine if cessation can be attempted as a possible way of reducing further recurrences.

Antibiotic therapy or prophylaxis damages the colonic flora and allows C. *difficile* to flourish, if it is already present or is subsequently acquired before gut bacteria return to normal. It is likely that the antibiotic resistance phenotype of the infecting or colonizing C. *difficile* strain is also a factor in determining CDI risk. Gut model experiments show that when the concentration of an antibiotic decreases below the MIC for a C. *difficile* strain, this is a stimulus for C. *difficile* spore germination with subsequent toxin production (Freeman *et al.*, 2005; Saxton *et al.*, 2009) Most published studies that have examined the risk of CDI associated with different antibiotics are flawed because of failure to control for potential confounding factors. Exposure to C. *difficile*, antimicrobial polypharmacy and duration of antibiotics are frequently not addressed as causes of bias. These flaws mean that it is difficult to be certain which antibiotics constitute high-, medium- and low-risk agents in terms of propensity to induce CDI. Reporting bias may complicate matters here. Despite these difficulties, it is clear that interventions to alter antibiotic prescribing qualitatively or quantitatively can be successful in reducing the risk of CDI. The number of antimicrobial agents prescribed, the number of doses, and the duration of administration have all been associated with increased risk of CDI. Excessive doses of prophylactic antibiotics also increase the risk of CDI (Kreisel *et al.*, 1995). In view of the potential for confounding variables to hinder the accurate assessment of which antibiotics are driving an outbreak or increased incidence of CDI in a healthcare setting, initial interventions should focus on reducing overall antimicrobial use. The repeated observation that antibiotics are over-prescribed reinforces this preventative approach.

Almost any antibiotic may induce CDI, but broad-spectrum cephalosporins (in particular third-generation cephalosporins), broad-spectrum penicillins and clindamyin are most frequently implicated. Fluoroquinolones have also been identified as possible risk factors for CDI, although there are conflicting data (Loo *et al.*, 2005; Valiquette *et al.*, 2007), which may relate to the increased prevalence of fluoroquinolones-resistant C. *difficile* strains (including C. *difficile* ribotype 027). Fluoroquinolone-resistant C. *difficile* strains are not a new phenomenon and clusters of cases crucially imply sub-optimal adherence to infection control procedures. Furthermore, C. *difficile* strains are multiply resistant and thus may be promoted by several antibiotics in use within an institution. Conversely, ureidopenicillins (with or without β-lactamase inhibitors) appear to have low propensity to induce CDI. In general, narrow spectrum antibiotics, such as penicillin, trimethoprim, rifampicin, fusidic acid and nitrofurantoin appear to have low CDI risk. However, if combinations of antibiotics or multiple antibiotic courses are prescribed in an individual patient, the benefits associated with the use of narrow-spectrum agents may not be realized. There are few published reports associating co-amoxiclav with C. *difficile* infection, which is noteworthy because of the widespread usage of this combination antimicrobial agent. However, data from the *Clostridium difficile* Ribotyping Network for England show that co-amoxiclav was the second most commonly named antibiotic associated with CDI cases (Health Protection Agency, 2008). There are conflicting data about the CDI risk associated with carbapenems, which possibly relates to the variable susceptibility of C. *difficile* to these agents. A recent prophylaxis study noted an excess of CDI cases associated with perioperative ertapenem versus cefotetan (Rani *et al.*, 2006).

A recent Cochrane systematic review examined the effectiveness of interventions to improve antibiotic prescribing practices for hospital inpatients (Davey *et al.*, 2005). The best evidence to improve patient outcome was for multidisciplinary measures that include restrictive measures to reduce antibiotic prescribing and so decrease the risk of CDI. Such measures include automatic stop dates, electronic prescribing, restriction of specific antibiotic classes, education and local prescribing policies. Regular feedback of antibiotic usage data and CDI rates to prescribers should be used routinely in high-risk settings. Current interventional data support the restriction of cephalosporins and clindamycin in such patients. Piperacillin–tazobactam, in preference to cephalosporins, has been associated with lower CDI risk in prospective and sur- veillance studies (Settle *et al.*, 1998; Wilcox *et al.*, 2004). Data are lacking to support the usefulness of antimicrobial restriction for other antibiotics/classes. Older fluoroquinolones (including ciprofloxacin and levofloxacin) have poor antianaerobic activity, whereas new agents, such as moxifloxacin and gatti- floxacin have significantly increased activity. However, fluoroquinolone resist- ance in C. *difficile* affects old and new drugs, and it remains unclear whether CDI risk differs between these antibiotics (Saxton *et al.*, 2009).

Specific prophylaxis against *C. difficile* infection

It should be noted that there is no evidence of a benefit of using metronidazole or vancomycin to prevent CDI (in patients receiving antibiotic therapy); indeed, this approach may actually increase risk. Probiotic bacteria and/or yeasts have been examined for the prevention or treatment of CDI, but without convincing evidence of benefit. *Saccharomyces boulardii*, in particular, has been extensively studied, with conflicting results. It is commercially available as a freeze-dried preparation, but batch-to-batch variation in terms of microbial virulence has been reported. Also, cases of fungaemia have been described in immunocom- promised and immunocompetent patients following administration of *S. boulardii*. Cases of cross-infection have been reported (i.e. from a *S. boulardii*-treated patient), highlighting the potential virulence of this yeast in humans. *Lactobacillus* GG has attracted interest, but trials in acute diarrhoea have reported conflicting results. Most studies of biotherapy have been uncontrolled or poorly designed. A recent randomized, double-blind, placebo-controlled trial showed a beneficial effect of using a proprietary yoghurt as prophylaxis in patients receiving antibiotics (Hickson *et al.*, 2007), but suffered from major methodological flaws threatening the validity and generalizability of the study (Wilcox and Sandoe, 2007). In summary, two systematic reviews have not shown sufficient evidence to support the use of probiotics either for the preven- tion or treatment of CDI (Dendukuri *et al.*, 2005; Pillai and Nelson, 2008).

TREATMENT OF *C. DIFFICILE* INFECTION

The first approach in the treatment of CDI should be to stop the precipitating antibiotic whenever possible. Spontaneous improvement in symptoms may occur in the minority (about 15 per cent of patients). In practice, it is rarely possible to stop only the CDI-inducing antibiotic, not least because it is not possible to predict who will spontaneously improve and who will have pro- tracted and/or worsening symptoms. The use of more rapid C. *difficile* toxin detection methods has exacerbated this issue, as cytotoxin testing affords a greater opportunity to determine whether diarrhoea is continuing. However, the emergence of more virulent C. *difficile* strains has also meant that CDI-specific treatment should be started as soon as possible, unless there is a strong clinical suspicion that diarrhoea is due to some other cause. Patients with CDI, especially the elderly, who have a raised white cell count (>15–20×10^9/L), renal impairment, sepsis or marked signs, such as abdominal pain with evidence of colonic dilatation, may be more likely to develop a severe infection. Serum lactate >5 mmol/L is associated with very poor outcome.

There are two main specific treatments for CDI: oral vancomycin 125 mg qds for 7–10 days, and metronidazole 400–500 mg tds for 7–10 days. Early studies examining the relative efficacy of these antimicrobials in treating CDI suggested little difference in initial response or time to resolution of diarrhoea. However, recent data have suggested that metronidazole may be inferior to vancomycin, particularly in treating severe disease (Ellames *et al.*, 2007; Zar *et al.*, 2007; Al-Nassir *et al.*, 2008). In the only reported study to date, higher dosages of vancomycin were not more effective (Fekety *et al.*, 1989), but dosage-ranging studies for metronidazole have not been published. Metronidazole should be used as first-line treatment only if there is no evidence of severe CDI, in which case oral vancomycin is preferred. Reduced susceptibility to metronidazole has recently been reported, which warrants close attention given the relatively poor antibiotic concentrations that are achieved in the colonic lumen (Kuijper and Wilcox, 2008). Adjunctive treatment such as oral rifampicin has not been shown to be of proven benefit. A prospective, randomized, double-blind trial study of oral metronidazole vs oral fusidic acid (250 mg tds) showed similar clinical outcome (Wullt and Odenholt, 2004). However, a high rate of fusidic acid resistance developed, which means that this drug should not be favoured in CDI. About a quarter of symptom-free patients continue to excrete C. *difficile* in their faeces, meaning that there is no sense in microbiological follow-up of such cases.

Severe *C. difficile* infection

The optimal treatment of severe CDI is unclear. Several groups have recently reported poorer clinical response rates in CDI, possibly associated with C. *difficile* ribotype 027 (Pépin *et al.*, 2006, 2007). High vancomycin faecal levels (64–760 mg/L on day 2) are maintained throughout the duration of treatment, unlike those seen with metronidazole treatment, where the average antibiotic concentration falls from 9.3 mg/L in watery stools to 1.2 mg/L in formed stools (Bolton and Culshaw, 1986). Metronidazole was undetectable in the stools of asymptomatic C. *difficile* carriers. Unresolved issues include the place of intravenous metronidazole (500–750 mg tds) and/or high dosage (500 mg qds) oral vancomycin in acutely ill patients. For patients with ileus or those with megacolon, intravenous metronidazole can be supplemented by vancomycin administered via a nasogastric tube (which is then clamped for 1 hour) and/or by rectal instillation of vancomycin (500 mg in 100 ml of normal saline administered 6 hourly via a Foley catheter inserted per rectum). Pooled intravenous immunoglobulin (400 mg/kg) has been used in some patients, but no controlled trials have been performed. In severe cases with caecal dilatation >10 cm or uncontrolled sepsis surgical intervention should be considered. Results have been better following total or subtotal colectomy compared with hemicolectomy or caecostomy.

Recurrent *C. difficile* infection

Up to one-third of patients receive repeat treatment courses for CDI. Administration of other antibiotics during or after the initial treatment of CDI increases the risk of recurrent CDI. A recent US study noted that albumin level <25 g/L and intensive care unit stay were also predictors of failure of metronidazole therapy for CDI (Fernandez et al., 2004). Notably, in recent outbreaks of CDI in Canada, it was reported that symptomatic recurrence rates, particularly in the elderly, increased (from 29 per cent between 1991 and 2002 to 58 per cent during 2003–2004; Pépin et al., 2006, 2007). DNA fingerprinting studies have shown that symptomatic recurrences are often re-infections with different strains (Wilcox et al., 1998). Recurrent CDI is significantly more common in patients with a poor humoral response to toxin A, but this assay is not available other than as a research tool. These data suggest that the common practice of switching metronidazole to vancomycin and vice versa in patients with symptomatic recurrences is not logical. Similarly, there is little justification for using experimental treatment regimens for a first recurrence of CDI. In practice, in the absence of severe symptoms or signs (see above), the first recurrence is usually treated with oral metronidazole.

Approximately two-thirds of patients with a first recurrence of CDI resolve following either metronidazole or vancomycin treatment. Patients with multiple recurrences of CDI are very difficult to manage. Other antibiotic exposure should be avoided if at all possible. Approximately two-thirds of such cases may respond to pooled intravenous immunoglobulin therapy (400 mg/kg given as a stat dose and repeated once at 72–96 hours if no improvement), although controlled data are lacking. In the absence of debilitating or severe symptoms, consideration should be given to managing cases who have failed multiple treatment courses conservatively under supervision, in order to allow the gut flora to recover. Courses of 4–6 weeks with tapering and pulsed doses of vancomycin have been used in theory first to kill the vegetative bacteria, to allow spores to germinate and then be killed. However, the success of this regimen may be due to the prolonged antibiotic course, preventing reacquisition of C. *difficile* during the susceptible period when patients' bowel flora remain ineffectual against opportunistic bacterial colonization. The probiotic option *Saccharomyces boulardii* is discussed above. Faecal transplants given via rectal or nasogastric tubes have been used in small series of patients with good results, but the logistics of such therapy are considerable.

As yet unproven alternatives to metronidazole and vancomycin include nitazoxanide and rifaximin. Nitrothiazolide is marketed in some countries for the treatment of intestinal parasites, and is active against C. *difficile* with high colonic levels achieved following oral administration. In a small prospective, randomized, double-blind study nitazoxanide treatment produced similar response and recurrence rates to metronidazole therapy. Eight patients with multiple C. *difficile*-associated diarrhoea recurrences were given a 2-week course of rifaximin therapy when they were asymptomatic, immediately after completing their last course of vancomycin therapy (Johnson *et al.*, 2007). Seven of the eight patients experienced no further diarrhoea recurrence. Tolevamer is a non-antibiotic polymer that binds to C. *difficile* toxins A and B; unfortunately, in two recent phase III trials, it was inferior to metronidazole and vancomycin (Louie *et al.*, 2007; Bouza *et al.*, 2008). Several other new agents including a toxoid vaccine (Acambis) and Par-101 (Optimer Pharmaceuticals) are undergoing clinical trials, but it is unlikely that any of these will reach market before 2010.

Resistant Gram-negative rods

Peter M Hawkey and Savita Gossain

INTRODUCTION

The 1950s and 1960s saw a rise in hospital-acquired infections caused by Gram-negative bacilli and while infections caused by antibiotic resistant E. *coli* and other Enterobacteriaceae (e.g. *Klebsiella* and *Enterobacter* spp) increased, other environmental Gram-negative bacteria, particularly *Pseudomonas aeruginosa*, were also identified as causing outbreaks in specialized medical settings, such as burns units and in patients treated with cytotoxic agents. In parallel with this increasing occurrence of clusters of hospital-acquired infection caused by multi-resistant Gram-negative bacilli (MRGNB), a number of newer antibiotics active against this group of bacteria were introduced, such as aminoglycosides (gentamicin) and extended-spectrum cephalosporins (e.g. cefotaxime, ceftazidime). The widespread use of these agents in turn selected resistance, particularly as a ready mechanism for the dissemination of antibiotic resistance via plasmids and transposons existed in Gram-negative bacilli. The further development of medical practice created patients highly vulnerable to infections (advanced intensive care units, bone marrow transplantation, prolongation of life in cystic fibrosis, etc.) and enabled a broader range of environmental bacteria with low pathogenicity in immunocompetent individuals to become important causes of nosocomial infections (e.g. *Acinetobacter baumanii, Burkholderia cenocepacia,* and *Stenotrophomonas maltophilia*). Recently there has been a massive rise in the prevalence of extended-spectrum beta-lactamase (ESBL)-producing Enterobacteriaceae, particularly of the CTX-M type(Livermore and Hawkey, 2005). Because of rising carriage rates in the normal population, these individuals may, particularly under antibiotic treatment, act as sources for the further dissemination of a community-acquired bacterium to cause outbreaks of infection in both the hospital and the elderly care-home setting. In order to effect efficient control of such nosocomial infections, an understanding of the epidemiology of the bacterium concerned is essential and we have sub-divided this chapter according to the different bacterial families involved. The epidemiology of *A. baumanii*, which has exceptional resistance to drying, is very different from that of *P. aeruginosa* on an intensive care unit (ICU), where contamination of the wet environment is by contrast much more significant. However, many of the control measures are common to all MRGNB and these are listed in Table 12.1.

Table 12.1 Infection control interventions that may be applied to MRGNB (including ESBL) in healthcare facilities

Intervention	Comments	Examples of successful control
SURVEILLANCE		
Routine clinical susceptibility tests	Early identification of clusters	Landman *et al* 2007
Patient screening[a]		
i. All admissions to high risk areas (e.g. ITU)	Early identification of cross-infection	Macrae *et al* 2001; Webster *et al* 1998
ii. During outbreak	Important to identify spread to new areas/efficacy of control	Mammina *et al* 2007
Molecular typing		
i. host bacterium (PFGE or rapid PCR methods)	Enables cross-infection to be confirmed and confounding unrelated isolation of same species to be discounted	McNeil, 2001
ii. resistance determinant	Common phenotype (e.g. ESBL) may conceal genetically unrelated resistance mechanisms with different origins and patterns of spread	M'Zali *et al* 1997
ISOLATION		
Contact precautions with gloves and apron	Essential intervention to interrupt transmission	
Single room isolation if possible, otherwise cohort		Laurent *et al* 2008; Warren *et al* 2008

Table 12.1 Infection control interventions that may be applied to MRGNB (including ESBL) in healthcare facilities – *contd*

Intervention	Comments	Examples of successful control
TRANSMISSION		
Hand washing		Casewell & Phillips 1977; Hobson *et al* 1996; Wilks *et al* 2006; Zarrilli *et al* 2007
Safe disposal of highly contaminated source fluids (e.g. urine, sputum)		
Disinfection of contaminated equipment and aqueous products in patient contact (e.g. gels)		Gaillot *et al* 1998; Gastmeier *et al* 2003; Macrae *et al* 2001; Hobson *et al* 1996
Cleaning and disinfection of the environment, particularly post discharge of single rooms	May be supported by directed environmental sampling and molecular typing of isolates	
Reduce patient movements, and staff movements if cohorting used		Laurent *et al* 2008
ANTIBIOTIC POLICY		
Restriction or removal of likely selecting antibiotics (e.g. 3rd generation cephalosporins, quinolones for ESBL, and fluoroquinolones and carbapenems for *P. aeruginosa*))		Furtado *et al* 2008; Kim *et al* 2008; Rossolini & Matengoli 2005
Surveillance of antibiotic use by antimicrobial management team with feedback to prescribers		
COMMUNICATION & AUDIT		
Minimum weekly meetings with clinical/nursing staff during outbreaks		Laurent *et al* 2008
Feedback daily of new cases and cumulative cases to clinical areas using process control charts		Paterson & Bonomo 2005
Identify impact on healthcare economy of outbreaks/endemic transmission of MDRGNB		Conterno *et al* 2007

[a] usually by plating rectal swabs on antibiotic containing media (e.g. marker antibiotic – cefpodoxime, meropenem, etc.)

ENTEROBACTERIACEAE (e.g. *E. COLI, KLEBSIELLA PNEUMONIAE*, etc.)

This family comprises over 20 genera and more than 100 species of which at least half are definitely or probably associated with human disease. A wide range of resistance genes have been identified in Enterobacteriaceae, which are frequently mobile via plasmids/transposons. It is the identification and characterization of these genes that is frequently part of investigations of cross-infection caused by MRGNB. Resistance phenotypes of particular interest are aminoglycoside resistance, ESBL production, plasmidic AmpC production, and carbapenemase production (Hawkey, 2008). Some of these phenotypes present difficulties of identification, in particular ESBL and carbapenemase production. ESBL detection is most frequently made by demonstrating the protection of labile substrates, such as cefpodoxime by clavulanic acid, either in an agar diffusion test or in a broth microdilution test in an automated system. Some automated systems are relatively poor at detecting ESBLs and the use of supplementary testing for those isolates that show an intermediate susceptibility by breakpoint determination is recommended (e.g. CLSI criteria; Clinical Laboratory Standards Institute, 2006); see http://www.hpa-standard-methods.org.uk/documents/qsop/pdf/qsop51.pdf for UK standard methods. The chromosomal cephalosporinase *AmpC* may become de-repressed and confer high-level resistance to extended-spectrum cephalosporins (typically *Enterobacter* spp or *Citrobacter* spp) or become mobilized on plasmids with consequent derepression (Philippon *et al.*, 2002), presenting a similar cross-infection problem to ESBL. Very recently, *K. pneumoniae* strains carrying the carbapenamase gene bla_{KPC} have emerged and spread rapidly, particularly in the north east of the USA and Israel (Landman *et al.*, 2007). As with other carbapenamases, which are seen less frequently in Enterobacteriaceae (e.g. IMP and VIM), problems may be experienced in detecting strains carrying such genes; the use of supplementary testing using either broth microdilution (Anderson *et al.*, 2007) or differential media containing selecting antibiotics, such as the CHROMagar KPC followed by confirmation using a specific polymerase chain reaction assay (PCR), is needed (Samra *et al.*, 2008).

The epidemiology of Enterobacteriaceae reflects their role as gut commensals of mammals that are capable of surviving in the environment for limited periods of time. This is particularly true of *Klebsiella* and *Enterobacter*, which may replicate in moist environments in a hospital setting (e.g. distilled water, multi-dose vials; Dalben *et al.*, 2008). Typically patients are the source of these organisms and gut carriage is frequently identified (Laurent *et al.*, 2008), although occasionally outbreaks are reported in which respiratory colonization with *Klebsiella* as a source spread by direct contact is more important (Hollander *et al.*, 2001). Cross-infection in ICUs has been particularly noted for *Klebsiella* and to a lesser extent *Enterobacter*, with a variety of resistance markers mostly, ESBL and aminoglycoside. *Serratia marcescens* colonizes the neonatal gut and, although this organism is found frequently in normal neonates, colonized babies in neonatal ICUs may become significant sources with spread via the hands of staff to colonize and infect other babies. The earliest report of successful control of such an outbreak was when faecal screening and ward closure were used (Lewis *et al.*, 1983). Secondary contamination of ultrasound gels, hand creams and other moist environmental sources have been shown to perpetuate outbreaks of *S. marcescens* in neonatal units. Other *Enterobacteriaceae* have also been identified in cross-infection episodes in neonatal ICUs, such as *Enterobacter cloacae* when patient colonization and secondary colonization of other aqueous vectors have also been identified (Dalben *et al.*, 2008). Plasmids and mobile genetic elements carrying ESBL genes can spread rapidly amongst different bacterial strains and species leading to the development of a complex epidemiology as was described on an oncology ward for TEM ESBLs (Hibbert-Rogers *et al.*, 1995). The control of MRGNB has been further complicated by the emergence in the community of widely distributed strains of *E. coli* carrying $bla_{\text{CTX-M}}$ genes, particularly belonging to sequence type 131, leading to gut colonization with CTX-M-producing strains of Enterobacteriaceae (Lau *et al.*, 2008). The introduction of these organisms into hospitals and their subsequent spread by cross-infection adds a new dimension to the control of MRGNB infections, particularly as *E. coli* has not been considered to be a common nosocomial pathogen (Conterno *et al.*, 2007; Warren *et al.*, 2008).

Outbreak control

Nosocomial outbreaks are usually recognized when a rise of a particular species of Enterobacteriaceae coupled with a particular antibiotic resistance profile are noted as part of routine surveillance. In endemic settings, the recognition of cross-infection is much more difficult than those with low incidence. Investigation involves plotting clinical cases as an outbreak curve and then instituting detailed surveillance on the affected wards to identify particularly faecal carriers and likely environmental sources, e.g. non-disposable cloths, liquid medications and cleaning agents. Molecular sub-typing is most important and this may be accomplished by referral to a reference laboratory for pulse-field gel electrophoresis (PFGE) analysis of restriction fragment length polymorphisms (RFLPs) in genomic deoxyribonucleic acid (DNA), which is the most widely used technique. Newer techniques using repetitive sequence typing, which are available in an automated commercial format (e.g DiversiLab™) can be of use.

Identification of carriers of MRGNB by rectal swabbing has been reported as an important control measure, particularly if isolates are subjected to molecular sub-typing (Pena *et al.*, 1998; Macrae *et al.*, 2001; Laurent *et al.*, 2008). The institution of barrier precautions often poses problems owing to the large number of cases occurring in clusters; however, cohorting has been described to be successful (Laurent *et al.*, 2008; Warren *et al.*, 2008). The presumed route of transmission of these organisms is via hands and seminal early work (Casewell and Phillips, 1977) showed clearly for gentamicin-resistant *K. pneumoniae* that the introduction of chlorhexadine hand wash resulted in a marked decrease in the incidence of gentamicin-resistant *K. pneumoniae*. The selective pressure of antimicrobial administration is an important driver of endemic nosocomial cross-infection by MRGNB. A number of studies have shown that restriction, particularly of extended-spectrum cephalosporins and to a lesser extent quinolones will result in marked reductions in ESBL cross-infection (Rice *et al.*, 1996; Kim *et al.*, 1998; Pena *et al.*, 1998; Furtado *et al.*, 2008).

The Swedish Strategic programme against antibiotic resistance produced guidelines in November 2007 utilizing a range of control measures in the hope that the proportion of ESBL-producing *E. coli/K. pneumoniae* will be maintained at 1 per cent (http://en.strama.se).

BURKOLDERIA CEPACIA COMPLEX

This group of bacteria is widely distributed in the environment and grows readily on most bacteriological media. The original species description was applied to bacteria that caused slippery skin in onions but modern taxonomic methods identify nine formally named genomovars by RFLP analysis of the *recA* gene (Mahenthiralingam *et al.*, 2001). Specific PCRs can also be used to identify genomovars (Whitby *et al.*, 2000). Since 2004, a further four new *recA* phylotypes have been identified (Mahenthiralingam *et al.*, 2008). Ease of growth in the absence of complex nutrients and intrinsic resistance to multiple antibiotics and disinfectants ensure that bacteria of the *Burkholderia* complex are widely distributed in both the natural and hospital environment (Mahenthiralingam *et al.*, 2008). The complex is particularly associated with disease in patients with cystic fibrosis. Genomovar III (*B. cenocepacia*) accounts for 60–70 per cent of all infections, the remainder usually being caused by genomovar II (*B. multivorans*) (Pitt and Simpson, 2005). Infections in other clinical settings are mostly seen in immunocompromised patients and in ICUs, where they may frequently be related to contamination of pharmaceutical and cosmetic products. One particularly large outbreak was associated with contaminated alcohol-free mouthwash used in ICUs (Kutty *et al.*, 2007). As with cystic fibrosis, *B. cenocepacia* and *B. multivorans* are most frequently encountered, the remaining 10 per cent being caused by a wide range of genomovars (Mahenthiralingam *et al.*, 2008).

Outbreak control

Clinical disease caused by *B. cenocepacia* in patients with cystic fibrosis is very varied, from asymptomatic carriage to septicaemia. A wide range of infection control interventions have been instituted, including identifying cystic fibrosis patients carrying *B. cenocepacia* and segregating them from other non-colonized patients (Saiman and Siegel, 2004). Cross-infection to patients without cystic fibrosis, in an ICU, has been identified and single-room isolation should be applied to patients infected or colonized with *B. cenocepacia* (Holmes *et al.*, 1999). *B. cenocepacia* is particularly effective at degrading parabens (para-hydroxybenzoic acid esters), which are frequently used as antibacterial preservatives, that property being specifically implicated in a number of outbreaks including one involving contaminated ultrasound gel (Hutchinson *et al.*, 2004). Infection control precautions rely heavily on standard precautions with hand hygiene, and the use of gloves and plastic aprons or gowns to protect clothing from becoming contaminated, but also must extend to decontamination of the local environment when lockers, beds and equipment associated with respiratory therapy (e.g. nebulizers, spirometers and bronchoscopes) should be carefully disinfected. Multi-dose vials of medication may also become contaminated, the organism growing in the presence of antibacterial preservatives (Saiman and Siegel, 2004). Outbreaks should be investigated by matching patient isolates with those from the environment and from likely fomites using molecular typing for which ribotyping has been found to be of value (Holmes *et al.*, 1999). PFGE following RFLP analysis has also been used as well as a number of rapid PCR typing methods (Pitt and Simpson, 2005). Multi-locus sequence typing has also been applied to strains to elucidate the global epidemiology of *B. multivorans* (Baldwin *et al.*, 2008).

STENOTROPHOMONAS MALTOPHILIA

This bacterium is widely distributed in nature and has been isolated from soil, water and milk. In the clinical laboratory, it is probably the most frequently isolated non-fermentative Gram-negative rod after *P. aeruginosa*, although its pathogenicity is low and patients who have been given broad-spectrum antibiotics frequently acquire colonization from the healthcare environment. The epidemiology is similar to *Burkholderia* spp and has been reviewed in detail elsewhere (Denton and Kerr, 1998). Typically *S. maltophilia* is resistant to carbapenems by producing a chromosomally encoding carbapenemase (L1) and has intrinsic resistance to many other antimicrobial agents (Denton and Kerr, 1998). Infections in patients with cystic fibrosis are well recognized, which may be attributable to the widespread use of broad-spectrum antibiotics including carbapenems. The environment is much more frequently a source of infection with *S. maltophilia* than *B. cenocepacia* and hospital outbreaks have recorded a wide range of sources, such as taps, showers, ice-making machines and nebulizers (Denton and Kerr, 1998). *S. maltophilia* can cause infection in patients in ICUs and has a poor outcome, independent risk factors being the duration of prior treatment with antibiotics and the presence of chronic obstructive pulmonary disease (Nseir *et al.*, 2006). In addition, patients with cancer, particularly when immunosuppressed, are increasingly infected by *S. maltophilia*, even those who have not received carbapenems or have other recognized risk factors (Safdar and Rolston, 2007). Patients with cystic fibrosis can carry strains acquired from other patients but there may be a correlation between environmental strains and the wide variety of *S. maltophilia* strain types seen in patients with cystic fibrosis. This suggests that the environment can be the source for primary acquisition, with secondary spread from patient to patient being relatively rare compared with *B. cenocepacia* infections (Denton *et al.*, 1998).

Outbreak control

Measures are very similar to those used for *Burkholderia* spp but should particularly concentrate on eliminating environmental sources. Sometimes simple interventions may prevent cross-infection such as the introduction of water filters to prevent the contamination of nebulizer equipment in a cystic fibrosis unit (Woodhouse *et al.*, 2008). Molecular typing is by PFGE; ribotyping has also been found to be useful (Denton and Kerr, 1998).

MISCELLANEOUS AEROBIC GRAM-NEGATIVE BACILLI

A variety of environmental bacteria may be associated with hospital-acquired infection; the two most frequently encountered belong to the genus *Chryseobacterium* (formerly *Flavobacterium*) and *Achromobacter*, now known as *Alcaligenes*. *Alcaligenes xylosoxidans* is the most frequently encountered species of the genus, typically colonizing the aqueous environment and is marked by having substantial resistance to disinfectant compounds, such as quaternary ammonium compounds and alcohols in which the organisms may grow to act as a source. Contaminated water may also be a source and outbreaks have been described involving deionized water in haemodialysis systems (Reverdy *et al.*, 1984). *A. xylosoxidans* typically causes infection in immunocompromised patients in ICU settings but it is very often considered a colonizing organism rather than a primary pathogen. It has also been identified in respiratory tract specimens from patients with cystic fibrosis.

Outbreak control

Control is directed at identifying the source, particularly avoiding multi-use disinfectant solutions and interrupting transmission by identifying infected/colonized patients and using isolation with handwashing (Schoch and Cunha, 1988).

Chryseobacterium meningosepticum and *C. multivorans* are the dominant species observed in clinical infection. *C. meningosepticum* is readily identified by commercial phenotypic tests such as API20NE and may be sub-typed using PFGE/RFLP analysis using the restriction endonuclease *Apa*1 (Hoque *et al.*, 2001). *C. meningosepticum* is best known for causing outbreaks of cross-infection from environmental sources in neonatal units when meningitis is a common infection. Outbreaks may be persistent and require careful attention to environmental control and cross-infection practice (Ceyhan *et al.*, 2008).

Both *Alcaligenes* spp and *Chryseobacterium* spp are resistant to multiple antibiotics and therapy will be determined by antimicrobial susceptibility testing of isolates.

ACINETOBACTER SPP

Acinetobacter spp are a group of Gram-negative bacilli, usually of low pathogenicity in normal individuals, which have emerged as important pathogens in healthcare-associated infections, particularly for patients in ICUs or those undergoing invasive clinical procedures. Their innate resistance to many antibiotics and ability to acquire transmissible resistance elements rapidly contributes to their importance as nosocomial pathogens, with *A. baumanii* being the most frequent species associated with infections in the healthcare setting. More common clinical infections include nosocomial and ventilator-associated pneumonia, urinary tract infection, wound infection and bacteraemia. *A. baumanii* can be important in traumatic wound infections in returning military personnel from Iraq and Afghanistan, probably acquired during hospitalization rather than at the time of injury (Calhoun *et al.*, 2008). Infections caused by multi-drug-resistant *Acinetobacter* spp have also been described in patients in long-term care facilities (Bonomo, 2000).

Acinetobacter spp are commonly found in soil and water, and may also be part of the normal commensal flora of normal skin, throat, respiratory and gastrointestinal tracts in healthy humans. *Acinetobacter lwoffi*, *A. johnsonii*, *A. radioresistens* and genospecies 3 are the most common species colonizing both patients and the normal population, whereas *A. baumanii* and genospecies 13 most commonly infect and colonize hospital inpatients, being rarely seen in the non-hospitalized population (Seifert *et al.*, 1997). The ability of *A. baumanii* to survive desiccation (Jawad *et al.*, 1998) is an important characteristic that enables it to survive for prolonged periods in the environment, behaving more like a Gram-positive bacterium.

Reliable identification to species level (i.e. differentiation of *A. baumanii*) requires DNA-based methods, which often require specialist referral, although amplified 16s ribosomal ribonucleic acid (rRNA) DNA restriction analysis requires only PCR amplification and digestion with restriction endonucleases (Peleg *et al.*, 2008).

Antimicrobial resistance in *Acinetobacter* species has significantly increased in the last ten years (Lockhart *et al.*, 2007) and treatment options are therefore frequently limited. Selection of these multi-drug-resistant (MDR) strains may be due to increasing antibiotic usage as well as healthcare-associated transmission. The definition of MDR *Acinetobacter* spp varies in the literature; two of the most frequently used are the presence of carbapenem resistance or resistance to more than three different classes of antimicrobials (Falagas *et al.*, 2006). Most MDR *Acinetobacter* in the UK are highly clonal and belong to the South

East clone (SE clone), or OXA-23 clone 1 lineages, both of which are endemic in many hospitals. Similar spread of clones across European countries have occurred with European clones I, II and III recognized as well as intercontinental spread (Peleg *et al.*, 2008).

In healthcare settings where *Acinetobacter* species have been implicated in outbreaks of infection, there is often widespread environmental contamination including of curtains (Das *et al.*, 2002), respiratory equipment (Bernards *et al.*, 2004), items of shared medical equipment (Villegas and Hartstein, 2003; Bernards *et al.*, 2004; Maragakis *et al.*, 2004; Wilks *et al.*, 2006), and door handles and computer keyboards (Wilks *et al.*, 2006). Once contaminated, *Acinetobacter* may survive for long periods in these sites and may act as reservoirs for spread via hands of healthcare staff.

Outbreak control

Routine surveillance methods will enable detection of a nosocomial outbreak of *Acinetobacter* but this is more difficult when it is endemic. Comparison of phenotypic profiles, antibiograms and molecular typing of clinical/screening isolates will assist in outbreak definition. The most effective methods are molecular and include: ribotyping (Biendo *et al.*, 1999); PFGE of restriction endonuclease-digested genomic DNA (Gouby *et al.*, 1992); repetitive extragenic palindromic sequence-based PCR (REP-PCR; Snelling *et al.*, 1996); and random amplified polymorphic DNA analysis (Levidiotou *et al.*, 2002). All show good discrimination, although there is currently no agreed standard method. REP-PCR is simple to perform, reproducible and more discriminatory than ribotyping (Snelling *et al.*, 1996).

Control measures include the reinforcement of hand hygiene, strict use of gloves and aprons and regular cleaning of the environment (Wilks *et al.*, 2006; Zarrilli *et al.*, 2007). Other outbreaks have required more stringent interventions including cohorting of infected/colonized patients with active surveillance cultures (Urban *et al.*, 2003), closure of wards and deep cleaning prior to reopening (Aygun *et al.*, 2002; Zanetti *et al.*, 2007). The long-term persistence of *Acinetobacter* in the ICU environment has also been described (Webster *et al.*, 1998) and, therefore, consideration should be given to long-term surveillance after termination of outbreaks. Antibiotic stewardship with broad-spectrum antibiotic restriction is an important outbreak-control measure, although successful control of *Acinetobacter* outbreaks tends to involve multiple interventions, making it difficult to evaluate individual measures.

PSEUDOMONAS AERUGINOSA

Pseudomonas aeruginosa is the main human pathogen of the genus, which is widely distributed in the natural environment. *P. aeruginosa* is present in soil and water, and is frequently recovered from fresh vegetables, flowers and plants, from which strains carrying infection may be derived (Romling *et al.*, 1994). *P. aeruginosa* is resistant to many disinfectants including quarternary ammonium compounds.

Pseudomonas aeruginosa is an infrequent colonizer of the human gut, the faecal carriage rate being between 2 and 10 per cent in healthy individuals, although the carriage increases following administration of antibiotics and hospitalization, particularly in ICUs and burns units. Colonization of body sites is often in moist areas, such as the ear, axilla and perineum; the respiratory tract of ventilated patients and the gastrointestinal tract of patients receiving chemotherapy for malignancy (Rossolini and Mantengoli, 2005). This predilection for moist environments allows *P. aeruginosa* to survive in areas of the hospital environment such as sink traps, water, ice packs, mops, ventilator tubing and water reservoirs (Muscarella, 2004).

Pseudomonas aeruginosa is an opportunistic pathogen. In hospitalized patients, it is one of the commonest causes of ventilator-associated and hospital-acquired pneumonia. Urinary and surgical-site infections in the hospital setting are also important causes of morbidity (McNeil *et al.*, 2001) and burns may become infected, resulting in secondary septicaemia. Cystic fibrosis patients are a special group in whom *P. aeruginosa* is a major pathogen. Most patients will become infected at some stage of their illness, usually through acquisition from the environment or via cross-infection from other cystic fibrosis or non-cystic fibrosis patients in healthcare or summer camps (Govan and Nelson, 1992). Long-term colonization of the respiratory tract follows, unless there is a concerted effort to eradicate the organism on first infection. *P. aeruginosa* is also beginning to be recognized as a cause of chronic infections in patients with chronic obstructive airways disease (Martinez-Solano *et al.*, 2008).

Pseudomonas aeruginosa is intrinsically resistant to a number of antimicrobials by virtue of resistance mechanisms, including chromosomally encoded AmpC beta-lactamase and the presence of multi-drug efflux systems (Paterson, 2006). Resistance genes, such as plasmid-mediated beta-lactamases and metalloenzymes of the IMP and VIM types, may be present, which, with resistance to other antibiotics, leads to 'pan'-resistant clones(Paterson, 2006).

Continuous surveillance of antimicrobial susceptibility of clinical isolates of *P. aeruginosa* is necessary to determine local policy for empirical treatment of infections in high-risk units and also enables the early detection of outbreaks of infection.

Outbreak control

Typing of isolates is essential to determine whether outbreaks are multi-source or single-source of a clonal nature. This is reliant on molecular techniques, of which RFLP/PFGE of chromosomal DNA is most frequently used (Pitt and Simpson, 2005).

As with most outbreaks of MRGNB, the reinforcement of hand hygiene (Widmer *et al.*, 1993) and standard infection control precautions is central to achieving control. Healthcare staff with skin or nail lesions as a point source should also be considered in clonal outbreaks (McNeil *et al.*, 2001). The ability of *P. aeruginosa* to survive in moist areas of the hospital environment, and in tap water especially (Muscarella, 2004), gives rise to cross-infection. Any aqueous solution used in healthcare could potentially be contaminated (e.g. irrigation fluids, disinfectants, soaps, eye drops, dialysis fluids). It may also contaminate respiratory therapy equipment, ventilator tubing and bronchoscopes in ICUs, and thereby spread between patients (Teres *et al.*, 1973; Srinivasan *et al.*, 2003). *P. aeruginosa* may also be found on flowers, plants and in flower water such that, in units housing patients highly susceptible to pseudomonal infections (ICUs, haematology/oncology wards and burns units), flowers and plants are not advised.

Patient isolation for colonized/infected patients is commonly used to achieve control and is one of the measures used in cystic fibrosis centres, where those infected with *P. aeruginosa* are treated on different days and in separate areas to those who are not colonized (Festini *et al.*, 2006).

Antibiotic restriction is an essential part of controlling *P. aeruginosa* outbreaks, particularly if identified as multi-clonal. Interventions based on rotation of antimicrobials and restriction of certain classes (e.g. fluoroquinolones and carbapenems) may be used (Rossolini and Mantengoli, 2005).

CJD

Donald J Jeffries

INTRODUCTION

Human transmissible spongiform encephalopathies

Creutzfeldt–Jakob disease (CJD) is a name used to describe several types of transmissible spongiform encephalopathies (TSEs) or prion diseases, which are rare, fatal, neurodegenerative diseases of humans. The TSEs of humans and other species are listed in Box 12.1. TSEs are believed to be caused by infectious proteins called prions and the apparent absence of nucleic acid means that they have very different properties to 'orthodox' infectious agents such as bacteria and viruses (Prusiner, 2001). Diseases caused by prions are due to the accumulation in the body of a modified form of the host prion protein. The highest levels of protein deposition, and infectivity, occur in the brain and posterior eye. The normal form of prion protein (PrPc) is present in a wide range of species and its function has not been clearly defined. In TSEs, the protein

Box 12.1 Transmissible spongiform encephalopathies (TSEs; prion diseases) of animals and humans (listed in order of discovery)

ANIMAL DISEASE

- Scrapie: sheep and goats
- Transmissible mink encephalopathy (TME): mink
- Wasting disease: deer and elk
- Bovine spongiform encephalopathy[a] (BSE): cattle
- TSE of wild ruminants[a]: Arabian oryx, scimitar-horned oryx, nyala, eland, gemsbok, ankole, bison, kudu
- Feline spongiform encephalopathy[a]: domestic cat, cheetah, tiger, puma, ocelot
- 'Atypical scrapie': sheep and goats

HUMAN DISEASE

- Kuru
- Sporadic Creutzfeldt–Jakob disease (CJD)
- Familial CJD[b]
- Gerstmann–Straüssler–Scheinker syndrome[b]
- Fatal familial insomnia[b]
- Variant CJD[a]

[a]Caused by the same agent.
[b]Genetic forms of the disease.

undergoes post-translational misfolding to an isoform with an increased beta-sheet structure. This abnormal isoform (PrPtse) is resistant to degradation by proteases and a wide range of physicochemical agents (Taylor, 2000; Box 12.2) and is associated with infectivity. As the infectious agent is identical chemically, but not structurally, to the host protein, it is not recognized as foreign by the host and hence there is no significant form of inflammatory, interferon or immune response.

A consistent feature of TSEs is the development of spongiform change (vacuolation) in the cerebral cortex and this is associated with deposition of prion protein in the brain, sometimes in the form of amyloid plaques (De Armond and Prusiner, 2003). The commonest form of CJD is sporadic CJD and, as listed in Box 12.1, there are several types of genetically determined TSEs which are associated with mutations or insertions in the prion protein gene (*PRNP*). TSEs are experimentally transmissible by inoculation and in some cases orally. Once clinical signs appear, all TSEs are progressive and fatal (Collins *et al.*, 2004). Infection can be confirmed by immunochemical staining of brain or other infected tissue, for example tonsil in variant CJD (vCJD) and there is

---

Box 12.2 Chemical disinfectants and processes ineffective in removing prion infectivity. Adapted with modification from annex C, ACDP (2006)

Chemical disinfectant	Gaseous disinfectant	Physical process
Alcohols	Ethylene oxide	Dry heat
Ammonia	Formaldehyde	Ionizing, ultraviolet, microwave radiation
Beta-propiolactone		Autoclaving 121°C (NB Autoclaving at 134°C cannot be guaranteed to remove all infectivity)
Chlorine dioxide		
Formalin		
Glutaraldehyde and other aldehydes (e.g. OPA)		
Hydrochloric acid		
Hydrogen peroxide		
Iodophors		
Peracetic acid		
Phenolics		
Sodium dichloroisocyanurate		
10 000 ppm sodium hypochlorite		

---

currently no blood test or other detection system applicable to individuals in the pre-clinical phase. No prophylaxis or effective treatment is available for prion diseases. There has been no confirmed instance of occupational transmission of any form of TSE, human or animal, despite careful investigation of the history of confirmed cases and follow-up of those exposed in the workplace.

Studies are in progress in the UK to assess the prevalence of infection with variant CJD in apparently well individuals in the community. If a latent carrier state of vCJD exists, the individuals concerned may have a normal life expectancy but, if the agent in their tissues is infectious, there is a possibility that iatrogenic transmission by blood, tissue and organs, or via contaminated surgical instruments, could lead to a self-sustaining epidemic. Although the global distribution of vCJD highlights the need for the UK to introduce interventions to counter this threat, the growing numbers of other countries reporting cases of vCJD (Table 12.2) indicates the need to introduce measures to make tissue donation and surgical procedures safer on a worldwide basis.

Sporadic CJD

With a mean age of onset in the sixth decade, sporadic CJD typically presents as a rapidly progressive dementia, often accompanied by cerebellar ataxia and myoclonus, with death in an akinetic-mute state after a median duration of 4–5

Table 12.2 Variant Creutzfeldt–Jakob disease cases worldwide, July 2006

UK	162
France	20 (19)
Republic of Ireland	4 (2)
Italy	1 (1)
USA	2
Canada	1
Saudi Arabia	1 (1)
Japan	1
Netherlands	2 (2)
Portugal	1 (1)
Spain	1 (1)

NB Numbers in brackets represent cases with no obvious geographical link with the UK

months. It occurs in all countries with an annual incidence of 1.0–1.5 per million population (Masters *et al.*, 1979; Ladogana *et al.*, 2005).

Iatrogenic CJD

Creutzfeldt–Jakob disease has been transmitted horizontally by healthcare procedures including neurosurgery, use of intracerebral electrodes, corneal grafting, injection of growth hormone and gonadotrophin derived from cadaver pituitary glands and dura mater used for reconstruction in neurosurgery (Brown *et al.*, 2006). Current numbers of recorded cases of iatrogenic CJD are given in Table 12.3.

Variant CJD

Variant CJD was first reported in 1996 (Will *et al.*, 1996) and laboratory studies have confirmed that it is the same agent as that causing bovine spongiform encephalopathy (BSE; Bruce *et al.*, 1997; Hill *et al.*, 1997). In marked contrast to sporadic CJD, vCJD presents at a much younger age (median age at death 29 years) and the clinical effects are usually heralded by psychiatric disturbance (anxiety, insomnia, withdrawal) and unpleasant sensory experiences leading to

Table 12.3 Iatrogenic Creutzfeldt–Jakob disease (CJD), July 2006

Source	No. of cases	Incubation period (months)
Neurosurgery	4	12–28
Intracerebral electrodes	2	16–20
Corneal transplant	2	16–320
Dura mater graft	196	18–216
Cadaveric growth hormone	194	50–456
Cadaveric gonadotrophin	4	144–192
Blood components[a]	2	78–94

[a]Two probable transmissions of variant CJD from transfusion of red blood cells. A third transmission of infection to an individual who was heterozygous for methionine/valine at codon 129 on the prion gene did not present as clinical variant CJD.

ataxia, tremor and involuntary movements (Collins *et al.*, 2004). To date there have been 192 cases of vCJD with the majority (162) occurring in the UK. Information on cases of vCJD reported in other countries (Table 12.2) reveals that an increasing number have had no history of residence in, or other obvious links with, the UK.

Genetically determined TSE

The three main genetically determined types of CJD are familial CJD, Gerstmann–Straüssler–Scheinker syndrome and fatal familial insomnia. All are inherited in an autosomal dominant pattern and the presence of one of a number of mutations, or insertions, in the *PRNP* gene may predispose to a high likelihood of disease in affected individuals (Collins *et al.*, 2004).

DISTRIBUTION OF INFECTIVITY IN HUMANS

Transmissible spongiform encephalopathy agents are not uniformly distributed in the tissues of infected humans and other species (World Health Organisation, 2006). In the clinical stages of all human prion diseases the highest infectivity titres are found in the central nervous system reaching levels of 8 logs (100 million infectious units) per gram in the brain and posterior eye, and 6 logs (one million infectious units) per gram in the spinal cord. Other regions, specifically the anterior eye and olfactory mucosa, are known to contain lower levels of infectivity. This pattern of distribution of infectivity is found in the later stages of the incubation period and during the clinical disease of sporadic CJD. On the basis of present knowledge, this same pattern of distribution of infectivity is assumed to occur in all other human TSEs except variant CJD. In vCJD, in addition to the concentration of infectivity in the central nervous system, eye and olfactory mucosa as seen in sporadic CJD and other forms of human TSEs, the agent is detectable outside the nervous system in the later stages of the incubation period and during the clinical illness (Bruce *et al.*, 2001). Tissues consistently positive for abnormal prion by immunohistochemistry and/or infectivity include the tonsils, spleen and gastrointestinal lymphoid tissue (Wadsworth *et al.*, 2001). The pattern of distribution of abnormal prion may vary in different individuals depending on the genetic sequence of their *PRNP* gene and possibly on the route of infection with the vCJD agent. At present, all cases of clinical vCJD have been homozygous for methionine at codon 129 in their *PRNP* gene (Ironside *et al.*, 2006). One of three cases probably infected by blood transfusion in the UK, who was a methionine/valine heterozygote at codon 129, died from a cause unrelated to vCJD (Peden *et al.*, 2004). At post mortem, the patient had abnormal prion in the spleen and one cervical lymph node, with none detectable in the brain, spinal cord, tonsils or gastrointestinal lymph nodes. Concern about the possibility of undetected carriers of vCJD in the UK has led to the screening of anonymized collections of stored appendix and tonsil material, and prospective studies are now in progress. Of a total of 12 700 samples reported as tested to date, three have stained positively for abnormal prion in lymph nodes associated with the appendix (Hilton *et al.*, 2004). Two of these samples were available for genotyping and both were found to be homozygous for valine at codon 129 (Ironside *et al.*, 2006). On the basis of study of patients with iatrogenic CJD, the genetic variability at codon 129 has been shown to influence the duration of incubation of the disease (Collinge *et al.*, 1991). If it proves also to influence the tissue distribution, there may be clinical presentations of vCJD that are different from those currently recognized in methionine homozygotes. It is not inconceivable that patients could present with non-neurological diseases. The status and prognosis of individuals harbouring valine homozygotes cannot be investigated owing to the anonymization of the archived samples. Further studies currently in progress should help to determine the prevalence of infection in residents in the UK.

MANAGEMENT OF THE RISKS OF CREUTZFELDT–JAKOB DISEASE IN HEALTHCARE

In 2006 the incidence of BSE in cattle in the UK was at a very low level and the numbers of cases of vCJD continues to decline year by year. It is to be hoped that this signifies the decline in human infections resulting from dietary exposure to the BSE agent but, as all clinical cases of vCJD to date have been methionine homozygotes at codon 129, there is concern that the longer incubation periods likely to occur in valine homozygotes and in methionine/valine heterozygotes may be associated with future increases in incidence of the disease. Long-term surveillance of kuru in New Guinea has revealed cases with incubation periods likely to be of 56 years or more (Collinge *et al.*, 2006). Over the 16 years of enhanced surveillance coordinated by the National CJD Surveillance Unit, there has been no significant increase in sporadic, iatrogenic or familial forms of CJD in the UK other than what might be expected by the generation of increased awareness promoted by the publicity surrounding the BSE epidemic and the appearance of vCJD. With the success in controlling the likelihood of dietary exposure to BSE, it is critically important to reduce to a minimum the likelihood of transmission of the agents by healthcare procedures. With the probability that vCJD has been transmitted by blood transfusion and the belief that there may be several thousand asymptomatic carriers of vCJD in the UK, measures have been introduced to enhance the safety of blood transfusion. Recipients of blood components and plasma products who have been identified as having received donations from individuals who have subsequently developed vCJD are informed of their status and advised to take precautions to protect public health. These precautions include self-exclusion from donating blood, tissues and organs, and alerting surgeons and dentists to the fact that they may present a risk of carrying the vCJD agent. This approach is consistent with measures previously recommended in the UK for those identified as a possible risk of transmitting other forms of human prion diseases (pituitary-derived human growth hormone and dura mater graft recipients, members of families with evidence of familial CJD, etc.). Several important measures to improve the safety of the UK blood supply have been introduced in recent years. Along with advice to use blood components sparingly and only if the need is unavoidable, the specific interventions are listed in Table 12.4.

With the knowledge that iatrogenic CJD transmission has been associated with brain surgery and use of intracerebral electrodes, the UK Spongiform Encephalopathy Advisory Committee (SEAC) commissioned the Department of Health to carry out a risk assessment for surgical transmission of vCJD. This risk assessment was published on the Department of Health website in February 2000 and concluded that 'surgical transmission cannot be ruled out as a risk to public health' (Department of Health, 2001). A further risk assessment of possible risks from surgical transmission of vCJD was published on the Department of Health website in March 2005 (Department of Health, 2005). This allowed consideration and incorporation of recent research findings and also included the results of studies of efficacy of protein removal by Sterile Supply Departments in the UK. These studies of instruments sampled from Sterile Supply Departments have since been published (Baxter et al., 2006; Murdoch et al., 2006). The findings of this interim review indicate that 'overall, the risks of vCJD transmission via surgery still appear significant. Though achieving high standards of decontamination remains of critical importance, the limitations of current technology mean that instruments used on an infective patient could still be at significant risk of passing on vCJD.'

Table 12.4 Measures introduced by the UK National Blood Service to reduce the possible risk of transmission of variant Creutzfeldt–Jakob disease (vCJD) by blood and plasma. Based on a press release from the UK National Blood Service 20 July 2005

1997	Withdrawal and recall of any blood components, plasma derivatives or tissues obtained from any individual who later develops vCJD
1999	Import of plasma from the USA for fractionation to manufacture plasma derivatives
	Leucodepletion of all blood components
2004	Importation of clinical fresh-frozen plasma from the USA for patients born on or after 1 January 1996
	Exclusion of donors who have received a blood transfusion in the UK since 1 January 1980
2005	Importation of clinical fresh-frozen plasma from the USA for patients up to the age of 16 years
Continuing	Promotion of appropriate use of blood and tissues and alternatives throughout the National Health Service

The most important way of reducing risks of transmission via surgical instruments and endoscopes is to ensure that decontamination is as effective as possible. As the agent of vCJD is particularly thermostable and reductions of infectivity of more than 1000-fold are unlikely to be achieved by autoclaving (at any temperature) great reliance must be placed on thorough cleaning (Taylor, 2004). The lack of suitable disinfectants able to reduce the infectivity of prions on fibreoptic endoscopes emphasizes the need for meticulous cleaning of all forms of endoscope together with the introduction of single-use accessories and cleaning brushes where possible (Advisory Committee on Dangerous Pathogens; ACDP, 2006, Annex F).

With levels of infectivity that can exceed 8 logs (100 million) infectious units per gram of tissue, the brain and posterior eye are likely to carry the highest risk of transmitting CJD. In addition, operations that involve the lymphoreticular system, anterior eye and olfactory mucosa are likely to present some risk of transmission via the instruments.

MANAGEMENT OF INCIDENTS OCCURRING IN HEALTHCARE

As the number of cases of vCJD increased during the latter part of the 1990s, it became clear that potential problems were likely when patients with known or suspected vCJD required surgery, endoscopy or dentistry. Concern was focused particularly on the risks to individuals, and public health in general, if surgical instruments and endoscopes used on patients infected with the agent of vCJD were to be used on other patients. These concerns were emphasized by the realization that, at present, we cannot be certain that the infectious moiety of prions can be removed by washing or by normal agents used in decontamination, including autoclaving or disinfectants. On the recommendation of the ACDP/SEAC TSE Joint Working Group, the CJD Incidents Panel was established for the UK in 2000. This Panel of experts from many specialties includes ethicists and lay members, and has advised on incidents relating to surgery, blood component transfusion and plasma product administration involving all forms of human prion disease. In addition to the establishment of the CJD Incidents Panel, the ACDP/SEAC TSE Joint Working Group (now reconstituted as the ACDP Working Group) also recommended strongly that usage details and tracking of surgical instrument sets (and, if possible, single instruments) should be introduced to allow investigation of subsequent use and thus protection of public health by identifying those at risk following an incident involving a patient with known or suspected TSE infection. Similarly, endoscopy units were alerted to the need to record routinely the serial numbers of all fibreoptic endoscopes in case the need arose to follow up the subsequent use of an endoscope used on a patient with suspected TSE infection. The basis of operation of the CJD Incidents Panel, the Panel framework document, minutes of its meetings and annual reports are available on the Health Protection Agency website

(2006). The Panel framework document provides the details of modelling carried out to estimate the numbers of patients who should be alerted to public health risks following different types of surgery on patients considered at risk of CJD. In addition to regular meetings of the entire CJD Incidents Panel to review management of incidents in healthcare, the Panel also acts on a real-time basis to advise on management of cases as they occur and, if necessary, recommend the quarantining (and on occasion removal from use) of instruments, and the notification of patients deemed to have been at risk of infection and hence of potential danger to public health. The introduction of a traceability system for surgical instruments, endoscopes and reusable accessories will help to avoid unnecessary quarantining or removal of items from use.

PROSPECTS FOR THE FUTURE

There is an urgent need for improvements to decontamination processes that will allow a confident statement that we can remove or inactivate all forms of prion infectivity on stainless steel instruments and from other instruments, particularly endoscopes. Modern day-approaches to decontamination of surgical instruments by sending them for processing in large centralized decontamination centres, while possibly allowing better standardization and use of large equipment, may be counter-productive if protein on the instruments is allowed to dry in transit, thus reducing the efficiency of removing it. Marked improvements in protein removal from instruments may be achievable either by applying a preliminary wash immediately after use on the operating table, or by keeping them moist all the way to the Decontamination Unit. This is currently under review.

At present, there are very few disinfectants that can be recommended for decontamination of prion infectivity in healthcare (ACDP, 2006, Annex C). The two best characterized, molar sodium hydroxide and sodium hypochlorite (20 000 ppm available chlorine), are caustic and are likely to be too destructive to use routinely on stainless steel or endoscope materials. Newer preparations are currently being produced with claims for effective inactivation of prion infectivity; some of these substances have achieved CE marking and are going into production and marketing. Before attempting to introduce these newer products to decontamination processes, it will be important to ensure that the following important criteria are met.

1 Are the agents active in reducing prion infectivity within a suitable time period?
2 Have they been assessed against relevant strains of TSE agents? Some laboratory strains of TSE agent are much more easily destroyed in model systems than the agents of BSE/CJD.
3 If the agent has an effect on human prions, what is the nature of any residual infectious prion after treatment? Has the TSE agent been changed in any way either to alter its behaviour in animal systems or possibly to

make it more resistance to further decontamination? We know that application of protein fixatives (e.g. aldehydes) stabilizes infectivity and renders it more difficult to remove in future.

4 Is the decontamination agent being considered compatible for use in current surgical instrument or endoscope decontamination cycles? As well as being practical, it must be shown not to compromise decontamination of more orthodox infectious agents.

Several agencies in the UK have stated publicly that, unless and until the above criteria have been satisfied, health care establishments should continue to follow existing guidelines as available on the Department of Health website (ACDP, 2006).

Clearly, continuation of measures already introduced to enhance the safety of blood together with meaningful interventions to improve the safety of surgical and endoscopic instrumentation is likely to reduce or remove the risk of a sustained epidemic relating to healthcare procedures, and to increase safety for individual patients. There is a distinct possibility that sensitive tests (probably based on markers in blood) will allow the identification of carriers of the infection(s) before they become symptomatic. Introduction of such tests is itself likely to be problematic, as it will probably take several years before the significance of a positive result becomes clear. As with other blood tests, any shortfall in specificity is likely to produce many potentially worried individuals for whom the significance of the test may be unknown.

Research in progress to try to identify therapies and/or prophylaxis to treat or prevent prion disease may add additional purpose to the identification of individuals at risk from blood transfusion or surgery/endoscopy as well as those found to be positive on blood testing for the agents.

ACKNOWLEDGEMENT

The author is grateful to Professor James W. Ironside, National CJD Surveillance Unit, University of Edinburgh, for assistance during the preparation of this section of the chapter and for providing up-to-date information on numbers of cases of variant and iatrogenic CJD.

Tuberculosis

Adam Fraise and E Grace Smith

BACKGROUND

Tuberculosis (TB) is caused by the bacterium *Mycobacterium tuberculosis* and is predominantly a disease of the lungs (pulmonary TB), but can also affect other parts of the body (extrapulmonary TB). Non-pulmonary forms of TB are rarely infectious and, therefore, from an infection control point of view, the pulmonary form of TB disease is the most important. Transmission occurs through coughing of infectious droplets and usually requires close contact with an infectious case, with the greatest risk being for those with prolonged household contact. People who have live mycobacteria visible on microscopy of stained sputum (smear-positive cases) are the most infectious.

Globally about nine million new cases of TB, and nearly two million deaths from TB, are estimated to occur every year. TB is the leading cause of death among curable infectious diseases and the World Health Organisation declared TB a global emergency in 1993. About 8000 new cases of TB are currently reported each year in the UK with most cases occurring in major cities, particularly in London.

GUIDELINES

Recent guidelines were published by the UK's National Institute for Health and Clinical Excellence (National Collaborating Centre for Chronic Conditions, 2006) whereas US guidelines for the prevention of transmission of *Mycobacterium tuberculosis* in healthcare settings were published in 1994 (updated 2005) and published in the *Morbidity and Mortality Weekly Report* (Centers for Disease Control and Prevention, 1994, 2005). Both these documents give detailed advice on the organizational and practical aspects of preventing and controlling TB, with specific guidance for the healthcare sector.

ISOLATION

Since the most infectious patients are those who are smear-positive sputum, it is appropriate to nurse all patients with clinically suspected pulmonary TB in a single room. They should stay in this isolation room until three separate sputum samples are negative on microscopy (i.e. no acid-fast bacilli seen) in which case they are deemed to be of low infectivity and can be taken out of isolation. However, it is important to recognize that patients with pulmonary TB who are smear-negative may still transmit the infection (Behr *et al.*, 1999) and therefore should not share a ward with HIV-positive or immunosuppressed patients, as such patients are highly susceptible to infection with mycobacteria.

Patients with TB should have a risk assessment for drug resistance and, should the risk be high, they will need special infection control precautions; see later section on 'Multi-drug resistant tuberculosis'(MDRTB). Patients who are smear positive (on any of the three sputum specimens taken after admission) should stay in a single room until successful completion of 14 days treatment or until discharge from hospital, whichever is the earlier.

PERSONAL PROTECTIVE EQUIPMENT

There is no requirement for healthcare workers to wear special personal protective equipment (masks or gowns) when dealing with patients with TB unless MDRTB is suspected (see later) or procedures that generate aerosols are being performed. It is also advisable to use masks and gowns when caring for patients who generate their own aerosols by profuse coughing. In the case of patients with suspected or known MDRTB, staff and visitors who are in contact with a potentially infective patient should wear masks conforming to the FFP3 standard.

When patients are transported around the hospital, it is rarely practical for all staff who come in contact with the patient to wear protective equipment. In the case of non-MDRTB, this is not a problem unless the patient is actively coughing, in which case he or she should wear a standard surgical mask. This will prevent large droplets from contaminating the environment but is not a replacement for FFP3 masks. If the patient has MDRTB, movement around the hospital should be avoided if at all possible. Where this cannot be avoided, FFP3 masks must be worn by all staff who come into contact with the patient.

VENTILATION

Any procedures which may generate aerosols (such as chest physiotherapy to induce sputum) should take place in an area with appropriate ventilation. This should ideally include dedicated supply and extract ventilation. The room should be under negative pressure compared with the outside and any attached ward areas or corridors. A lobby allows maximum safety by reducing the risk of viable mycobacteria being transferred to nearby areas and example layouts are given in the UK Department of Health publication HBN4 Supplement 1 (NHS Estates, 2005). Access and cleaning hatches should be avoided, if possible, and extract filters, which require regular maintenance with associated risk to maintenance staff, are not required as long as the air discharges 3 m above the roof of the building. If this cannot be achieved, filters should be in a 'safe change' housing and mounted outside the building.

MANAGEMENT OF AN OUTBREAK

When two or more cases of TB appear to be epidemiologically linked, this may be considered to be an outbreak. In this instance, the Infection Control Doctor will usually request for an outbreak committee meeting to be held (see Chapter 2). If the outbreak was identified in a hospital environment, then a representative of senior management should attend the committee. It is also wise to invite the individual with responsibility for infection control in the community, the Consultant in Communicable Disease Control (CCDC) in the UK, as well as a physician with experience in managing TB. A plan for managing patients who have acquired TB as part of the outbreak needs to be formulated, the patients' family doctors need to be informed and media aspects need to be actively managed. It is very helpful to have an experienced media professional involved to ensure that the press and other media are correctly informed, and also to avoid any misinformation causing panic and distress to patients and relatives.

CONTACT TRACING IN HOSPITAL

The names of all close patient contacts of a case of sputum-positive tuberculosis should be notified to the appropriate CCDC and to the general practitioner. Staff contacts are reported to the hospital occupational health department and their immune status is checked. Household contacts are defined as those who share a bedroom, kitchen, bathroom or sitting room with the index case. A risk assessment should be undertaken to identify those at highest risk of contracting the infection, and this assessment should cover length of contact, proximity of contact, degree of infectivity of the index case and susceptibility of the contact to infection. Tuberculin tests, interferon gamma tests or chest X-rays may be indicated for household contacts or close contacts in long-stay wards and also in neonatal, paediatric (under 3 months) or immunocompromised close contacts. It is recommended that patient contacts at lower risk should be informed of the exposure to a sputum-positive case by letter, copied to their consultant and GP. This will raise awareness to the diagnosis should symptoms develop in the contact, and may be used to enhance case finding if transmission has occurred readily to close contacts.

STAFF SCREENING

All staff in UK hospitals should have a pre-employment assessment (see Chapter 11), which will include some screening questions for symptoms of TB (weight loss, chronic cough) and may include a request for evidence of a visible BCG (bacille Calmette–Guérin) scar.

When a case of open TB has been identified on a hospital ward, staff who have had prolonged exposure to the index patient may be at risk of acquiring the infection. It is therefore wise to inform the staff member as well as their family doctor to consider TB as a possible cause of symptomatic illness in the future.

MULTI-DRUG RESISTANT TUBERCULOSIS

Drug resistance is an important issue, as patients infected with resistant strains of TB may be infectious for longer period than those infected with sensitive strains, resulting in a greater risk of transmission. Furthermore, the mortality is higher and the cure rate is lower than for sensitive strains. MDRTB is characterized by being resistant to isoniazid and rifampicin, although some strains may be resistant to other drugs as well.

The main factors which can be used to identify patients at high risk of being infected with MDRTB include: a history of prior treatment for TB, birth in a country with a high incidence of TB (especially sub-Saharan Africa or the Indian sub-continent), presence of HIV infection, residence in cities with a high incidence of MDRTB, age between 25 and 44 years and male gender. The treatment regimens for MDRTB are outside the scope of this book and should always be chosen in discussion with a physician experienced in the treatment of these cases.

Patients with suspected or proven MDRTB should be nursed in a negative pressure isolation room (conforming to HBN4 Supplement 1 or similar guidance) and staff should wear masks conforming to the FFP3 standard. In contrast to patients infected with sensitive strains, these masks should be worn whenever in contact with the patient (not just when aerosol-generating procedures are performed).

When MDRTB patients are discharged from hospital, it is important to discuss the case with the officer responsible for infection control in the community (the CCDC in the UK) to ensure that the public are adequately protected from potential infection and to set in place adequate arrangements for the secure administration of anti-TB medication.

SURVEILLANCE

All countries should consider the need for a national surveillance system for the incidence and prevalence of TB. An effective surveillance system is important so that national policy on BCG immunization and other control measures can be implemented on a sound basis. Surveillance systems can also be used to monitor the effectiveness of control measures and to identify outbreaks. However, some countries with a low incidence of the disease, high immigration or generalized use of BCG will find such a surveillance system impractical. For this reason, many countries monitor TB-related morbidity rather than TB incidence *per se*. Some countries, such as the UK, have a statutory notification system, which allows monitoring of clinically diagnosed cases of TB (not just those that are microbiologically proven).

TYPING

High-quality surveillance at local and national level requires the development and implementation of protocols for the public health use of laboratory techniques such as DNA fingerprinting and molecular typing, and the establishment of a central database linking fingerprinting and epidemiological data. These are also the tools that can enhance the national collection and analysis of information on incidents and outbreaks, to learn from them and develop more consistent responses, as more is learnt about the clinical behaviour and transmissibility of particular molecular types.

Typing methods have been of great use in the past to confirm that patients with epidemiological links share the same strain of TB. The evidence from other European TB typing programmes suggests that, to detect links between patients early enough to interrupt transmission, rather than merely to detect past events, all strains should be typed as they are isolated and the information made available to TB teams as they carry out their epidemiological investigations (Lambregts-van Weezenbeek et al., 2003). The health gains from such a strategy have been evident for meningococcal disease and for a number of enteric infections. Proactive application of TB typing has been hampered in the past by the slow techniques available, but newer techniques, related to those used for human DNA fingerprinting, have made it possible to provide timely information and make a contribution to individual patient care.

Internationally, mycobacterial interspersed repetitive unit–variable number tandem repeat (MIRU-VNTR) (Mazars et al., 2001; Supply et al., 2006) typing is replacing or being used alongside older methods, such as random fragment length polymorphism insertion sequence 6110 (RFLP IS6110) or the less discriminatory spacer oligonucleotide typing (Spoligotyping). MIRU-VNTR typing is robust, reproducible and may be delivered as a digitized result within 2–4 weeks of the growth of a culture of TB, as part of a routine service. Further developments are needed to increase the discrimination of typing methods for particular groups of strains, but it is also important to link results to epidemiological and clinical information for maximum effect. Use of 15 locus MIRU-VNTR typing in parts of the UK since 2003 has assisted with recognition of clustered cases (Drobniewski et al., 2003; Evans et al., 2007) with detection of approximately 3 per cent of cultures as falsely positive, usually as a result of laboratory cross-contamination, and has helped to focus and monitor contact tracing.

ATYPICAL MYCOBACTERIA

Most mycobacterial species have an environmental reservoir and are referred to as atypical mycobacteria, to distinguish them from members of the *Mycobacterium tuberculosis* complex, which includes the human and animal pathogens *M. tuberculosis*, *M. africanum* and *M. bovis*. Atypical mycobacterial species cause pulmonary, cutaneous or lymph node infections in humans. Disseminated infections, with *M. avium*, for example, are recognized in severely immune compromised patients but there is no clear evidence of person-to-person transmission. Patients do not need to be isolated once infection with an atypical species is confirmed, but mixed infection with TB occurs rarely.

Specimens may be contaminated with an atypical species from an environmental source, so invasive infection should not be assumed without repeated isolation from non-sterile sites and a consistent clinical picture.

Atypical mycobacteria in clinical specimens will also be smear positive, and unnecessary treatment or contact tracing and notification may be avoided by seeking rapid molecular identification for respiratory specimens or cultures from patients with pre-existing lung damage, who may be colonized with atypical mycobacteria. Contaminated endoscopy rinse water, usually with *M. chelonae*, can also be a source of false-positive diagnosis from microscopy of bronchoalveolar lavage specimens.

Possible person-to-person transmission is a matter of some concern for patients with cystic fibrosis (Olivier *et al.*, 2003), who may be colonized and then infected with a variety of atypical mycobacteria (Smith *et al.*, 1984; Torrens *et al.*, 1998; Quittell, 2004; Pierre-Audigier *et al.*, 2005). *M. abscessus* is a long-term colonizer, is difficult to treat and causes clinical deterioration, but transmission has not been demonstrated in reports from a number of studies of isolates with epidemiological links (Bange *et al.*, 2001; Sermet-Gaudelus *et al.*, 2003; Jönsson *et al.*, 2007). In part, this may be due to the lack of good typing methods for atypical mycobacteria.

For further information, see Griffith *et al.* (2007), Subcommittee of the Joint Tuberculosis Committee.

Legionnaire's disease (*Legionella* pneumonia)

Christina Bradley and Adam Fraise

Legionnaire's disease is a potentially severe respiratory infection first recognized in 1976. It is caused by a Gram-negative bacillus, *Legionella pneumophila*, and several other related species. The organism is widely distributed in nature and is commonly found in soil and surface waters. It multiplies over a temperature range varying from 20°C to over 40°C. Colonization of static water is likely, and the organism may commonly be found in the hot-water systems of large buildings, such as hospitals, hotels and offices, usually without any evidence of infection among staff or patients. Outbreaks have originated from air-conditioning systems, particularly their associated cooling towers. Hot-water systems and showers have also been recognized as sources of infection (Bartlett *et al.*, 1986; Fallon, 1994); however, the exact source of the outbreak is often far from easy to establish. Outbreaks in the UK have been reported in hospitals, usually new ones, and occasionally in hotels and other large buildings with cooling towers. Sporadic cases also occur in the community, with no recognizable source. Although some aspects of the epidemiology of the disease remain obscure, there is no evidence of person-to-person spread, nor is infection thought to be acquired by ingestion. It is believed that the pneumonia is acquired by inhaling fine aerosols consisting of *Legionella*-containing particles about 5 μm in diameter, which are able to find their way into the lung alveoli. From this it also follows that some mechanism for generating a fine spray of *Legionella*-contaminated water should be sought as a possible source of any outbreak (e.g. cooling-tower drift, showers, 'whirlpools', etc.). The elderly, especially those with pre-existing chronic respiratory tract disease, and the immunosuppressed are particularly susceptible, but the disease can occur at any age. The organism has probably been one of the causes of pneumonia, particularly in the elderly, for many years, and the risk of acquiring *Legionella*, as distinct from other pneumonias (e.g. pneumococcal pneumonia) has been exaggerated. *Legionella* has been reported to be responsible for 2–7 per cent of community-acquired pneumonia.

CLINICAL DIAGNOSIS

Early detection of cases of infection is of major importance, and is usually based initially on clinical suspicion by the clinician or microbiologist. Sputum, if obtainable, is usually mucoid, and shows scanty neutrophils and no predominant organism. *Legionella* can sometimes be identified by direct immunofluorescence and by culture of sputum, but usually additional techniques, such as trans-tracheal or bronchial aspiration or lung biopsy, are required. The commonest and most useful method for diagnosis of legionnaire's disease is by the detection of antigen in urine. Antibody levels in the acutely ill are often of little help, but diagnosis can be made at a later stage if a fourfold increase is obtained, or a single high titre (>128), particularly if specific immunoglobulin M is detected. Serotyping of the *Legionella* strain may be useful if an epidemiological investigation is required. Isolation of the patient is unnecessary for infection control purposes, but may be indicated because of the severity of the established disease and the untoward publicity associated with it.

OUTBREAKS

If the patient has been in hospital for 10 days or more, it is likely that infection was acquired in hospital, and enquiries may reveal other possible cases, which can be confirmed by antibody tests. However, further investigation is not usually warranted following a sporadic case, as legionellas are commonly found in hospital water supplies. These are rarely associated with infection, and control measures could be excessive and unnecessarily expensive.

Two or more cases warrant further investigation, which would include case–control studies, antibody testing and sampling of possible environmental sources. If there is evidence of a community-acquired outbreak, or if an extensive investigation is likely, the Health Protection Agency should be asked for assistance as soon as possible. The outbreak committee should be convened and the hospital engineer should be co-opted.

MICROBIOLOGICAL MONITORING

If environmental sampling is required, this should be done before any control measures are instituted (Health and Safety Executive, 2000; Department of Health, 2006). Five-litre samples of water should be collected from all known potential sources (e.g. hot- and cold-water systems and cooling towers). Samples should be taken from the mains supplies, holding tanks, calorifiers, hot and cold taps, and showers. Temperatures should be recorded at hot-water taps both at the time of sampling and 3 min later. If a cooling tower is a possible source, samples should be taken from various points in the pipework, the cooling water return at the top, and from the pond.

Routine microbiological monitoring of the water supplies is not recommended, except possibly:

- in wards for immunosuppressed patients;
- when an outbreak is suspected and as a follow-up for a limited period after measures have been introduced to control an outbreak;
- in water systems, control levels for treatment (e.g. temperature, biocide concentration) are reduced or not consistently achieved.

The elimination of legionellas from a water supply depends on chlorination or raising the temperature.

MAINTENANCE OF WATER SYSTEMS

Chlorination of a cooling tower may be achieved by addition of a hypochlorite solution or tablets to give a level of available chlorine of 5 mg/L (ppm) for a period of several hours followed by cleaning and re-chlorination. Higher levels of available chlorine (e.g. up to 50 mg/L) have been recommended. Levels of 50 mg/L are also suggested in header tanks for disinfection of hot- or cold-water supply systems. Continuous chlorination to give levels of 1–2 mg/L available chlorine is an expensive alternative. Moreover, metal corrosion may be a long-term consequence of continuous or repeated chlorination. Commercial systems that dispense chlorine dioxide at 0.5 mg/L into water systems are now available. Ionization, ozone and ultraviolet treatments have also been described (Health and Safety Executive, 2000).

It is also recommended that hot water should be stored in tanks (calorifiers at 60°C and distributed to taps at 52°C ± 2°C). These temperatures are not always easy to achieve in practice, nor can they be relied upon to destroy the organism. In addition, patients, particularly the elderly and confused, must be protected from accidental scalding.

Good maintenance of equipment is the main preventative measure (Health and Safety Executive, 2000; Department of Health, 2006).

Hospital engineers should ensure that water systems are correctly designed and adequately maintained. For example, storage tanks should have an adequate flow rate and have well-fitted covers, calorifiers should have facilities for easy drainage and cleaning, and stratification should be minimized; 'dead legs' should be avoided, water pipes should be lagged to prevent incidental heating of cold-water pipes and loss of temperature from hot-water pipes, and washers should be replaced as necessary with approved types that do not support the growth of *Legionella*. Cooling towers should be cleaned at least twice yearly, and treated with appropriate biocides and corrosion inhibitors. Cold-water supplies should be maintained at 20°C or less.

OTHER SOURCES

Legionnaire's disease can also be transmitted by whirlpools, humidifiers and nebulizers. This equipment should be treated with a chlorine-releasing agent or, if nebulizers are used for respiratory therapy, they can either be disposable or disinfected by heat (e.g. low-temperature steam), although occasionally chemical disinfection may be required. *Legionella* is widely distributed, and it is not known why infection occurs on some occasions and not others. In the absence of infection it is not recommended that expensive additional measures are introduced. However, careful surveillance of patients to detect cases is necessary in hospitals, particularly in units for immunosuppressed patients.

REFERENCES

Acar J, Casewell M, Freeman J. *et al.* (2000) Avoparcin and virginiamycin as animal growth promoters: a plea for science in decision-making. *Clinical Microbiology and Infection* **6**, 477.

Advisory Committee on Dangerous Pathogens (2006) *Transmissible spongiform encephalopathy agents: safe working and the prevention of infection.* Guidance from the Advisory Committee on Dangerous Pathogens and the Spongiform Encephalopathy Advisory Committee. London: Department Health. Available online at: http://www.advisorybodies.doh.gov.uk/acdp/tseguidance/Index.htm.

Al-Nassir WN, Sethi AK, Nerandzic MM *et al.* (2008) Comparison of clinical and microbiological response to treatment of *Clostridium difficile*-associated disease with metronidazole and vancomycin. *Clinical Infectious Diseases* **47**, 56.

Anderson KF, Lonsway DR, Rasheed JK *et al.* (2007) Evaluation of methods to identify the *Klebsiella pneumoniae* carbapenemase in Enterobacteriaceae. *Journal of Clinical Microbiology* **45**, 2723.

Anon. (1986) Guidelines for the control of methicillin-resistant *Staphylococcus aureus*. Report of a combined working party of the Hospital Infection Society and British Society for Antimicrobial Chemotherapy. *Journal of Hospital Infection* **7**, 193.

Appelbaum PC (2006) The emergence of vancomycin-intermediate and vancomycin-resistant *Staphylococcus aureus*. *Clinical Microbiology and Infection* **12**, 16.

Austin DJ, Bonten MJ, Weinstei RA *et al.* (1999) Vancomycin-resistant enterococci in intensive-care hospital settings: transmission dynamics, persistence, and the impact of infection control programs. *Proceedings of the National Academy of Sciences of the United States of America* **96**, 6908.

Aygun G, Demirkiran O, Utku T *et al.* (2002) Environmental contamination during a carbapenem-resistant *Acinetobacter baumannii* outbreak in an intensive care unit. *Journal of Hospital Infection* **52**, 259.

Baldwin A, Mahenthiralingam E, Drevinek P *et al.* (2008) Elucidating global epidemiology of *Burkholderia multivorans* in cases of cystic fibrosis by multilocus sequence typing. *Journal of Clinical Microbiology* **46**, 290.

Bange FC, Brown A, Smacny C, Wallace RJ Jnr and Bottger EC (2001) Lack of transmission of *Mycobacterium abscessus* among patients with cystic fibrosis attending a single clinic. *Clinical Infectious Diseases* **32**, 1648.

Barna JC and Williams DH (1984) The structure and mode of action of glycopeptide antibiotics of the vancomycin group. *Annual Review of Microbiology* **34**, 339.

Bartlett CLR, Macrae AD and Macfarlane JD (1986) Legionella *infections*. London: Edward Arnold.

Baxter RL, Baxter HC, Campbell GA *et al.* (2006) Quantitative analysis of residual protein contamination on reprocessed surgical instruments. *Journal of Hospital Infection* **63**, 439.

Behr MA, Warren SA, Salamon H *et al.* (1999) Transmission of *Mycobacterium tuberculosis* from patients smear-negative for acid-fast bacilli. *Lancet* **353**, 444.

Bernards AT, Harinck HI, Dijkshoorn L, van der Reijden TJ.and van den Broek PJ (2004) Persistent *Acinetobacter baumannii*? Look inside your medical equipment. *Infection Control and Hospital Epidemiology* **25**, 1002.

Biendo M, Laurans G, Lefebvre JF, Daoudi F.and Eb F (1999) Epidemiological study of an *Acinetobacter baumannii* outbreak by using a combination of antibiotyping and ribotyping. *Journal of Clinical Microbiology* **37**, 2170.

Bolton RP and Culshaw MA (1986) Faecal metronidazole concentrations during oral and intravenous therapy for antibiotic associated colitis due to *Clostridium difficile*. *Gut* **27**, 1169.

Bonomo RA (2000) Multiple antibiotic-resistant bacteria in long-term-care facilities: an emerging problem in the practice of infectious diseases. *Clinical Infectious Diseases* **31**, 1414.

Bonten MJM, Hayden MK, Nathan C *et al.* (1996) Epidemiology of colonisation of patients and environment with vancomycin-resistant enterococci. *Lancet* **348**, 1615.

Bouza E, Dryden M, Mohammed R, *et al.* (2008) Results of a phase III trial comparing tolevamer, vancomycin and metronidazole in patients with *Clostridium difficile*-associated diarrhoea. *Programs and Abstracts of the 18th European Congress of Clinical Microbiology and Infectious Diseases, Barcelona, Spain*. Basel: European Society of Clinical Microbiology and Infectious Diseases, Abstract O464.

Boyce JM., Opal SM, Chow JW *et al.* (1994) Outbreak of multidrug-resistant *Enterococcus faecium* with transferable *vanB* class vancomycin resistance. *Journal of Clinical Microbiology* **32**, 1148.

Brown AR, Amyes SGB, Paton R *et al.* (1998) Epidemiology and control of vancomycin-resistant enterococci (VRE) in a renal unit. *Journal of Hospital Infection* **40**, 115.

Brown DFJ and Walpole E (2003) Evaluation of selective and enrichment media for isolation of glycopeptide-resistant enterococci from faecal specimens. *Journal of Antimicrobial Chemotherapy* **51**, 289.

Brown DFJ, Brown NM, Cookson BD *et al.* (2006) National glycopeptide-resistant enterococcal bacteraemia surveillance working group report to the Department of Health, August 2004. *Journal of Hospital Infection* **62**, S1.

Brown DFJ, Edwards DI, Hawkey PM *et al.* on behalf of the Joint Working Party of the British Society for Antimicrobial Chemotherapy, Hospital Infection Society and Infection Control Nurses Association (2005) Guidelines for the laboratory diagnosis and susceptibility testing of methicillin-resistant *Staphylococcus aureus* (MRSA). *Journal of Antimicrobial Chemotherapy* **56,** 1000.

Brown P, Brandel JP, Preece M and Sato T (2006) Iatrogenic Creutzfeldt–Jakob disease: the waning of an era. *Neurology* **67,** 389.

Bruce ME, Will RG, Ironside JW *et al.* (1997) Transmissions to mice indicate that 'new variant' CJD is caused by the BSE agent. *Nature* **389**, 498.

Bruce ME, McConnell I, Will RG and Ironside JW (2001) Detection of variant Creutzfeldt–Jakob disease infectivity in extra-neural tissues. *Lancet* **358**, 208.

Calhoun JH, Murray CK and Manring MM (2008) Multidrug-resistant organisms in military wounds from Iraq and Afghanistan. *Clinical Orthopaedics and Related Research* **466**, 1356.

Casewell M and Phillips I (1977) Hands as route of transmission for *Klebsiella* species. *British Medical Journal* **2**, 1315.

Centers for Disease Control and Prevention (1993) Nosocomial enterococci resistant to vancomycin – United States. MMWR **42**, 597.

Centers for Disease Control and Prevention (1994) Guidelines for preventing the transmission of *Mycobacterium tuberculosis* in health-care facilities. *MMWR* **43**(RR13), 1.

Centers for Disease Control and Prevention (1999) National Nosocomial Infections Surveillance (NNIS) System report, data summary from January 1990–May 1999, issued June 1999. *American Journal of Infection Control* **27,** 520.

Centers for Disease Control and Prevention (2005) Guidelines for the investigation of contacts of persons with infectious tuberculosis. *MMWR* **54**(RR15), 1.

Ceyhan M, Yildirim I, Tekeli A *et al.* (2008) A *Chryseobacterium meningosepticum* outbreak observed in 3 clusters involving both neonatal and non-neonatal pediatric patients. *American Journal of Infection Control* **36**, 453.

Clinical Laboratory Standards Institute (2006) *Performance standards for antimicrobial susceptibility testing*, 16th Informational Supplement M100-S/6. Wayne, PA: CLSI.

Coia JE, Duckworth GJ, Edwards DI *et al.* for the Joint Working Party of the British Society of Antimicrobial Chemotherapy, the Hospital Infection Society, and the Infection Control Nurses Association (2006) Guidelines for the control and prevention of methicillin-resistant *Staphylococcus aureus* (MRSA) in healthcare facilities. *Journal of Hospital Infection* **63**(Suppl 1), 1.

Collinge J, Palmer MS and Dryden AJ (1991) Genetic predisposition to iatrogenic Creutfeldt–Jakob disease. *Lancet* **337**, 1441.

Collinge J, Whitfield J, McKintosh E *et al.* (2006) Kuru in the 21st century-an acquired human prion disease with very long incubation periods. *Lancet* **367**, 2068.

Collins SJ, Lawson VA and Masters CL (2004) Transmissible spongiform encephalopathies. *Lancet* **363**, 51.

Conterno LO, Shymanski J, Ramotar K, Toye B, Zvonar R and Roth V (2007) Impact and cost of infection control measures to reduce nosocomial transmission of extended-spectrum beta-lactamase-producing organisms in a non-outbreak setting. *Journal of Hospital Infection* **65**, 354.

Cookson BD, Macrae MB, Barrett SP *et al.* (2006) Combined Working Party of the Hospital Infection Society and Infection Control Nurses Association. Guidelines for the control of glycopeptide-resistant enterococci in hospitals. *Journal of Hospital Infection* **62**, 6.

Cooper BS, Stone SO, Kibbler CC *et al.* (2003) Systematic review of isolation policies in the hospital management of methicillin-resistant *Staphylococcus aureus*: a review of the literature with epidemiological and economic modelling. *Health Technology Assessment* **7**, 1.

Cosgrove SE, Sakoulas G, Perencevich EN, Schwaber MJ, Karchmer AW, Carmeli Y (2003) Comparison of mortality associated with methicillin-resistant and methicillin-susceptible *Staphylococcus aureus* bacteremia: a meta-analysis. *Clinical Infectious Diseases* **36**, 53.

Courvalin P. (2006) Vancomycin resistance in Gram-positive cocci. *Clinical Infectious Diseases* **42**, S25.

Cox RA, Mallaghan C, Conquest C, King J (1995) Epidemic methicillin-resistant *Staphylococcus aureus*: controlling the spread outside hospital. *Journal of Hospital Infection* **29**, 107.

Dalben M, Varkulja G, Basso M *et al.* (2008) Investigation of an outbreak of *Enterobacter cloacae* in a neonatal unit and review of the literature. *Journal of Hospital Infection* **70**, 7.

Das I, Lambert P, Hill D, Noy M, Bion J.and Elliott T (2002) Carbapenem-resistant *Acinetobacter* and role of curtains in an outbreak in intensive care units. *Journal of Hospital Infection* **50**, 110.

Davey P, Brown E, Fenelon L *et al.* (2005) Interventions to improve antibiotic prescribing practices for hospital inpatients. *Cochrane Database of Systematic Reviews* **4**, CD003543.

De Armond CI and Prusiner SB (2003) Perspectives on prion biology, prion disease pathogenesis, and pharmacologic approaches to treatment. *Clinical Laboratory Medicine* **23**, 1.

Dendukuri N, Costa V, McGregor M and Brophy JM (2005) Probiotic therapy for the prevention and treatment of *Clostridium difficile*-associated diarrhea: a systematic review. *Canadian Medical Association Journal* **19**, 167.

Denton M and Kerr KG (1998) Microbiological and clinical aspects of infection associated with *Stenotrophomonas maltophilia*. *Clin.Microbiol.Rev*, **11**, 57.

Denton M, Todd NJ, Kerr KG, Hawkey PM and Littlewood JM (1998) Molecular epidemiology of *Stenotrophomonas maltophilia* isolated from clinical specimens from patients with cystic fibrosis and associated environmental samples. *Journal of Clinical Microbiology* **36**, 1953.

Department of Health (2001) *Risk assessment for surgical transmission of variant CJD.* Available online at: http://www.doh.gov.uk/en/PublicationsandStatistics/Publications/PublicationsPolicyAndGuidance/DH_4075387.

Department of Health (2004) Bloodborne MRSA infection rates to be halved by 2008 – Reid (press release 4 November). London: Department of Health Available at:

http://www.dh.gov.uk/PublicationsAndStatistics/PressReleases/PressReleasesNotices/fs/en?CONTENT_ID=4093533&chk=MY per cent2BkD/.

Department of Health (2005) *Assessing the risk of vCJD transmission via surgery: an interim review*. Available online at: https://www.dh.gov.uk/en/PublicationsandStatistics/Publications/PublicationsPolicyAndGuidance/DH_4113541/DH_4115311.

Department of Health (2006) Health Technical Memorandum 04-01: *The control of Legionella, hygiene, 'safe' hot water, cold water and drinking systems. Part A Design, installation and testing. Part B Operational management*. London: Department of Health.

DiazGranados CA, Zimmer SM, Klein M and Jernigan JA (2005). Comparison of mortality associated with vancomycin-resistant and vancomycin-susceptible enterococcal bloodstream infections: a meta-analysis. *Clinical Infectious Diseases* **41**, 327.

Drobniewski FA, Gibson A, Ruddy M, Yates MD (2003) Evaluation and utilization as a public health tool of a national molecular epidemiological tuberculosis outbreak database within the United Kingdom from 1997 to 2001. *Journal of Clinical Microbiology* **41**, 1861.

Duckworth G, Cookson B, Humphreys H, Heathcock R (1998) Revised methicillin-resistant *Staphylococcus aureus* infection control guidelines for hospitals. Report of a working party of the British Society for Antimicrobial Chemotherapy, the Hospital Infection Society and the Infection Control Nurses Association. *Journal of Hospital Infection* **39**, 253.

Dufour P, Gillet Y, Bes M *et al.* (2002) Community-acquired methicillin-resistant *Staphylococcus aureus* infections in France: emergence of a single clone that produces Panton–Valentine leukocidin. *Clinical Infectious Diseases* **35**, 819.

Ellames D, Wilcox MH, Fawley WN *et al.* (2007) Comparison of risk factors and outcome of cases of *Clostridium difficile* infection due to ribotype 027 vs. other ribotypes. *Programs and Abstracts of the 47th Interscience Conference on Antimicrobial Agents and Chemotherapy, Chicago, IL*. Washington, DC: American Society for Microbiology, p. 337.

Endtz HP, van den BN, van Belkum A. *et al.* (1997) Fecal carriage of vancomycin-resistant enterococci in hospitalized patients and those living in the community in The Netherlands. *Journal of Clinical Microbiology* **35**, 3026.

Enright MC, Robinson DA, Randle G *et al.* (2002) The evolutionary history of methicillin-resistant *Staphylococcus aureus* (MRSA). *Proceedings of the National Academy of Sciences of the United States of America* **99**, 7687.

European Antimicrobial Resistance Surveillance System (2005) *Annual Report 2004*. Bilthoven: RIVM. Available online at: http://www.rivm.nl/earss/result/Monitoring_reports/

Evans JT, Smith EG, Banerjee A *et al.* (2007) Cluster of human tuberculosis caused by *Mycobacterium bovis*: evidence for person-to-person transmission in the UK. *Lancet* **14**, 1270.

Falagas ME, Koletsi PK.and Bliziotis IA (2006) The diversity of definitions of multidrug-resistant (MDR) and pandrug-resistant (PDR) *Acinetobacter baumannii* and *Pseudomonas aeruginosa*. *Journal of Medical Microbiology* **55**, 1619.

Fallon RJ (1994) How to prevent an outbreak of Legionnaires disease. *Journal of Hospital Infection* **27**, 247.

Fawley WN, Underwood S, Freeman J *et al.* (2007) Efficacy of hospital cleaning agents and germicides against epidemic *Clostridium difficile* strains. *Infection Control and Hospital Epidemiology* **28**, 920.

Fekety R, Silva J, Kauffman C *et al.* (1989) Treatment of antibiotic-associated *Clostridium difficile* colitis with oral vancomycin: comparison of two dosage regimens. *American Journal of Medicine* **86,** 15.

Fernandez A, Anand G and Friedenberg F (2004) Factors associated with failure of metronidazole in Clostridium difficile-associated disease. *Journal of Clinical Gastroenterology* **38,** 414.

Festini F, Buzzetti R, Bassi C *et al.* (2006) Isolation measures for prevention of infection with respiratory pathogens in cystic fibrosis: a systematic review. *Journal of Hospital Infection* **64,** 1.

Fraise AP (1996) The treatment and control of vancomycin resistant enterococci. *Journal of Antimicrobial Chemotherapy* **38,** 753.

Freeman J, Baines SD, Jabes D and Wilcox MH (2005) Comparison of the efficacy of ramoplanin and vancomycin in both *in vitro* and *in vivo* models of clindamycin-induced *Clostridium difficile* infection. *Journal of Antimicrobial Chemotherapy* **56,** 717.

Freeman J, Baines SD, Saxton K and Wilcox MH (2007) Effect of metronidazole on growth and toxin production by epidemic *Clostridium difficile* PCR ribotypes 001 and 027 in a human gut model. *Journal of Antimicrobial Chemotherapy* **60,** 83.

French GL (1998) Enterococci and vancomycin resistance. *Clinical Infectious Diseases* **27**(Suppl 1), S75.

French GL (2005) Clinical impact and relevance of antibiotic resistance. *Advanced Drug Delivery Reviews* **57,** 1514.

Frieden TR, Munsiff SS, Low DE *et al.* (1993) Emergence of vancomycin-resistant enterococci in New York city. *Lancet* **342,** 76.

Furtado GH, Perdiz LB, Santana IL, Camargo MM, Parreira FC, Angelieri DB and Medeiros EA (2008) Impact of a hospital-wide antimicrobial formulary intervention on the incidence of multidrug-resistant gram-negative bacteria, *American Journal of Infection Control* **36,** 661.

Gemmell CG, Edwards DI, Fraise AP, Gould FK, Ridgway GL, Warren RE on behalf of the Joint Working Party of the British Society for Antimicrobial Chemotherapy, Hospital Infection Society and Infection Control Nurses Association (2006) Guidelines for the prophylaxis and treatment of methicillin-resistant *Staphylococcus aureus* (MRSA) infections in the UK. *Journal of Antimicrobial Chemotherapy* **57,** 589.

Goldmann D (2006) System failure versus personal accountability – the case for clean hands. *New England Journal of Medicine* **355,** 121.

Gonzales RD, Schreckenberger PC, Graham MB *et al.* (2001) Infections due to vancomycin-resistant *Enterococcus faecium* resistant to linezolid. *Lancet* **357,** 1179.

Goossens H (1998) Spread of vancomycin-resistant enterococci: differences between the United States and Europe. *Infection Control and Hospital. Epidemiology* **19,** 546.

Gouby A, Carles-Nurit MJ, Bouziges N, Bourg G, Mesnard R.and Bouvet PJ (1992) Use of pulsed-field gel electrophoresis for investigation of hospital outbreaks of *Acinetobacter baumannii. Journal of Clinical Microbiology* **30,** 1588.

Govan JR and Nelson JW (1992) Microbiology of lung infection in cystic fibrosis. *British Medical Bulletin* **48,** 912.

Griffith DE, Aksamit T, Brown-Elliott BA, Catanzaro A *et al.* (2007) An official ATS/IDSA statement: diagnosis, treatment, and prevention of nontuberculous mycobacterial diseases. *American Respiratory Critical Care Medicine* **175,** 367.

Grundmann H, Tami A, Hori S, Halwani M and Slack R (2002) Nottingham

Staphylococcus aureus population study: prevalence of MRSA among elderly people in the community. *British Medical Journal* **324,** 1365.

Hawkey PM (2008) The growing burden of antimicrobial resistance. *Journal of Antimicrobial Chemotherapy* 62(Suppl 1), pi1.

Health and Safety Executive (2000) *Legionnaire's disease. The control of legionella bacteria in water systems. Approved Code of Practice and guidance.* London: The Stationery Office.

Health Protection Agency (2006). Available at: http://www.hpa.org.uk/webw/ HPAweb&Page&HPAwebAutolistName/Page/1225960587688?p=1225960587688.

Health Protection Agency (2008) *Surveillance of healthcare associated infections report 2008.* London: Health Protection Agency. Available at: http://www.hpa.org.uk/ web/HPAwebFile/HPAweb_C/1216193833496 (last accessed 22 August 2008)

Hibbert-Rogers LC, Heritage J, Gascoyne-Binzi DM, Hawkey PM, Todd N, Lewis IJ and Bailey C (1995) Molecular epidemiology of ceftazidime resistant Enterobacteriaceae from patients on a paediatric oncology ward. *Journal of Antimicrobial Chemotherapy* **36,** 65.

Hickson M, D'Souza AL, Muthu N *et al.* (2007) Use of probiotic *Lactobacillus* preparation to prevent diarrhoea associated with antibiotics: randomised double blind placebo controlled trial. *BMJ* **335,** 80.

Hill AF, Desbruslais M, Joiner S *et al.* (1997) The same prion strain causes vCJD and BSE. *Nature* **389,** 448.

Hilton D, Ghani A, Conyers L *et al.* (2004) Prevalence of lymphoreticular prion protein accumulation in UK tissues. *Journal of Pathlogy* **203,** 733.

Holden MT, Feil EJ, Lindsay JA *et al.* (2004) Complete genomes of two clinical *Staphylococcus aureus* strains: evidence for the rapid evolution of virulence and drug resistance. *Proceedings of the National Academy of Sciences of the United States of America* **101,** 9786.

Hollander R, Ebke M, Barck H.and von Pritzbuer E (2001) Asymptomatic carriage of *Klebsiella pneumoniae* producing extended-spectrum beta-lactamase by patients in a neurological early rehabilitation unit: management of an outbreak. *Journal of Hospital Infection* **48,** 207.

Holmes A, Nolan R, Taylor R *et al.* (1999) An epidemic of *Burkholderia cepacia* transmitted between patients with and without cystic fibrosis. *Journal of Infectious Disease* **179,** 1197.

Hoque SN, Graham J, Kaufmann ME and Tabaqchali S (2001) *Chryseobacterium (Flavobacterium) meningosepticum* outbreak associated with colonization of water taps in a neonatal intensive care unit. *Journal of Hospital Infection* **47,** 188.

Hospital Infection Control Practices Advisory Committee (1995) Recommendations for preventing the spread of vancomycin resistance. *Infection Control and Hospital. Epidemiology* **16,** 105–113. [Erratum, *Infection Control and Hospital. Epidemiology* **16,** 498].

Hutchinson J, Runge W, Mulvey M *et al.* (2004) *Burkholderia cepacia* infections associated with intrinsically contaminated ultrasound gel: the role of microbial degradation of parabens. *Infection Control and Hospital Epidemiology* **25,** 291.

Ieven M, Vercauteren E, Descheemaeker P *et al.* (1999) Comparison of direct plating and broth enrichment culture for the detection of intestinal colonization by glycopeptide-resistant enterococci among hospitalized patients. *Journal of Clinical Microbiology* **37,** 1436.

Ironside JW, Bishop MT, Connolly K *et al.* (2006) Variant Creutzfeldt–Jakob disease: prion protein genotype analysis of positive appendix tissue samples from a retrospective prevalence study. *BMJ* **332**, 1189.

Itani KM, Wilson SE, Awad SS *et al.* (2006) Ertapenem versus cefotetan prophylaxis in elective colorectal surgery. *New England Journal of Medicine* **355**, 2640.

Jönsson BE, Gilljam M, Lindblad A, Ridell M, Wold AE and Welinder-Olssen C (2007) Molecular epidemiology of *Mycobacterium abscessus*, with focus on cystic fibrosis. *Journal of Clinical Microbiology* **45**, 1497.

Jawad A, Seifert H, Snelling AM, Heritage J and Hawkey PM (1998) Survival of *Acinetobacter baumannii* on dry surfaces: comparison of outbreak and sporadic isolates. *Journal of Clinical Microbiology* **36**, 1938.

Jevons MP (1961) Celbenin-resistant staphylococci. *British Medical Journal* **i**, 124.

Johnson S, Schriever C, Galang M *et al.* (2007) Interruption of recurrent *Clostridium difficile*-associated diarrhea episodes by serial therapy with vancomycin and rifaximin. *Clinical Infectious Diseases* **44**, 846.

Kim J, Kwon Y, Pai H, Kim JW and Cho DT (1998) Survey of *Klebsiella pneumoniae* strains producing extended-spectrum beta-lactamases: prevalence of SHV-12 and SHV-2a in Korea. *Journal of Clinical Microbiology* **36**, 1446.

Kirst HA, Thompson DG and Nicas TI (1998) Historical yearly usage of vancomycin. *Antimicrobial Agents and Chemotherapy* **42**, 1303.

Kreisel D, Savel TG, Silver AL and Cunningham JD (1995) Surgical antibiotic prophylaxis and *Clostridium difficile* toxin positivity. *Archives of Surgery* **130**, 989.

Kuijper EJ and Wilcox MH (2008) Decreased effectiveness of metronidazole for the treatment of *Clostridium difficile* infection? *Clinical Infectious Diseases* **47**, 63.

Kuijper EJ, Coignard B, Brazier JS *et al.* Update of *Clostridium difficile*-associated disease due to PCR ribotype 027 in Europe. *Euro Surveillance* **12**, E1-2.

Kutty PK, Moody B, Gullion JS *et al.* (2007) Multistate outbreak of *Burkholderia cenocepacia* colonization and infection associated with the use of intrinsically contaminated alcohol-free mouthwash. *Chest* **132**, 1825.

Ladogana A, Puopolo M, Croes EA *et al.* (2005) Mortality from Creutzfeldt–Jakob disease and related disorders in Europe, Australia and Canada. *Neurology* **64**, 1586.

Lambregts-van Weezenbeek CS, Sebek MM, van Gerven PJ *et al.* (2003) Tuberculosis contact investigation and DNA fingerprint surveillance in The Netherlands: 6 years' experience with nation-wide cluster feedback and cluster monitoring. *International Journal of Tuberculosis and Lung Disease* **7**(Suppl 3), S463.

Landman D, Bratu S, Kochar S *et al.* (2007) Evolution of antimicrobial resistance among *Pseudomonas aeruginosa*, *Acinetobacter baumannii* and *Klebsiella pneumoniae* in Brooklyn, NY. *Journal of Antimicrobial Chemotherapy* **60**, 78.

Lau SH, Kaufmann ME, Livermore DM *et al.* (2008) UK epidemic *Escherichia coli* strains A-E, with CTX-M-15 β-lactamase, all belong to the international O25:H4-ST131 clone. *Journal of Antimicrobial Chemotherapy* **62**, 1241.

Laurent C, Rodriguez-Villalobos H, Rost F *et al.* (2008) Intensive care unit outbreak of extended-spectrum beta-lactamase-producing *Klebsiella pneumoniae* controlled by cohorting patients and reinforcing infection control measures. *Infection Control and Hospital Epidemiology* **29**, 517.

Leclercq R, Derlot E, Duval J *et al.* (1988) Plasmid-mediated resistance to vancomycin and teicoplanin in *Enterococcus faecium*. *New England Journal of Medicine* **319**, 157.

Leclerq R and Courvalin P (1997) Resistance to glycopeptides in enterococci. *Clinical Infectious Diseases* **24**, 545.

Leonard J, Marshall JK and Moayyedi P (2007) Systematic review of the risk of enteric infection in patients taking acid suppression. *American Journal of Gastroenterology* **102**, 2047.

Levidiotou S, Galanakis E, Vrioni G, Papamichael D, Nakos G and Stefanou D (2002) A multi-resistant *Acinetobacter baumannii* outbreak in a general intensive care unit. *In Vivo* **16**, 117.

Lewis DA, Hawkey PM, Watts JA, Speller, DC, Primavesi RJ, Fleming PJ and Pitt TL (1983) Infection with netilmicin resistant *Serratia marcescens* in a special care baby unit, *British Medical Journal (Clinical Research Ed)* **287**, 1701.

Livermore DM and Hawkey PM (2005) CTX-M: changing the face of ESBLs in the UK. *Journal of Antimicrobial Chemotherapy* **56**, 451.

Lockhart SR, Abramson MA, Beekmann SE *et al.* (2007) Antimicrobial resistance among Gram-negative bacilli causing infections in intensive care unit patients in the United States between 1993 and 2004. *Journal of Clinical Microbiology* **45**, 3352.

Loo VG, Poirier L, Miller MA *et al.* (2005) A predominantly clonal multi-institutional outbreak of *Clostridium difficile*-associated diarrhea with high morbidity and mortality. *New England Journal of Medicine* **353**, 2442.

Louie T, Gerson M, Grimard D *et al.* (2007) Results of phase III trial comparing tolevamer, vancomycin and metronidazole in patients with *Clostridium difficile*-associated diarrhoea (CDAD). *Programs and Abstracts of the 47th Interscience Conference on Antimicrobial Agents and Chemotherapy, Chicago, IL*. Washington, DC: American Society for Microbiology, p. 212, Abstract K-425a,

Macrae MB, Shannon KP, Rayner DM, Kaiser AM, Hoffman PN and French GL (2001) A simultaneous outbreak on a neonatal unit of two strains of multiply antibiotic resistant *Klebsiella pneumoniae* controllable only by ward closure. *Journal of Hospital Infection* **49**, 183.

Mahenthiralingam E, Baldwin A and Dowson CG (2008) *Burkholderia cepacia* complex bacteria: opportunistic pathogens with important natural biology. *Journal of Applied Microbiology* **104**, 1539.

Mahenthiralingam E, Vandamme P, Campbell ME *et al.* (2001) Infection with *Burkholderia cepacia* complex genomovars in patients with cystic fibrosis: virulent transmissible strains of genomovar III can replace *Burkholderia multivorans*. *Clinical Infectious Diseases* **33**, 1469.

Maragakis LL, Cosgrove SE, Song X *et al.* (2004) An outbreak of multidrug-resistant *Acinetobacter baumannii* associated with pulsatile lavage wound treatment. *JAMA* **292**, 3006.

Martinez-Solano L, Macia MD, Fajardo A, Oliver A and Martinez JL (2008) Chronic *Pseudomonas aeruginosa* infection in chronic obstructive pulmonary disease. *Clinical Infectious Disease* **47**, 1526.

Masters CL, Harris JO, Gadjusek DC *et al.* (1979) Creutzfeldt–Jakob disease: patterns of worldwide occurrence and the significance of familial and sporadic clustering. *Annals of Neurology* **5**, 177.

Mazars E, Lesjean S, Banuls AL *et al.* (2001) High-resolution minisatellite-based typing as a portable approach to global analysis of *Mycobacterium tuberculosis* molecular epidemiology. *Proceedings of the National Academy of Sciences USA* **98**, 1901.

McNeil SA, Nordstrom-Lerner L, Malani, PN, Zervos, M and Kauffman CA (2001) Outbreak of sternal surgical site infections due to *Pseudomonas aeruginosa* traced to a scrub nurse with onychomycosis, *Clinical Infectious Diseases* **33**, 317.

Moellering RC (1992) Emergence of enterococcus as a significant pathogen. *Clinical Infectious Diseases* **14**,1173.

Montecalvo MA, de Lencastre H, Carraher M *et al.* (1995) Natural history of colonization with vancomycin-resistant *Enterococcus faecium. Infection Control and Hospital. Epidemiology* **16**, 680.

Munoz-Price LS, Lolans K and Quinn JP (2005) Emergence of resistance to daptomycin during treatment of vancomycin resistant *Enterococcus faecalis* infection. *Clinical Infectious Diseases* **41**, 565.

Murdoch H, Taylor D, Dickenson J *et al.* (2006) Surface decontamination of surgical instruments: an ongoing dilemma. *Journal of Hospital Infection* **63**, 432.

Murray BE (1990) The life and times of the enterococcus. *Clinical Microbiology Reviews* **3**, 46.

Murray BE (2000) Vancomycin-resistant enterococcal infections. *New England Journal of Medicine* **342**, 710.

Muscarella LF (2004) Contribution of tap water and environmental surfaces to nosocomial transmission of antibiotic-resistant *Pseudomonas aeruginosa. Infection Control and Hospital Epidemiology* **25**, 342.

Muto CA, Jernigan JA, Ostrowsky BE *et al.* (2003) SHEA guideline for preventing nosocomial transmission of multidrug-resistant strains of *Staphylococcus aureus* and Enterococcus. *Infection Control and Hospital Epidemiology* **24**, 362.

National Collaborating Centre for Chronic Conditions (2006) *Tuberculosis: clinical diagnosis and management of tuberculosis, and measures for its prevention and control.* London: Royal College of Physicians.

NHS Estates (2005) *Isolation facilities in acute settings.* Health Building Note 4, supplement 1. London: The Stationary Office.

Noble WC, Viran Z and Cree RGA (1992) Co-transfer of vancomycin and other resistance genes from Enterococcus faecalis NCTC 12201 to *Staphylococcus aureus. FEMS Microbiology Letters* **93**, 195.

Nseir S, Di Pompeo C, Brisson H *et al.* (2006) Intensive care unit-acquired *Stenotrophomonas maltophilia*: incidence, risk factors, and outcome. *Critical Care* **10**, pR143.

Office for National Statistics (2008) *Clostridium difficile* deaths. Available at: http://www.statistics.gov.uk/CCI/nugget.asp?ID=1735&Pos=1&ColRank=1&Rank=192 (last accessed 22 August 2008).

Oh WS, Ko KS, Song J *et al.* (2005) High rate of resistance to quinupristin–dalfopristin in *Enterococcus faecium* clinical isolates from Korea. *Antimicrobial Agents and Chemotherapy* **49**, 5176.

Olivier K, Weber DJ, Wallace RJ *et al.* (2003) Nontuberculous mycobacteria I: multicenter prevalence study in cystic fibrosis. *American Journal of Respiratory and Critical Care Medicine* **167**, 828.

Pépin J, Routhier S, Gagnon S and Brazeau I (2006) Management and outcomes of a first recurrence of *Clostridium difficile*-associated disease in Quebec, Canada. *Clinical Infectious Diseases* **42**, 758.

Pépin J, Valiquette L, Gagnon S *et al.* (2007) Outcomes of *Clostridium difficile* associated disease treated with metronidazole or vancomycin before and after the emergence of NAP1/027. *American Journal of Gastroenterology* **102**, 2781.

Paterson DL (2006) The epidemiological profile of infections with multidrug-resistant *Pseudomonas aeruginosa* and *Acinetobacter* species. *Clinical Infectious Diseases* **43**(Suppl 2), pS43.

Peden AH, Head MW, Ritchie DL *et al.* (2004) Preclinical vCJD after blood transfusion in a PRNP codon 129 heterozygous patient. *Lancet* **364**, 527.

Peleg AY, Seifert H and Paterson DL (2008) *Acinetobacter baumannii*: emergence of a successful pathogen, *Clinical Microbiology Reviews* **21**, 538.

Pena C, Pujol M, Ardanuy C *et al.* (1998) Epidemiology and successful control of a large outbreak due to *Klebsiella pneumoniae* producing extended-spectrum beta-lactamases, *Antimicrobial Agents and Chemotheapy* **42**, 53.

Philippon A, Arlet G and Jacoby GA (2002) Plasmid-determined AmpC-type beta-lactamases. *Antimicrobial Agents and Chemotherapy* **46**, 1.

Pierre-Audigier C, Ferroni A, Sermet-Gaudelus I. *et al.* (2005) Age-related prevalence and distribution of nontuberculous mycobacterial species among patients with cystic fibrosis. *Journal of Clinical Microbiology* **43**, 3467.

Pillai A and Nelson R (2008) Probiotics for treatment of *Clostridium difficile* associated colitis in adults. *Cochrane Database of Systematic Reviews* **1**, CD004611.

Pitt TL and Simpson AJ (2005) *Pseudomonas* and *Burkholderia* spp. In: Gillespie SH and Hawkey PM (eds) *Principles and practice of clinical microbiology*, 2nd edn. Chichester: John Wiley and Sons.

Prusiner SB (2001) Shattock lecture: neurodegenerative diseases and prions. *New England Journal Medicine* **334**, 1516.

Quittell L (2004) Management of non-tuberculous mycobacteria in patients with cystic fibrosis. *Paediatric Respiratory Reviews* **5**(Suppl A), S217.

Reacher MH, Shah A, Livermore DM *et al.* (2000) Bacteraemia and antibiotic resistance of its pathogens reported in England and Wales between 1990 and 1998: trend analysis. *British Medical Journal* **320**, 213.

Reverdy ME, Freney J, Fleurette J *et al.* (1984) Nosocomial colonization and infection by *Achromobacter xylosoxidans*. *Journal of Clinical Microbiology* **19**, 140.

Reynolds PE (1989) Structure, biochemistry and mechanism of action of glycopeptide antibiotics. *European Journal of Clinical Microbiology and Infectious Diseases* **8**, 943.

Rice LB, Eckstein EC, DeVente J and Shlaes DM (1996) Ceftazidime-resistant *Klebsiella pneumoniae* isolates recovered at the Cleveland Department of Veterans Affairs Medical Center. *Clinical Infectious Diseases* **23**, 118.

Ridwan B, Mascini E, van der Reijden N *et al.* (2002) What action should be taken to prevent spread of vancomycin resistant enterococci in European hospitals. *British Medical Journal* **324**, 666.

Roghmann M, Qaiyumi S, Johnson JA *et al.* (1997) Recurrent vancomycin-resistant *Enterococcus faecium* bacteremia in a leukemia patient who was persistently colonized with vancomycin-resistant enterococci for two years. *Clinical Infectious Diseases* **24**, 514.

Romling U, Wingender J, Muller H and Tummler B (1994) A major *Pseudomonas aeruginosa* clone common to patients and aquatic habitats. *Applied and Environmenal Microbiology* **60**, 1734.

Rossolini GM and Mantengoli E (2005) Treatment and control of severe infections caused by multiresistant *Pseudomonas aeruginosa*. *Clinical Microbiology and Infection* **11**(Suppl 4), 17.

Sabol K, Patterson JE, Le JS *et al.* (2005) Emergence of daptomycin resistance in *Enterococcus faecium* during daptomycin therapy. *Antimicrobial Agents and Chemotherapy* **49**, 1664.

Safdar A and Rolston KV (2007) *Stenotrophomonas maltophilia*: changing spectrum of a serious bacterial pathogen in patients with cancer. *Clinical Infectious Diseases* **45**, 1602.

Saiman L and Siegel J (2004) Infection control in cystic fibrosis. *Clinical Microbiology Review* **17**, 57.

Samra Z, Bahar J, Madar-Shapiro L, Aziz N, Israel S and Bishara J (2008) Evaluation of CHROMagar KPC for rapid detection of carbapenem-resistant Enterobacteriaceae. *Journal of Clinical Microbiology* **46**, 3110.

Saxton K, Baines SD, Freeman J, O'Connor R and Wilcox MH (2009) Effects of exposure of *Clostridium difficile* PCR ribotypes 027 and 001 to fluoroquinolones in a human gut model. *Antimicrobial Agents and Chemotherapy* **53**, 412.

Schaberg DR, Culver DH, Gaynes RP (1991) Major trends in the microbial etiology of nosocomial infection. *American Journal of Medicine* **91**(Suppl 3B), S72.

Schoch PE and Cunha BA (1988) Nosocomial *Achromobacter xylosoxidans* infections. *Infection Control and Hospital Epidemiology* **9**, 84.

Schouten MA, Hoogkamp-Korstanje JA, Meis JF *et al.* (2000) Prevalence of vancomycin-resistant enterococci in Europe. *European Journal of Clinical Microbiology and Infectious Diseases* **19**, 816.

Seifert H, Dijkshoorn L, Gerner-Smidt P, Pelzer N, Tjernberg I and Vaneechoutte M (1997) Distribution of *Acinetobacter* species on human skin: comparison of phenotypic and genotypic identification methods. *Journal of Clinical Microbiology* **35**, 2819.

Sermet-Gaudelus I, Le Bourgeois M, Pierre-Audigier C *et al.* (2003) *Mycobacterium abscessus* and children with cystic fibrosis. *Emerging Infectious Diseases* **9**, 1587.

Settle CD, Wilcox MH, Fawley WN *et al.* (1998) Prospective study of the risk of *Clostridium difficile* diarrhoea in elderly patients following treatment with cefotaxime or piperacillin–tazobactam. *Alimentary Pharmacology and Therapeutics* **12**, 1217.

Shanson DC (1981) Antibiotic-resistant *Staphylococcus aureus*. *Journal of Hospital Infection* **2**, 11.

Smith MJ, Efthimiou J, Hodson ME and Batten JC (1984) Mycobacterial isolations in young adults with cystic fibrosis. *Thorax* **39**, 369.

Snelling AM, Gerner-Smidt P, Hawkey PM *et al.* (1996) Validation of use of whole-cell repetitive extragenic palindromic sequence-based PCR (REP-PCR) for typing strains belonging to the *Acinetobacter calcoaceticus-Acinetobacter baumannii* complex and application of the method to the investigation of a hospital outbreak. *Journal of Clinical Microbiology* **34**, 1193.

Spicer WJ (1984) Three strategies in the control of staphylococci, including methicillin-resistant *Staphylococcus aureus*. *Journal of Hospital Infection* **5(A)**, 45.

Srinivasan A, Wolfenden LL, Song X (2003) An outbreak of *Pseudomonas aeruginosa* infections associated with flexible bronchoscopes. *New England Journal of Medicine* **348**, 221.

Supply P, Allix C, Lesjean S *et al.* (2006) Proposal for standardization of optimized mycobacterial interspersed repetitive unit-variable-number tandem repeat typing of *Mycobacterium tuberculosis*. *Journal of Clinical Microbiology* **44**, 4498.

Taylor DM (2000) Inactivation of transmissible degenerative encephalopathy agents: a review. *Veterinary Journal* **159**, 10.

Taylor DM (2004) Resistance of transmissible spongiform encephalopathy agents to decontamination. *Contributions to Microbiology* **11**, 136.

Teres D, Roizen MF and Bushnell LS (1973) Successful weaning from controlled ventilation despite high deadspace-to-tidal volume ratio. *Anesthesiology* **39**, 656.

Tokars JI, Satake S, Rimland D *et al.* (1999) The prevalence of colonization with vancomycin-resistant *Enterococcus* at a Veterans' Affairs institution. *Infection Control and Hospital Epidemiology* **20**, 171.

Tornieporth NG, Roberts RB, John J *et al.* (1996) Risk factors associated with vancomycin-resistant *Enterococcus faecium* infection or colonization in 145 matched case patients and control patients. *Clinical Infectious Diseases* **23**, 767.

Torrens JK, Dawkins P, Conway SP and Moya E (1998) Non-tuberculous mycobacteria in cystic fibrosis. *Thorax* **53**, 182.

Urban C, Segal-Maurer S and Rahal JJ (2003) Considerations in control and treatment of nosocomial infections due to multidrug-resistant *Acinetobacter baumannii*. *Clinical Infectious Diseases* **36**, 1268.

Uttley AH, Collins CH, Naidoo J *et al.* (1988) Vancomycin-resistant enterococci. *Lancet* **1**, 57.

Valiquette L, Cossette B, Garant MP *et al.* (2007) Impact of a reduction in the use of high-risk antibiotics on the course of an epidemic of *Clostridium difficile*-associated disease caused by the hypervirulent NAP1/027 strain. *Clinical Infectious Diseases* **45**(Suppl 2), S112.

van den Bogaard AE, Bruinsma N and Stobberingh EE (2000) The effect of banning avoparcin on VRE carriage in The Netherlands. *Journal of Antimicrobial Chemotherapy* **46**, 146.

van den Bogaard AE, Mertens P, London NH *et al.* (1997) High prevalence of colonization with vancomycin- and pristinamycin-resistant enterococci in healthy humans and pigs in The Netherlands: is the addition of antibiotics to animal feeds to blame? *Journal of Antimicrobial Chemotherapy* **40**, 454.

Verhoef J, Beaujean D, Blok H *et al.* (1999) A Dutch approach to methicillin-resistant *Staphylococcus aureus*. *European Journal of Clinical Microbiology and Infectious Disease* **18**, 461.

Villegas MV and Hartstein AI (2003) Acinetobacter outbreaks, 1977–2000. *Infection Control and Hospital Epidemiology* **24**, 284.

Wadsworth JD, Joiner S, Hill AF *et al.* (2001) Tissue distribution of protease resistant prion protein in variant Creutzfeldt–Jakob disease using a highly sensitive immunoblotting assay. *Lancet* **358**, 171.

Warren RE, Harvey G, Carr R, Ward D and Doroshenko A (2008) Control of infections due to extended-spectrum beta-lactamase-producing organisms in hospitals and the community. *Clinical Microbiology and Infectection* **14**(Suppl 1), 124.

Webster CA, Crowe M, Humphreys H and Towner KJ (1998) Surveillance of an adult intensive care unit for long-term persistence of a multi-resistant strain of *Acinetobacter baumannii. European Journal of Clinical Microbiology and Infectious Diseases* **17**, 171.

Wegener HC (1998) Historical yearly usage of glycopeptides for animals and humans: the American-European paradox revisited. *Antimicrobial Agents and Chemotherapy* **42**, 3049.

Whitby PW, Carter KB, Hatter KL, LiPuma JJ and Stull TL (2000) Identification of members of the *Burkholderia cepacia* complex by species-specific PCR. *Journal of Clinical Microbiology* **38**, 2962.

Widmer AF, Wenzel RP, Trilla A, Bale MJ, Jones RN and Doebbeling BN (1993) Outbreak of *Pseudomonas aeruginosa* infections in a surgical intensive care unit: probable transmission via hands of a health care worker, *Clinical Infectious Diseases* **16**, 372.

Wilcox MH and Sandoe JA (2007) Probiotics and diarrhea: data are not widely applicable. *BMJ* **335**, 171.

Wilcox MH, Fawley WN, Settle CD and Davidson A (1998) Recurrence of symptoms in *Clostridium difficile* infection – relapse or reinfection? *Journal of Hospital Infection* **38**, 93.

Wilcox MH, Freeman J, Fawley W *et al.* (2004) Long-term surveillance of cefotaxime and piperacillin–tazobactam prescribing and incidence of *Clostridium difficile* diarrhoea. *Journal of Antimicrobial Chemotherapeutics* **54**, 168.

Wilcox MH, Mooney L, Bendall R *et al.* (2008) A case-control study of community associated *Clostridium difficile* infection. *Journal of Antimicrobial Chemotherapy* **62**, 388.

Wilks M, Wilson A, Warwick S, Price E, Kennedy D, Ely A and Millar MR (2006) Control of an outbreak of multidrug-resistant *Acinetobacter baumannii-calcoaceticus* colonization and infection in an intensive care unit (ICU) without closing the ICU or placing patients in isolation. *Infection Control and Hospital Epidemiology* **27**, 654.

Will RG, Ironside JW, Zeidler M *et al.* (1996) A new variant of Creuzfeldt–Jakob disease in the UK. *Lancet* **347**, 921.

Woodford N, Johnson AP, Morrison D *et al.* (1995) Current perspectives on glycopeptide resistance. *Clinical Microbiology Reviews* **8**, 585.

Woodhouse R, Peckham DG, Conway SP and Denton M (2008) Water filters can prevent *Stenotrophomonas maltophilia* contamination of nebuliser equipment used by people with cystic fibrosis. *Journal of Hospital Infection* **68**, 371.

World Health Organisation (2006) *WHO guidelines on tissue infectivity distribution in transmissible spongiform encephalopathies.* Geneva: WHO Press.

Wullt M and Odenholt I (2004) A double-blind randomized controlled trial of fusidic acid and metronidazole for treatment of an initial episode of *Clostridium difficile*-associated diarrhoea. *Journal of Antimicrobial Chemotherapy* **54**, 211.

Zanetti G, Blanc DS, Federli I *et al.* (2007) Importation of *Acinetobacter baumannii* into a burn unit: a recurrent outbreak of infection associated with widespread environmental contamination. *Infection Control and Hospital Epidemiology* **28**, 723.

Zar FA, Bakkanagari SR, Moorthi KM and Davis MB (2007) A comparison of vancomycin and metronidazole for the treatment of *Clostridium difficile*-associated diarrhea, stratified by disease severity. *Clinical Infectious Diseases* **45,** 302.

Zarrilli R, Casillo R, Di Popolo A *et al.* (2007) Molecular epidemiology of a clonal outbreak of multidrug-resistant *Acinetobacter baumannii* in a university hospital in Italy. *Clinical Microbiology and Infection* **13,** 481.

PART THREE

Prevention

13 PREVENTION OF INFECTION IN WARDS AND OUTPATIENT DEPARTMENTS

Dawn Hill and Susan Millward

INTRODUCTION

There are various methods by which patients, healthcare staff and visitors can be protected from micro-organisms whilst in wards or outpatient healthcare facilities. A combination of well-designed buildings and the application of standard infection control precautions for all patients will assist in the prevention and control of infection. The application of transmission-based precautions when patients are managed with known infections will support the prevention of healthcare-associated infection. The safe management of wounds and invasive devices will also protect patients from unnecessary infections.

BUILDING DESIGN AND ENVIRONMENTAL HYGIENE

The environment within which healthcare is provided can have a significant impact on the prevention and control of infection. It is recognized that infection control advice must be an integral part of the design process for any building or developmental work to ensure that infection control is 'designed into' all healthcare builds (NHS Estates, 2002). Infection Control Teams (ICTs) need to be actively involved in all stages of a reconfiguration or new build to ensure that infection control issues are taken into account. National Healthcare Strategies reinforce the inclusion of infection prevention within building design together with the maintenance of a clean environment.

Wards and outpatients departments

Transmission of infection is more likely to occur in large open wards and departments and, therefore, consideration must be given to designing healthcare facilities, which will minimize this risk.

Infection Control Teams must ensure that all building work and environmental design takes account of national guidance (Health Facilities Note 30, NHS Estates, 2002). In particular, ICTs must ensure that national standards contained in guidance are included in build specifications. The areas, which often create challenges when a new build is planned, include the provision of sufficient space between beds, adequate storage for equipment, linen and waste and the provision of sufficient numbers of hand wash-basins. Therefore clinical staff and ICTs must ensure that these aspects are addressed at an early stage of planning. Bed groupings should be kept to the minimum number possible with inpatient bays having no more than four beds (DH Estates and Facilities Division, 2008). The number of single rooms should also reflect the developing nature of healthcare, antimicrobial resistance and patient expectations. The provision of sufficient numbers of single rooms within healthcare facilities is now seen as of paramount importance in the control of healthcare-associated infections (Noble, 2004).

Outpatient departments need to take account of the move towards the increased provision of healthcare in the primary care setting, with the likelihood that more patients will attend outpatient clinics for review. Consideration should therefore be given to the types of treatments and investigations that may be performed in such environments in the future along with any anticipated increased throughput of patients.

Isolation facilities

Patient placement can contribute to the prevention of transmission of micro-organisms (e.g. patient isolation). The design of single rooms needs to take account of the requirement for patient and staff visibility. This will ensure that the rooms are used appropriately with doors being closed when required to contain micro-organisms transmitted by the airborne route. Well-designed single rooms, which address the issue of visibility, assist with the need for communication between healthcare staff and patients, while minimizing risks of patient perception of loneliness and isolation.

Single rooms are required for patients with known or suspected airborne infections and those whose condition results in contamination of the environment, such as occurs with diarrhoea and vomiting, heavily discharging wounds, uncontrolled bleeding or heavy dispersal of skin scales owing to skin conditions or burns. Single rooms can act as a reminder in ensuring that staff adhere to standard precautions; however, without adherence to standard precautions, the placement in a single room alone will not prevent transmission by direct or indirect contact. Single rooms may also be required to protect patients who have an increased susceptibility to infection (e.g. those with very low neutrophil counts).

There is often competing demand for single-room facilities between patients with infections, those receiving palliative care, patients who create noise and patients who require one-to-one nursing care. Therefore, when the number of single rooms required is assessed, all uses should be taken into account.

Handwashing facilities

Handwashing is frequently stated to be the single most important factor in the prevention of healthcare-associated infection (Ayliffe et al., 2000). Compliance with hand hygiene is often poor and one of the contributory factors is the lack of (or inadequate) availability of hand wash-basins. Good departmental design with sufficient hand wash-basins appropriately placed can increase compliance. There must be sufficient basins to encourage and assist staff to conform to hand-hygiene protocols (Boyce *et al.*, 2000; Pittet, 2000).

Hand wash-basins should comply with HTM64 (NHS Estates, 2006) and they should be located to ensure that staff have immediate access to facilities, for example (NHS Estates, 2002):

- one hand wash-basin per bed in high-level care areas, such as intensive care and high-dependency units;
- one hand wash-basin per single ensuite room (this should be in addition to the patient's ensuite facilities);
- one hand wash-basin between four patients in acute, elderly and long-term settings with an additional facility at the entrance to multi-bedded bays;
- one hand wash-basin between six patients in low-dependency settings (e.g. mental health and learning disability units).

In primary care and outpatient settings, where clinical procedures or examination of patients/clients takes place, a hand wash-basin must be close to where procedures take place. A hand-wash facility should be available at the entrance to all main clinical areas/wards/floors to facilitate handwashing on entering and leaving these areas. The provision of alcohol hand rubs at the point of care is important to ensure that staff decontaminate hands between patients and procedures.

Flooring

Flooring must be able to withstand regular cleaning and the use of disinfectants (e.g. chlorine-releasing agent). Carpets are not recommended for use in or adjacent to any clinical environments (NHS Estates, 2002). Carpets are difficult to maintain, require enhanced cleaning during outbreaks of infection, and become stained and aesthetically unpleasing, often subsequently requiring removal and replacement at considerable cost and disruption to services. Attractive vinyl flooring materials are available, which can provide aesthetic appeal.

Environmental hygiene

Good hospital hygiene is an integral and important component of a strategy for preventing healthcare-associated infections in hospitals (Pratt *et al.*, 2006). There is limited scientific evidence to support the link between hospital cleanliness and rates of healthcare-associated infection. However, clinical evidence indicates that the hospital environment must be visibly clean, free from dust and dirt, and acceptable to patients, their visitors and staff (Pratt *et al.*, 2006).

National Standards of Cleanliness, such as those produced within the UK (e.g. Department of Health [DoH], 2001; Welsh Assembly Government, 2003; Scottish Executive 2004) should be applied within all healthcare establishments. There must be clear quality monitoring procedures in place supported by infection control audits of the environment (Infection Control Nurses Association [ICNA], 2004). There should be mechanisms in place to ensure that, where standards are not being met, action plans are generated and implemented. The hospital environment can become contaminated with micro-organisms that are responsible for healthcare-associated infection (Wilcox *et al.*, 2003; Barker *et al.*, 2004; Denton *et al.*, 2004). Increased levels of cleaning (using detergent and chlorine-releasing agent) should be considered in outbreaks of infection where the pathogen concerned survives in the environment (e.g. *Clostridium difficile*) and environmental contamination may be contributing to the spread (Chadwick *et al.*, 2000; Pratt *et al.*, 2006).

STANDARD PRECAUTIONS

Standard precautions are based upon a set of principles designed to minimize exposure to and transmission of a wide variety of micro-organisms. Since every patient is a potential infection risk, it is essential that standard precautions are used for all patients all of the time. The EPIC project, Developing National Evidence-based Guidelines for Preventing Healthcare Associated Infections (Pratt *et al.*, 2006), provides the evidence base for standard precautions.

Standard infection control precautions include:

• hand hygiene;
• protective clothing and equipment;
• the safe disposal of sharps, clinical waste and healthcare laundry;
• a clean environment;
• decontamination of equipment;
• management of exposure to blood and body fluids;
• patient placement.

Other fundamental issues that are required include:

• education of patients, carers and healthcare workers;
• immunization of healthcare workers.

Good practice involves monitoring implementation of standard precautions through the use of audit (ICNA, 2004). Some organizations have implemented an infection control link practitioner (ICLP) network to undertake audits of practice within clinical departments as a means of regularly monitoring clinical infection control standards. Audits undertaken by clinical teams at a local level, with support being provided by the ICT, can result in an increased ownership of the problems identified and subsequent action plan. ICLPs can provide a positive contribution in establishing an effective culture of infection prevention and control at a local level (Healthcare Commission, 2007).

Hand decontamination

Handwashing is a core element in the prevention of transmission of healthcare-associated infection. However, evidence suggests compliance to hand hygiene recommendations is poor (Boyce, 1999; Pittet, 2001). Reasons for poor compliance include poor handwashing facilities, lack of time, heavy workload and skin sensitivities. The National Patient Safety Agency (2004) launched the 'Cleanyourhands Campaign'. The campaign promotes effective hand decontamination and recommended the use of alcohol hand rubs at the point of care, as a suitable, effective alternative to traditional handwashing with soap and water, providing hands are visibly clean. Staff must be made aware of the fire risks associated with a high level of use and storage of alcohol products (NHS Estates, 2005a); alcohol hand rubs must not be placed near electrical sockets, switches or devices, and alcohol must be thoroughly rubbed in until dry before undertaking any clinical procedure. Training must be provided on the correct use of alcohol hand rubs: the alcohol hand rub should be applied to all surfaces of visibly clean hands and be rubbed to dryness. Hands should be washed with soap and water periodically between alcohol uses.

The promotion of hand hygiene requires a multi-modal strategy using a clear, robust and simple conceptual framework (Sax *et al.*, 2007). The fundamental reference points for hand hygiene 'My five moments for hand hygiene' provide a clear visual focus for staff in ensuring that hands are decontaminated appropriately. The five moments focus on: before patient contact, before an aseptic task, after body fluid exposure, after patient contact and after contact with patients' surroundings (Sax *et al.*, 2007).

In some instances, hands must be decontaminated using soap and water rather than alcohol hand rub. This includes when a patient is diagnosed/suspected with infection caused by spores or non-enveloped viruses (e.g. *Clostridium difficile* and Norovirus) as spores and some viruses are not effectively removed by alcohol.

To improve compliance with handwashing, provision of a good-quality, single-use, wall-mounted, cartridge-type soap (not antibacterial) and good-quality soft paper towels are important to ensure staff do not get sore, cracked or chapped hands. Provision and regular use of a hand moisturizer is also recommended. Hand moisturizers can be made available to staff in wall-mounted cartridge dispensers, thereby reducing the risks of transmission of infection associated with multi-use tubes and pots of creams.

The type of handwash technique and the products used will be determined by the practices or procedures to be carried out. Hand-decontamination methods used should be based on an assessment of the risk in each individual circumstance. Antimicrobial handwash preparations (e.g. chlorhexidine and triclosan) may be indicated in high-risk units, such as intensive care units. Alternatively hand disinfection can also be achieved by washing hands with soap and water, drying and then applying an alcohol hand rub. A surgical handwash is carried out prior to any surgical procedure and involves the use of antiseptic hand soap for 2–3 minutes, covering all areas of hands and forearms.

Handwashing should be carried out using a rigorous technique (see Figure 6.1, p. 139):

1 hands should be placed under warm running water before applying any solution;
2 solution is then applied to wet hands – manufacturers' instructions provide guidance regarding the volume of solution to be applied;
3 hands should be washed until a good lather is evident, this will take 10–15 seconds and should cover all areas of the hand;
4 lather should be rinsed off using running warm water;
5 taps should be turned off using a 'no touch' technique (e.g. elbows);
6 hands must be thoroughly dried using disposable soft paper towels, which must be discarded into an appropriate foot-operated waste container to avoid re-contamination of the hands;
7 a moisturizer can be applied providing it does not affect the action of the hand-cleansing solution.

Monitoring of hand-hygiene compliance within the clinical setting should be undertaken on an ongoing basis using hand-hygiene observational tools. Results of observations should be rapidly fed back to staff to assist in improving practice.

Nailbrushes are not recommended for social or hygienic handwashes. Where they are used for surgical handwash they should be single use. Short nails harbour fewer organisms, are easier to clean and are less likely to tear gloves. Artificial nails have been implicated in outbreaks of infection and must not be worn (Passaro et al., 1997; Parry et al., 2001). Rings, wristwatches and bracelets must be removed before working in a clinical environment, beginning any clinical procedure or surgical hand scrub (Boyce and Pittet, 2002; Kelsall et al., 2006).

Hair should be worn neatly in a style that does not require frequent re-adjustment as this could cause contamination of hands, which may result in cross-infection to patients.

Uniforms

Contamination of uniforms with micro-organisms including *Staphylococcus aureus*, *Clostridium difficile*, and glycopeptide-resistant enterococci (GRE), can occur in the clinical setting (Babb et al.,1983; Perry et al., 2001). Maximum contamination occurs in areas of greatest hand contact, for example, pocket and apron areas (Babb *et al.*, 1983; Loh *et al.*, 2000), which may lead to re-contamination of washed hands. Staff should wear short-sleeved shirts/blouses and avoid wearing white coats when providing patient care, as cuffs can become contaminated and are more likely to be in contact with patient's skin.

Uniform fabric must be capable of withstanding disinfection temperatures of at least 65°C and, where possible, a commercial laundry service should be used. If laundering facilities are not available on site, staff should be provided with written guidance on laundering uniforms, which must be agreed and approved by the ICT. If laundered at home, uniforms should be washed separately at disinfection temperatures (on a minimum 60°C cycle). This should be followed by a tumble dry and/or iron as hot air drying or ironing will further reduce any micro-organisms that may be present.

While there is no conclusive evidence that uniforms (or other work clothes) pose a significant hazard in terms of transmission of infection (DoH, 2007), there is increasing public awareness regarding infection prevention and a growing expectation that healthcare staff do not wear uniforms outside their organization (e.g. in food shops). This should be re-enforced by healthcare organizations, which must provide sufficient uniforms, and adequate laundering and changing facilities so staff can wear clean uniforms for each shift [Royal College of Nursing (RCN), 2005b].

Protective clothing

The main purpose of personal protective equipment (PPE) is to protect staff from the risk of exposure to blood and other body fluids, and reduce the opportunities for transmission of micro-organisms from staff to patient and vice versa. The use of protective clothing must be based on a risk assessment and published best practice guidelines (ICNA, 2002; National Institute of Clinical Excellence [NICE], 2003; Pratt *et al.*, 2006).

The use of protective clothing is underpinned by the Health and Safety at Work Act (1974), the Management of Health and Safety at Work Regulations (Health and Safety Executive, 1992a), Personal Protective Equipment at Work Regulations (Health and Safety Executive, 1992b) and the Control of Substances Hazardous to Health (COSHH) Regulations (Health and Safety Executive, 2002), where employers must provide PPE, and employees must comply with organizational policies relating to the use and wearing of PPE.

Disposable plastic aprons

Plastic aprons must be worn to reduce the level of contamination of uniforms/clothing when direct patient care is given (e.g. assisting patients with toileting, bathing or any activity that may result in the dispersal of pathogens, such as bed-making, and/or procedures causing splashing of blood and body fluids). Plastic aprons should be worn as single-use items for one procedure or episode of patient care before being discarded as clinical waste. The use of coloured aprons for different tasks, rooms and/or patients has been promoted for correct use and appropriate changing of aprons, for example, in intensive care units and critical care units.

Dispensers are available which can hold a selection of different sized gloves plus aprons and an alcoholic hand rub, and these may be particularly useful for ward corridors, consulting rooms and other areas where protective clothing may be required.

Gloves

Gloves are used to protect hands from contamination with organic matter and micro-organisms as well as reducing the risks of transmission of micro-organisms to both patients and staff. Gloves must, therefore, be worn when there is a likelihood of exposure to body fluids, the potential for contact with non-intact skin or mucous membranes, or if there is a need to maintain sterility. Gloves should not be worn unnecessarily or as a substitute for hand hygiene, as their prolonged and indiscriminate use may cause adverse reactions and skin sensitivity (Pratt et al., 2006).

Gloves must conform to European Community (CE) standards and must be available in all clinical areas. Glove choice should be based on individual assessment of risk (ICNA, 2002). This will involve identifying who is at risk (patient or healthcare practitioner), the type of procedure and potential for exposure to blood, body fluids, secretions and excretions, and whether sterile or non-sterile gloves are required.

Training on the correct procedure for donning sterile gloves must be provided for staff to prevent contamination of the outer surface of the glove. It is equally important to educate staff on the importance of washing hands after removal of gloves and ensuring glove removal is carried out using a technique that avoids contamination of the hands and the environment. Glove perforations can be minimized during surgical procedures by double gloving, even in low-risk surgery (Boyce and Pittet, 2002; Tanner and Parkinson, 2006). Use of a coloured under-glove shows increased awareness of glove perforation during surgery and this is now an accepted strategy for reducing risks of sharps injury (Parker, 2000).

Face and eye protection

Face and eye protection (e.g. mask and/or visor) should be considered where there is a risk of blood or body-fluid splashes. There appears to be little benefit from wearing surgical masks to protect patients during routine ward procedures such as wound dressing or invasive medical procedures (Pratt et al., 2006). Personal respiratory protection is required in certain respiratory diseases (e.g. TB, HIV-related or multiple-drug-resistant tuberculosis) and where patients who are severely immunocompromised are at an increased risk of infection. In these instances, surgical masks worn by staff are not effective protection and specialized respiratory protective equipment should be worn (e.g. a particulate filter mask; NICE, 2003; Pratt *et al.*, 2006). For further information, see Chapter 12, p. **281**.

Sharps

Sharps can be defined as needles, scalpels, stitch cutters, glass ampoules and any sharp instrument. The main risks associated with an inoculation (sharps) injury are hepatitis B, hepatitis C and HIV. A combination of training, safer working practices and, where appropriate, the use of medical devices incorporating sharps protection mechanisms can reduce the risk of needlestick and sharps injuries. Where safety needle devices are introduced into the clinical setting with appropriate training, the number of occupationally acquired needlestick injuries can be reduced (Adams and Elliott, 2006). Needle safety devices should, therefore, be considered where there are clear clinical indications that they will provide safer systems of working for healthcare personnel (NICE, 2003).

The emphasis on preventing sharps injuries must, however, focus on ensuring safe handling practices are in place. Guidance on the reduction of sharps injuries (ICNA, 2003; RCN, 2005a) identifies the following safe practices which minimize the risk of injury.

- Used sharps must be discarded into a sharps container at the point of use.
- Sharps must not be passed directly from hand to hand – a 'neutral zone' must be used with a tray or dedicated area (particularly applicable in operating theatres with passing of sharps instruments).
- Sharps handling must be kept to a minimum.
- Needles and syringes must not be disassembled by hand prior to disposal.
- Needles should not be recapped.
- Sharps containers should conform to UN3291 and BS 7320 standards.
- Sharps containers must not be filled above the mark indicating they are full.
- Sharps containers should be located in a safe position and, in public areas, must not be placed on the floor. Brackets to secure sharps containers are particularly useful in areas such as outpatient consulting rooms where there are likely to be children present.
- Temporary closure mechanisms should be used when sharps boxes are not in use.

While safe handling and disposal of sharps can minimize the risk of injury, it is essential that staff are aware of how to manage an injury should one occur. Staff must have access to occupational health services and be aware of their hepatitis B status in the event of a needlestick injury.

Management of clinical waste

Waste handling and disposal practices must take account of national guidance (Hazardous Waste Regulations, 2005; DoH, 2006). The 2005 waste regulations replace the Special Waste regulations 1996 and, along with the European Waste Catalogue (EWC; 2001) detail the categories of waste and methods of disposal. The EWC codes replace previous categories A–E.

It is imperative that staff receive waste disposal training in order that they segregate waste at clinical level. Correctly labelled bins should be sited appropriately to assist in correct disposal and segregation. Foot-operated, hands-free waste bins should be available to minimize contamination of hands during disposal of waste.

Handling of healthcare linen

Used linen is a potential source of infection, as it is likely to be contaminated with potentially pathogenic organisms. A disposable plastic apron should, therefore, be worn when handling used linen to prevent contamination of staff uniforms. Staff should avoid shaking linen, as this may result in dispersal of potentially pathogenic organisms into the environment. Used linen must not be carried against the body or carried through a ward/department, as this increases the risk of disseminating bacteria into the air and on to environmental surfaces as well as contaminating healthcare workers uniforms. To transport linen, a linen skip should be taken to the patient and linen placed into an appropriate coloured bag. Hands must always be washed after handling any used linen.

The linen bag should be no more than two-thirds full and appropriately sealed before being removed from the ward or department. Staff must ensure foreign objects such as needles; scissors, catheter bags, etc. are removed before linen is placed into linen bags, as failure to do so places linen personnel and other members of staff at unnecessary risk of injury.

Clean and contaminated linen must be kept separate at all times and ward/departmental linen storage areas must be dedicated for that purpose. There should be no inappropriate items in the clean linen store, such as patient equipment. Dirty linen should be segregated according to local and national policy (NHS Executive, 1995), ensuring used linen is disinfected at 65°C for not less than 10 minutes or 71°C for not less than 3 minutes.

Decontamination of patient equipment

Chapter 6 deals with methods of decontamination; this section focuses on communal patient equipment used in ward and outpatient areas.

Healthcare equipment can be a potential source of infection and up to one-third of healthcare-associated infections may be prevented by ensuring adequate cleaning of equipment (Schabrun and Chipase, 2006). repair of any piece of equipment will affect the ability to clean it is therefore essential that the integrity of re-usable equipm before being decontaminated appropriately between each patient.

Equipment used in the critical setting is more likely to have standard clean-ing protocols than that used in other settings and this can result in non-critical equipment being implicated in the transmission of infection. This will include equipment such as bed pans, commodes, blood pressure cuffs, stethoscopes, continuous passive movement machines, bath hoists and lifts (Schabrun and Chipase, 2006). Other equipment such as computer keyboards (Man *et al.*, 2002) may harbour potentially pathogenic organisms and must be included in cleaning schedules.

Equipment in outpatient departments warrants particular attention owing to the high throughput and limited time between patient consultations with sub-sequent risks of transmission of infection. Equipment such as sigmoidoscopes and ultrasound equipment (Sykes *et al.*, 2006) must be correctly decontami-nated between patients. Filters should be used on sigmoidoscopes to prevent backflow into the tubing.

In ward areas, the patient's bed is probably the most frequently used piece of equipment in the clinical area and high bed-occupancy rates leave little time for cleaning between patients (O'Connor, 2000). Beds and associated manual handling equipment can become contaminated with pathogenic bacteria (Bar-nett *et al.*, 1999) and have been implicated in outbreaks of infection (Catalano *et al.*, 1999). Responsibilities for cleaning patient equipment must be clearly defined in local policies and procedures, and the ICT must assist wards/depart-ments in the development of detailed cleaning schedules or A–Z lists of patient equipment and how they should be managed/decontaminated.

All staff must take responsibility for the areas in which they work and man-agers are responsible for ensuring compliance to cleaning protocols. Many items are now available as single-use disposable and these will reduce the risk of transmission of infection. When cleaning equipment, staff should wear protec-tive clothing (e.g. gloves and aprons). Staff must also decontaminate their hands. General-purpose detergent and/or disposable detergent wipes are rec-ommended for the cleaning of surfaces that are likely to come into contact only with healthy skin and are considered 'low risk' (Medicines and Healthcare Products Regulatory Agency, 2002), unless otherwise stated.

Where equipment requires disinfection following use on patients with infections or as a result of contamination with body fluids, the use of a disinfectant solution such as a chlorine-releasing agent (1000 ppm available chlorine) is advised. All equipment must be cleaned with a general-purpose detergent to remove organic matter prior to disinfection. Staff must be aware that some equipment is damaged by some disinfectants (e.g. mattresses by alcohol, stainless steel by chlorine) and it is therefore important to follow manufacturers' guidance for cleaning equipment and using disinfectant solutions.

Best practice is as follows:

- always check the integrity of equipment – check for damage, tears, etc.;
- always check equipment is clean prior to use;
- use disposable cleaning cloths;
- wear protective clothing when cleaning equipment;
- dilute solutions correctly;
- use fresh solutions – where these can be made up and stored, they should be labelled (e.g. name, date and strength) and changed as per manufacturers' instructions (usually every 24 hours);
- equipment should be stored in designated storage areas, off the floor on shelving or racking.

The importance of effective hand hygiene must also be emphasized, as the transfer of micro-organisms from surfaces to patients is largely considered to be through direct hand contact.

Isolation

Many different approaches have been used in identifying the need to isolate a patient in preventing the transmission of infection. These have included using isolation categories such as strict, standard and protective (Ayliffe *et al.*, 2000), disease-specific isolation precautions (Garner and Simmons, 1983) and also a combination of routine (universal or standard) and additional isolation precautions (Wilson, 2006). The combination approach has been incorporated into guidance produced within the USA (Garner, 1996) and provides a simple approach to isolation, with standard precautions being supported by additional transmission-based isolation precautions when the standard precautions alone are unlikely to prevent transmission of infection. For simplicity, the terms strict, standard and protective isolation will be used to describe the precautions required.

Strict isolation

Strict isolation is required only for infections which rarely occur (e.g. viral haemorrhagic fever). This type of isolation is undertaken within specialized Infectious Disease Units in most developed countries.

Standard isolation

Standard isolation involves the use of standard infection control precautions but also includes physical separation of the patient in a contained environment, such as a single room or, in the event of cohorting, a group of patients infected with the same micro-organisms in a double- or multi-bedded room. Isolation of patients in hospital who have a known or suspected infection is required to prevent cross-infection to other patients and in some cases staff. The common conditions, infections and micro-organisms requiring isolation in hospitals include unexplained diarrhoea and/or vomiting where an infective cause is possible, *Clostridium difficile* diarrhoea, viral gastroenteritis, e.g. norovirus, methicillin-resistant *Staphylococcus aureus* (MRSA), where transmission cannot be prevented through standard precautions alone; some multiple-resistant Gram-negative infections and untreated pulmonary tuberculosis. In addition, patients presenting with symptoms of communicable infections, such as mumps, measles and chickenpox, will require isolation during the infectious periods. Segregation of patients acts as a reminder to healthcare staff to implement effective precautions.

Protective isolation

This is required to protect immunocompromised patients who have an increased susceptibility to exogenous infection (e.g. those with very low neutrophil counts).

Accommodation

The type of room within which patients with infections are cared for can vary from a single room with natural ventilation provided by windows and doors to a fully equipped isolation suite with lobby. The presence of an ensuite facility (integral toilet and shower/bath) prevents the patients having to leave the room unnecessarily and limits the risk of transmission of enteric infections. The Interdepartmental Working group on Tuberculosis (DoH, 1998) and Centre for Disease Control and Prevention (1994) guidelines for preventing transmission of pulmonary tuberculosis have recommended negative-pressure facilities for patients with multi-drug-resistant tuberculosis.

Negative pressure is achieved when the air in the room is at a negative pressure in relation to the surrounding areas with 6–12 air changes per hour (Garner, 1996). The air discharged to the outside must be away from ventilation inlets or windows. The alternative is to use high-efficiency particle air (HEPA) filtration of room air before the air is circulated to other areas of the hospital; however, this would involve considerable expense and risk should the filters fail (DoH, 1998).

In newly designed facilities, standards for the design of isolation rooms are recommended in Health Building Note 4 Supplement 1 'Isolation facilities in acute settings' (NHS Estates, 2005b). This includes the following.

- an enhanced ensuite single room, without a lobby, with air extraction via the ensuite;
- an isolation suite with ensuite facilities (with extraction) and a ventilated lobby to which air is supplied under positive pressure, thereby discharging

to both corridor and bedroom, thus preventing air transfer between the corridor and the patient's room in either direction, providing source isolation and a degree of protective isolation; these rooms would be required only for a small number of patients, as the majority of patients requiring isolation can be cared for in enhanced single rooms as above;

- filtration of air with HEPA filters: advisable when there is a need to protect highly susceptible patients from all airborne pathogens (including fungal spores such as aspergilli), as in the case of patients undergoing bone marrow transplantation; high standards of infection control precautions are also required.

The use of rooms that can be switched from positive to negative pressure is not recommended because they rely on staff being able to assess the type of ventilation required and knowing how to select the correct ventilation mode. If set incorrectly, patients can be put at risk of infection (NHS Estates, 2005b).

The application of isolation precautions involves a combination of appropriate physical environment, correct healthcare policies and proper behaviour of healthcare staff (Masterton *et al.*, 2003) based upon a risk assessment. Isolation (transmission-based) precautions are aimed at minimizing the transmission of organisms from:

- patient to patient;
- patient to staff;
- staff to patient.

The transmission of infection to patients can be controlled by physical protection (single room isolation) in addition to implementation of standard precautions. Staff must understand that it is the micro-organism rather than the person that requires isolation, and precautions should be specifically directed at the route of transmission of the organism concerned (Wilson, 2006). A clear understanding of the 'chain of infection' is important to implementation of appropriate transmission-based precautions.

Transmission of infection involves:

- an infectious agent (pathogen);
- a reservoir where the organism can thrive;
- a host–patient(s) susceptible to the infection;
- an entry route, which may be through:
  - inhalation (e.g chickenpox, influenza)
  - ingestion (e.g. salmonella, norovirus)
  - inoculation/skin/sexual contact (e.g. hepatitis B, HIV);
- exit route – faeces, urine, blood, vomit, sputum, air;
- transmission route – this may be through either contact (direct or indirect) or the airborne or droplet route.

Risk assessment

A risk assessment must be used to determine the need for isolation and implementation of appropriate control measures that will minimize the risks of infection and transmission of infection. The decision about which isolation precautions are required will depend upon a variety of influential factors including:

- the organism involved and its route of spread (e.g. contact, airborne, droplet, enteric or bloodborne);
- the risk of spread to other patients and staff, and the patient's clinical environment;
- the potential severity of the infection;
- the safety of the patient;
- the availability of isolation rooms.

There is often limited availability of isolation rooms and/or operational needs that conflict with infection control needs (Wigglesworth and Wilcox, 2006). However, infection risks must be assessed, and the decision of whether to isolate or not must be documented in the patient's records.

Isolation (transmission-based) precautions

To ensure compliance with isolation precautions by healthcare staff and visitors, a notice at the entrance to a patient's room, or by the bed, should indicate any special precautions that are being observed, while maintaining confidentiality.

Where a single room is used for patients with airborne infections, the door should be kept closed to restrict the spread of infectious micro-organisms. However, when single rooms are being used to care for patients with infections transmitted by the contact route, the door can be left open. Subject to a suitable risk assessment, the patient can leave the room to take a walk if well enough, or to visit other departments for treatments, such as physiotherapy. In these circumstances, communication is required with the department to be visited to ensure the necessary standard precautions are applied.

Protective clothing should be readily available inside and outside the patient's room (Wilson, 2006). The use of wall-mounted protective clothing dispensers (for aprons and gloves) is recommended for ease of use and to prevent corridors being blocked by trolleys holding such equipment. Protective clothing should be worn when staff are in contact with the infective material and discarded before any contact with other patients, usually before leaving the patient's room. In the event that the healthcare staff need to remove contaminated equipment from the room, then the protective clothing should be removed once the procedure is completed. However, care must be taken not to contaminate the environment outside of the room in the process.

Wherever a patient is cared for, they should be allocated dedicated equipment (e.g. commode, blood pressure cuffs, monitors, etc., and these must be adequately decontaminated after use.

Staff should must have a clear understanding of the isolation precautions required to prevent transmission of infection and in some instances staff immunity to infection may need to be considered (e.g. in the event of chickenpox).

Visitors

Visitors should be asked to wash their hands before and after seeing patients. Visitors do not normally need to be excluded, but advice should be sought from staff caring for the patient. Visitors should not need to wear protective clothing, e.g. gloves and aprons (unless they are assisting in the physical care of the patient), as they are not providing care to subsequent patients.

Psychological effects of isolation

Mood disturbance is a significant consequence of isolation in a proportion of patients (Davies and Rees, 2000). Patients in isolation are often deprived of social contact and this can result in a loss of self-esteem, control and choice as well as depression and anxiety. Isolation rooms should be designed to allow visibility by both staff and patients, and encourage effective communication including an explanation of the reasons for isolation and what this involves; patient leaflets should be available for common infections (e.g. *Clostridium difficile* and MRSA). While the recommended period of isolation varies for each infection, it is important that staff regularly review patient care needs.

Care of the infected, deceased patient

Not all patients who die of an infection continue to present an infection risk after death. However, micro-organisms can continue to multiply in the body after death and it is important that measures are taken to protect people who may handle the deceased. Although the diagnosis of the deceased should remain confidential, it is the duty of those with knowledge of the case to ensure those who need to handle the body, including porters, post-mortem staff, etc., are aware of any risks (Cutter, 1999).

Contact tracing

Patients and staff who have been in contact with a patient who has a communicable infection may be at risk of acquiring an infection themselves. The ICT should be informed of such cases so that a list of contacts can be drawn up and, where appropriate, staff and/or patients followed up. Definitions of a contact will depend upon the infection involved and hospital infection control isolation policies should include this information.

INFECTION PREVENTION DURING HEALTHCARE INTERVENTIONS

The concept of 'care bundles', developed by faculty at the Institute for Healthcare Improvement, can be used as a way to describe a collection of evidence-based processes needed to care effectively for patients undergoing particular treatments with inherent risks. The use of care bundles in the prevention of healthcare-associated infection can support the implementation of reliable processes.. The implementation of the bundles should then be monitored.

Principles of asepsis

The principle of asepsis is to prevent the transmission of micro-organisms to and from wounds, from healthcare workers' hands and other susceptible sites, thereby reducing the risk of infection/cross-infection.

Aseptic techniques should be used when there is a break in skin integrity (e.g. a wound) or when natural defence mechanisms are bypassed (e.g. insertion of invasive devices). The susceptible site should not come into contact with any item that is not sterile. Any items that have been in contact with a wound or susceptible site may be contaminated and should be discarded safely or decontaminated (Wilson, 2006).

It is important that all healthcare establishments develop a policy and associated procedures for asepsis to be applied in practice. All healthcare staff who perform such procedures must be trained in asepsis and no-touch techniques, and their competency must be assessed. Asepsis should be practised for all invasive procedures. This section will deal with the application of asepsis in non-surgical procedures.

Aseptic technique

A clear clean field must be available to perform the procedure (e.g. a dressing trolley or tray). This area should be cleaned with detergent and water prior to use for an aseptic procedure, as these items are often used for many alternative purposes in the clinical setting.

In the healthcare setting, the application of a modified aseptic (clean) technique (Wilson, 2006), which is often used to dress wounds, healing by secondary intention, such as in leg ulcers, can be considered. The modified aseptic technique involves the use of non-sterile instead of sterile gloves and bathing of wounds in a leg bath using tap water, for example. However, the aim of both aseptic and clean procedures is to prevent the transmission of micro-organisms to and from wounds and other susceptible sites, thereby reducing the risk of infection. Therefore, either approach should be treated as a discrete procedure involving preparation of an appropriate surface to work from and decontamination of equipment between patients.

The use of an aseptic non-touch technique (Rowley, 2001) can be applied to invasive procedures. The underlying principles are to wash hands effectively, never contaminate key parts, to touch non-key parts with confidence and take appropriate standard precautions. (Key parts are defined as those which come into direct contact with the patient's wound, intravenous infusate and those parts which, if contaminated by micro-organisms, increase the risk of infection.)

Aseptic/modified aseptic procedure

1 Reassure patients and ensure they receive a full explanation of the procedure.
2 Prepare equipment required prior to the procedure.
3 Hands must be decontaminated using soap and water or a disinfectant hand rub (if the hands are clean). Clean hands can be disinfected using an alcohol hand rub.
4 Wear a disposable, single-patient-use plastic apron.
5 Select sterile or non-sterile gloves according to the procedure being undertaken (e.g. sterile gloves if any susceptible site is to be touched by the gloved hand, if the procedure is likely to be complex or prolonged, and if the key susceptible sites cannot be kept aseptic by the non-touch method (Rowley, 2001). Use non-sterile gloves if a no-touch technique is being used (e.g. if the key susceptible sites are not touched during a procedure; Rowley, 2001).
6 Use aseptic principles to ensure that only sterile items come into contact with the susceptible site and sterile items do not come into contact with non-sterile objects (Wilson, 2006). An exception to this will involve bathing a patient's leg ulcer in a leg bath with tap water.
7 Discard waste and contaminated fluids as clinical waste.
8 Dispose of sharps into a sharps bin at the point of use.
9 Decontaminate any equipment which may have become contaminated during the process (e.g. trolley, tray, leg bath, etc.).
10 Dispose of protective clothing and decontaminate hands.

Management of invasive devices

There is evidence to support the use of the principles of asepsis in the insertion and management of all invasive devices (DoH, 2003; Pratt et al., 2006). Invasive devices breach the body's natural defence mechanisms against infection and therefore they should be used in a considered manner (risk assessment) rather than as a matter of routine. Healthcare staff should therefore ensure that, before any invasive device is inserted, alternative approaches have been considered and, if used, the reason for use is clearly documented. The date of insertion and date of removal of all invasive devices must be documented in the clinical record as a matter of routine to ensure there is a clear record of the device being present. Guidelines have been developed to prevent infections associated with invasive devices (ICNA, 2001; DoH, 2003; NICE, 2003; Pratt *et al.*, 2006). The guidance is summarized in Table 13.1.

Urinary catheters

Infection is a well-recognized complication of urinary catheterization (Emmerson *et al.*, 1996; Plowman *et al.*, 2001) and, therefore, all alternative options for management of continence should be considered prior to urethral catheterization of a patient. Urinary catheters should be used only when there is no suitable alternative and even then the catheter should be kept in place for as short a time as possible (Garibaldi *et al.*, 1974; DoH, 2003). The duration of catheterization is strongly correlated with the risk of infection (Pratt *et al.*, 2006).

Insertion of urinary catheters must be undertaken using an aseptic technique with sterile equipment to prevent infection. The meatus should be cleansed prior to insertion and the use of a single-use lubricant or anaesthetic gel (Woodward, 2005) will minimize urethral trauma and subsequent infection.

The type of catheter used should be based on clinical experience, patient assessment and anticipated duration of catheterization (Pratt *et al.*, 2006). The use of coated or impregnated catheters (e.g. silver alloy, silver oxide, antibiotics and antiseptic agents) should be based on up-to-date clinical evidence and clinical experience. The catheter chosen should have the smallest gauge catheter that will allow free urinary outflow (Pratt *et al.*, 2006). The ongoing management of the catheterized patient must include the use of a closed system. Breaking the closed system will increase the risk of infection to the patient; therefore the connection between the catheter and the closed drainage system should be broken only when there is a clear clinical reason.

Urine sampling should be undertaken through a needleless port on the urinary drainage system using an aseptic technique. Hands may become heavily contaminated during this procedure and, therefore, the use of gloves and hand decontamination before and after the procedure are essential in the prevention of cross-infection.

Routine personal meatal hygiene using soap and water should be undertaken.

Peripheral intravenous devices

Intravenous therapy has become an essential part of clinical care (ICNA, 2001). Insertion of peripheral cannulae must be undertaken by trained and competent staff using an aseptic technique (DoH, 2003). Prior to insertion of a peripheral cannula, healthcare workers must decontaminate their hands and wear non-sterile gloves. The insertion site must be disinfected using a suitable skin disinfectant (e.g. 2 per cent chlorhexidine in 70 per cent alcohol). Alcohol-based skin disinfectants should be allowed to air dry. The cannula should be secured with a

Table 13.1 Summary of guidance for the care of commonly used invasive devices

Procedure	Peripheral cannula	Central venous catheter	Urinary catheter
Hand decontamination	Before and after all contact with the device and patient	Disinfect hands before and after all contact with the device and patient	Before and after all contact with the device and patient
Procedure for insertion	Aseptic (modified) technique using non-sterile gloves	Aseptic technique with surgical scrub, sterile gloves, gown, drapes. Mask and hat should be considered	Aseptic technique using sterile gloves and apron
Skin preparation prior to insertion of device	Disinfect skin with 2% chlorhexidine in 70% alcohol	Disinfect skin with 2% chlorhexidine in 70% alcohol or povidone iodine for skin sensitive to chlorhexidine	Clean meatus with sterile saline or sterile water
Securing device	Sterile dressing	Sterile dressing	The catheter tubing can be secured to the patient's leg to prevent movement
Procedure for subsequent care	Non-sterile gloves and disposable apron. 2% chlorhexidine in 70% alcohol should be used to disinfect key parts of the device, e.g. hubs and ports	Disposable apron. Sterile gloves if touching key parts. Non-sterile gloves if using a non-touch technique. 2% chlorhexidine in 70% alcohol should be used to disinfect key parts of the device, e.g., hubs and ports	Modified aseptic technique using non-sterile gloves for catheter care and changing catheter bags. Soap and water for meatal care. Obtain urine samples from needleless sampling port using modified aseptic technique. Position urine drainage bags on a stand below the level of the bladder
Documentation	Record insertion site, date and any complications. Record date of insertion on the cannula dressing. Lines must be labelled with date used. Check site each clinical shift and record condition in patient records. Score using the VIP score	Check site daily and record condition in patient records	Check catheter daily and record reason for ongoing need in patient records
Indications for removal	VIP score of three or more or if *in situ* for 72 hours or mechanical failure	Clinical signs of infection or mechanical failure	Based on individual patient assessment

VIP, visual phlebitis.

sterile dressing to prevent movement and introduction of micro-organisms. Peripheral venous cannula sites must be checked at every shift for signs of infection and the cannula removed, if infection is suspected. The use of a visual phlebitis score should be included in practice (Jackson, 2003) for ease and standardization of assessment of the peripheral cannula.

Central venous catheters

Central venous catheters are indispensable in modern-day clinical practice, particularly in critical care areas and with patients requiring long-term intravenous treatment. Although they provide necessary venous access, their use is associated with an increased risk to the patient of local and systemic infections (ICNA, 2001). Prevention of infection must be paramount to all staff handling these devices. Aseptic technique using sterile gloves must be used during insertion, dressing changes, accessing and removal of the central line.

Central venous catheter care

A number of risk factors for catheter-related infection (CRI) including the vessel used, skin preparation with antiseptics, surgical technique and surgical skill have been identified. Extent of use, degree of manipulation and care of exit site are additional factors associated with CRI.

Venous catheters can be placed in the subclavian, internal jugular or femoral vein. Most authorities recommend the subclavian site as this has a reduced risk of infection compared with the jugular or femoral site. Alcoholic chlorhexidine gluconate solution should be used to prepare the skin prior to insertion and allowed to dry to prepare the skin (if no known allergy). Catheter insertion should be carried out by only a limited number of experienced operators, following strict aseptic technique.

Recurrent audit of complications related to central venous catheters, including sepsis should be carried out; care bundles can be used for this process. Regular training should be arranged for medical and nursing staff in catheter care.

Surveillance of access-associated bacteraemia

Continuous surveillance, a programme of risk reduction, periodic multidisciplinary input, infection control, and a programme of increased awareness and training were employed and shown to reduce the rate of CRI significantly (George *et al.*, 2006). Use of a consistent scheme for surveillance would allow comparison of data between the units.

ACKNOWLEDGEMENT

The authors would like to thank Dr Muhammad Raza for his assistance with the sections on intravenous lines.

REFERENCES

Adams D and Elliott TSJ (2006) Impact of safety needle devices on occupationally acquired needle stick injuries; a four year prospective study. *Journal of Hospital Infection* **64**, 50.

Ayliffe GAJ, Babb JR and Quoraishi AH (1978) A test for hygienic hand disinfection. *Journal of Clinical Pathology* **31**, 923.

Ayliffe GAJ, Fraise AP, Geddes AM and Mitchell K (2000) *Control of hospital infection. A practical handbook*, 4th edn. London: Chapman and Hall Medical.

Babb JR, Davies JG and Ayliffe GA (1983) Contamination of protective clothing and nurses uniforms in an isolation ward. *Journal of Hospital Infection* **4**, 149.

Barker J, Vipond IB and Bloomfield DF (2004) Effects of cleaning and disinfection in reducing the spread of Norovirus contamination via environmental surfaces. *Journal of Hospital Infection* **58**, 42.

Barnett J, Thomlinson D, Perry C, Marshall R and MacGowan AP (1999) An audit of the use of manual handling equipment and their microbiological flora – implications for infection control. *Journal of Hospital Infection* **43**, 309.

Bouza E, Burillo A and Munoz P (2002) Catheter-related infections: diagnosis and intravascular treatment. *Clinical Microbiology and Infection* **8**, 265.

Boyce JM (1999) It is time for action: improving hand hygiene in hospitals. *Annals of Internal Medicine* **130**, 153.

Boyce JM and Pittet D (2002) Guideline for hand hygiene in health-care settings. *MMWR Recommendations and Reports* **51**(RR-16), 1.

Boyce J, Kelliher S and Vallande N (2000) Skin irritation and dryness associated with two hand hygiene regimes: soap and water hand washing versus hand antisepsis with an alcoholic hand gel. *Infection Control and Hospital Epidemiology* **21**, 443.

Catalano M, Quelle LS, Jeric PE, Di Martino A and Maimone SM (1999) Survival of *Acinetobacter baumannii* on bed rails during an outbreak and during sporadic cases. *Journal of Hospital Infection* **42**, 27.

Centers for Disease Control and Prevention (1994) Guidelines for preventing the transmission of tuberculosis in heath care facilities. *MMWR* **43**(RR13), 1.

Chadwick PR, Beards G, Brown D *et al.* (2000) Report of the Public Health Laboratory Service. Viral gastro-enteritis working group management of hospital outbreaks of gastro-enteritis due to small round structured viruses. *Journal of Hospital Infection* **45**, 1.

Cutter M (1999) In the bag. *Nursing Times* **95**, 55.

Davies H and Rees J (2000) Psychological effects of isolation nursing (1) mood disturbance. *Nursing Standard* **14**, 35.

Denton M, Wilcox MH, Parnell P *et al.* (2004) Role of environmental cleaning in controlling an outbreak of *Acinetobacter baumannii* on a neurosurgical unit. *Journal of Hospital Infection* **56**, 106.

Department of Health (1998) *The Interdepartmental Working Group on Tuberculosis. The prevention and control of tuberculosis in the United Kingdom: Recommendations for the prevention and control of tuberculosis at local level*. Annexe D of the guidance outlines features of a negative pressure room used for multi drug resistant tuberculosis. London: Department of Health.

Department of Health (2001) *National standards of cleanliness*. London: Department of Health.

Department of Health (2003) *Winning ways working together to reduce healthcare associated infection in England*. London: The Stationery Office.

Department of Health (2006) *HTM 07-01. Safe management of healthcare waste*. London: The Stationery Office.

Department of Health (2007) *Uniforms and work wear. An evidence base for developing local policy*. London: Department of Health.

DH Estates and Facilities Division (2008) *Adult in-patient facilities*. Health Building Note (HBN) 04-01. London: The Stationery Office.

Emmerson AM, Enstone JE, Griffin M *et al.* (1996) The second national prevalence survey of infection in hospitals – overview of the results. *Journal of Hospital Infection* **32**, 175.

European Waste Catalogue (2001) 2001/216/EC. Available at: http/europa.eu.int/eur-lex/en/lif/reg/en_register_15103030.html.

Garibaldi RA, Burke JP, Dickman ML *et al.* (1974) Factors predisposing to bacteruria during indwelling urethral catheterisation. *New England Journal of Medicine* **291**, 215.

Garner JS (1996) The Hospital Infection Control Practices Advisory Committee. Guidelines for isolation precautions in hospitals. *Infection Control Hospital Epidemiology* **17**, 53.

Garner JS and Simmons BP (1983) Guideline for isolation precautions in hospitals. *Infection Control* **4**(Suppl 4), 245.

George A, Tokars JI, Clutterbuck EJ, Bamford KB, Pusey C and Holmes AH (2006) Reducing dialysis associated bacteraemia, and recommendations for surveillance in the United Kingdom: prospective study. *BMJ* **332**,1435.

Hazardous Waste (England and Wales) Regulations (2005) Statutory Instrument No. 894. London: The Stationary Office.

Health and Safety at Work Act 1974. London: HMSO.

Health and Safety Executive (1992a) *Management of health and safety at work regulations* (amended in 1999). London: HMSO.

Health and Safety Executive (1992b) *Personal protective equipment at work regulations*. London: HMSO.

Health and Safety Executive (2002) *The control of substances hazardous to health regulations*, 4th edn. Sudbury: HSE Books.

Healthcare Commission (2007) *Healthcare associated infections: what else can the NHS do?* London: Commission for Healthcare Audit and Inspection.

Infection Control Nurses Association (2001) *Guidelines for preventing intravascular catheter related infection*. Bathgate: Fitwise.

Infection Control Nurses Association (2002) *Protective clothing: principles and guidance*. Bathgate: Fitwise.

Infection Control Nurses Association (2003) *Sharps injury: prevention and risk management*. Bathgate: Fitwise.

Infection Control Nurses Association (2004) *Audit tools for monitoring infection control standards*. Bathgate: Fitwise.

Jackson A (1998) Infection control: a battle in vein infusion phlebitis. *Nursing Times* **94**, 68.

Kelsall NKR, Griggs RKS, Bowker KE and Bannister GC (2006) Should finger rings be removed prior to scrubbing for theatres? *Journal of Hospital Infection* **62**, 450.

Loh W, Ng W and Holton J (2000) Bacterial flora on the white coats of medical students. *Journal of Hospital Infection* **45**, 65.

Man GS, Olapoju M, Chadwick MV *et al.* (2002) Bacterial contamination of ward-based computer terminals. Letter to the Editor. *Journal of Hospital Infection* **52**, 314.

Masterton RG, Mifsud AJ and Rao GG (2003) Hospital isolation precautions working group. Review of hospital isolation and infection control precautions. *Journal of Hospital Infection* **54**, 171.

Medicines and Healthcare Products Regulatory Agency (2002) *Sterilisation, disinfection and cleaning of medical equipment: guidance on decontamination from the Microbiology Committee to the Department of Health*. MAC Manual, Part 1: Principles. London: Medical Devices Agency.

National Health Service Executive (1995) *Hospital laundry arrangements for used and infected linen*. HSG(95)18. London: HMSO.

National Institute for Clinical Excellence (2003) *Infection control: prevention of healthcare associated infection in primary and community care*. London: NICE.

National Patient Safety Agency (2004) *Cleanyourhands Campaign*. London: NPSA.

NHS Estates (2002) *Infection control in the built environment: design and planning*. Health Facilities Note (HFN) 30, amended in 2005. London: The Stationary Office.

NHS Estates (2005a) *Alcohol based hand rub – potential fire risk*. Gateway 5084. London: NHS Estates.

NHS Estates (2005b) *In-patient accommodation: options for choice*. Health Building Note (HBN) 4 Suppl 1: *Isolation facilities in acute settings*. London: The Stationary Office.

NHS Estates (2006) *Health Technical Memorandum 64. Sanitary assemblies*. London: The Stationary Office.

Noble A (2004) The architecture of infection control. *British Journal of Infection Control* **5**, 26.

O'Connor H (2000) Decontaminating beds and mattresses. *Nursing Times* **96**, 2.

Parker L (2000) Biogel Reveal; a puncture indicator system from Regent Medical. *British Journal of Nursing* **9**, 1182.

Parry MF, Grabt B, Yukna M *et al.* (2001) Candida osteomyelitis and diskitis after spinal surgery: an outbreak that implicates artificial nails. *Clinical Infectious Diseases* **32**, 352.

Passaro DJ and Waring L, Armstrong R *et al.* (1997) Post operative *Serratia marcescens* wound infections traced to an out of hospital source. *Journal of Infectious Diseases* **75**, 992.

Perry C, Marshall R and Jones E (2001) Bacterial contamination of uniforms. *Journal of Hospital Infection* **48**, 238.

Pittet D (2000) Improved compliance with hand hygiene in hospitals. *Infection Control and Hospital Epidemiology* **21**, 381.

Pittet D (2001) Improving adherence to hand hygiene practice; a multi-disciplinary approach. *Emerging Infectious Disease* **7**, 234.

Plowman R, Graves N, Griffin M *et al.* (2001) The rate and cost of hospital-acquired infections occurring in patients admitted to selected specialities of a district general hospital in England and the national burden imposed. *Journal of Hospital Infection* **47,** 198.

Pratt RJ, Pellowe CM, Wilson J *et al.* (2006) *Final draft epic2 national evidence-based guidelines for preventing healthcare associated infections in NHS hospitals in England.* London: Thames Valley University, Richard Wells Research Centre.

Rowley S (2001) Theory to practice: aseptic non touch technique. *Nursing Times* **97,** vi.

Royal College of Nursing (2005a) *Good practice in infection prevention and control: guidance for nursing staff.* London: RCN.

Royal College of Nursing (2005b) *Guidance on uniforms and clothing worn in the delivery of patient care: MRSA Campaign; wipe it out.* London: RCN.

Sax H, Allegranzia B, Uckay I, Larson E, Boyce J and Pittet D (2007) 'My five moments for hand hygiene': a user-centered design approach to understand, train, monitor and report hand hygiene. *Journal of Hospital Infection* **67,** 9.

Schabrun S and Chipase L (2006) Healthcare equipment as a source of nosocomial infection: a systematic review. *Journal of Hospital Infection* **63,** 239.

Scottish Executive (2004) *NHS Scotland National Cleaning Services Specification Scotland: Health Care associated Infection Task Force.* Edinburgh: Scottish Executive.

Sykes A, Appleby M, Perry J and Gould K (2006) An investigation of the microbiological contamination of ultrasound equipment. *British Journal of Infection Control* **7,** 16.

Tanner J and Parkinson H (2006) *Double gloving to reduce surgical cross-infection. Cochrane Database of Systematic Reviews*: Reviews Issue 3. Chichester: John Wiley & Sons Ltd.

Welsh Assembly Government (2003) *National standards of cleanliness for NHS Trusts. Performance sssessment (toolkit).* Cardiff: National Assembly for Wales.

Wigglesworth N and Wilcox MH (2006) Prospective evaluation of hospital isolation room capacity. *Journal of Hospital Infection* **63,** 156.

Wilcox MH, Fawley WN, Wigglesworth N *et al.* (2003) Comparison of the effect of detergent versus hypochlorite on environmental contamination and incidence of *Clostridium difficile* infection. *Journal of Hospital Infection* **54,** 109.

Wilson J (2006) *Infection control in clinical practice.* London: Baillière Tindall,

Woodward S (2005) Use of lubricant in female urethral catheterisation. *British Journal of Nursing* **14,** 1022.

14 PREVENTION OF INFECTION IN SPECIAL WARDS AND DEPARTMENTS

Richard PD Cooke, Michael A Cooper, Adam Fraise, Alison Hames, Peter Hoffman, Julie Hughes, Manjusha Narayanan, Muhammad Raza, Eric W Taylor, Michael J Weinbren

Paediatrics

Adam Fraise

SPECIAL PROBLEMS OF INFECTION

Healthcare-associated infections are a major problem in paediatric populations (Raymond and Aujard, 2000). Many children are admitted to hospital with (or incubating) community-acquired infections, some of which (e.g. respiratory virus infections, severe gastroenteritis and infected skin lesions) are difficult to control and may spread rapidly. Children are also more susceptible than adults to community-acquired diseases, as many of them have not developed immunity to the common infectious diseases. Furthermore, most children's wards may contain patients who are particularly susceptible (e.g. those with blood disorders or receiving steroids). The increase in the use of invasive techniques is associated with more infections, including the emergence of coagulase-negative staphylococci as a significant pathogen. Patient discipline is understandably rather lax in children's departments, and care must be taken to avoid the escape of children from isolation cubicles and misguided generosity in the sharing of toys, dummies, etc.

ISOLATION

As many of the infections seen on paediatric wards are transmitted via the airborne route, the availability of isolation facilities is of particular importance. Isolation facilities are needed for up to 50 per cent of general paediatric cases, and this proportion should be increased in specialist or tertiary referral units (particularly if there are many immunosuppressed patients). These isolation facilities should be used for any child with symptoms of diarrhoea or with a suspected or proven diagnosis of a transmissible infection such as open tuberculosis or varicella-zoster infection.

MAIN PATHOGENS IN CHILDREN

The organisms that may be involved in cross-infection are numerous and include respiratory viruses, varicella-zoster virus, viruses causing gastroenteritis (such as rotavirus); bacteria (such as Group A streptococci, enteropathogenic *Escherichia coli*, *Campylobacter* species); fungi (such as *Candida albicans*); dermatophytes that affect the scalp, and even skin or intestinal parasites (such as cryptosporidium). Specialist units may have particular problems with resistant micro-organisms; for example *Pseudomonas aeruginosa*, *P. cepacia* and *Staphylococcus aureus* occasionally cross-infect children suffering from cystic fibrosis.

GASTROINTESTINAL INFECTIONS

Gastrointestinal infections are common in children and range from mild viral infections, such as rotavirus, to potentially life-threatening conditions, such as bacillary dysentery or salmonellosis. Infection with *Shigella sonnei* is generally mild but is transmitted via the faecal–oral route and can be easily transmitted within a paediatric ward environment. As diagnosis of the cause of the diarrhoea commonly takes 2–3 days, it is important that all symptomatic children are isolated until they are asymptomatic or a non-infectious cause for their diarrhoea has been identified.

RESPIRATORY INFECTIONS

One of the commonest respiratory tract infection in children is respiratory syncytial virus (RSV), although infections from adenovirus, influenza and parainfluenza virus are also important. RSV infection is more common in winter and the disease is more severe in younger children. Infants with chronic pulmonary disease or congenital heart disease are at risk of severe or even fatal infection with RSV. RSV can easily spread from patient to patient and the incidence of hospital-acquired infection can be as high as 30 per cent (Leclair *et al.*, 1987). Transmission of RSV is by either direct contact with respiratory droplets or the hands of healthcare workers. Prevention of spread is very difficult as, during outbreaks, there are rarely sufficient isolation rooms to contain the infectious cases. Hospital-acquired pneumonia from bacterial pathogens is less common in children than in adults but is still an important condition, especially in the ventilated patient (Craven and Steger, 1989).

VARICELLA-ZOSTER (CHICKENPOX)

Varicella-zoster virus infection is common in childhood with about 80 per cent of cases occurring in the under-5 year age group. This infection can be particularly severe in the immunocompromised individual and there is a danger of severe neonatal varicella resulting in neonatal death, if infection is acquired by a mother around the time of delivery. The highest risk period is from 1 week before to 1 week after delivery.

Infection in early pregnancy is associated with a small risk that the fetus may become infected (the risk of congenital varicella syndrome is approximately 1 per cent in the first 12 weeks, and around 2 per cent from weeks 13–20; Health Protection Agency, 2008). Because of these risks, strict isolation is advisable for patients with varicella-zoster infection and staff on paediatric and maternity wards should be immune to varicella-zoster virus. Most staff will be immune due to previous infection; however, in the absence of natural immunity, this can be achieved by vaccination.

TUBERCULOSIS

Outbreaks of tuberculosis (TB) occasionally occur in paediatric wards. Infections are usually contracted from staff, but a parent whose child had 'closed' TB was implicated in one large outbreak. It is safest to isolate children with 'closed' TB, as well as 'open' TB, until the source is identified. Chapter 13 is particularly relevant to paediatric departments, and procedures are suggested for the management of children admitted with community-acquired infections.

BLOODSTREAM INFECTIONS

Hospital-acquired bloodstream infections are common, accounting for 10–20 per cent of all healthcare-associated infections in children (Welliver and Mclaughlin, 1984; Ford-Jones et al., 1989). Intravenous cannulation is a major risk factor for primary bloodstream infections and it is important to avoid prolonged catheter placement (Pratt et al., 2007). It is widely recommended that these devices should be removed when they are no longer indicated and should not remain in situ for more than 72 hours unless there are specific contraindications to changing them (e.g. if venous access is particularly difficult).

Central venous catheters are frequently used in patients with malignancy or those requiring parenteral nutrition and represent a major risk for device-associated bacteraemia. Skin preparation using a suitable disinfectant (e.g. 2 per cent chlorhexidine in alcohol) and fastidious line care are important means of reducing this risk and all hospitals should have clear procedures for the insertion and maintenance of these lines.

MENINGITIS

Although meningitis from *Haemophilus influenzae* type b (Hib) is less common in many developed countries as a result of the administration of Hib vaccine, meningitis caused by *Neisseria meningitidis* or viruses is still an important cause for admission to a paediatric unit. Close contacts of children with meningococcal or *Haemophilus* meningitis must be given chemoprophylaxis. Ciprofloxacin is the preferred agent but can only be given to adults. Children who have been in contact with the index case should be given rifampicin.

Neonatal meningitis is distinct from meningitis in older children because different pathogens are involved. The commonest organisms are beta-haemolytic streptococci of Lancefield group B and *E. coli*. These organisms are not commonly acquired by cross-infection and therefore there are no specific infection control implications. However, if meningitis from Gram-negative organisms is part of an outbreak, then the organisms may be present in the environment and environmental cleaning may be indicated (Gantz and Godofsky, 1996).

NEONATAL UNITS

Modern management of high-risk pregnancies has resulted in a significant number of premature infants surviving. The care of premature and low-birth-weight infants is undertaken in neonatal units (sometimes called special care baby units or SCBUs) where the risk of nosocomial infection is particularly high owing to the very susceptible nature of the infants (Grohskopf *et al.*, 2002). Babies in these units are usually managed in incubators, and many will require mechanical ventilation and intravenous therapy. Artificially ventilated infants are at high risk of ventilator-associated pneumonia, and intravenous therapy increases the risk of line-associated bacteraemia.

STAPHYLOCOCCUS AUREUS IN NEONATAL UNITS

Staphylococci are particularly likely to be transferred on the hands of staff. If an outbreak occurs, all babies should be treated with hexachlorophane powder (e.g. Ster-Zac) at each napkin change or twice daily, if this is not already routine procedure (Allen *et al.*, 1994). The buttocks, groins, lower abdomen, umbilicus and axilla should be powdered. Infected babies should be bathed daily with chlorhexidine–detergent solution. A 4 per cent chlorhexidine–detergent solution, or 70 per cent alcohol solution rubbed to dryness, should be used for all handwashing by the staff. Staff should wear gloves and a gown or apron when handling babies during an outbreak. Routine screening of staff for *S. aureus* is not necessary but, in an outbreak, carriers of the epidemic strains should be treated (Crossley *et al.*, 1979). General control methods should be applied, especially isolation of infected babies.

GRAM-NEGATIVE INFECTIONS IN NEONATAL UNITS

Because of the high risk of infection and the difficulty in making an accurate diagnosis, babies on neonatal units frequently need to be treated with empirical antimicrobial regimens. This in turn increases the risk of colonization and infection with resistant micro-organisms such as *Klebsiella*, *Enterobacter* and *Serratia*. Reports of outbreaks of these resistant organisms are frequent, and infection control teams need to be constantly on the lookout for cross-infection or outbreaks.

PREVENTION OF INFECTION

The number of nursing staff and the quality of their training are the major factors in controlling the spread of infection. Because of the risks of gastroenteritis, no more than four infants should be in any one room, and they should preferably be in cubicles with one or two cots only. Adequate washing facilities must be available in each cubicle, and each cubicle should have its own weighing machine. Older children should not be in wards with adults.

Hand hygiene is particularly important in preventing the transmission of infections. Rotavirus infection is associated with heavy environmental contamination and the large numbers of organisms may be difficult to remove from the hands. The use of gloves is recommended when handling excreta or contaminated materials. Alcoholic hand rubs should be available for use by staff and visitors, as these are effective against many pathogens including RSV. It is important to remember that alcohol is not active against norovirus or *Clostridium difficile* and, if patients infected with these organisms are present, handwashing with soap and water should be emphasized. Prevention of RSV spread to staff is important and, in addition to hand hygiene, they should be advised to avoid touching the nose and eyes. The use of goggles that cover the nose and eyes of staff has been associated with a reduction in infection, although the acceptability of this device remains uncertain.

The increase in intravenous site infections, often caused by coagulase-negative staphylococci, is mainly associated with central venous catheterization and parenteral feeding. Efficient skin disinfection (ideally with 2 per cent chlorhexidine in alcohol) and care of the site are important requirements (see Chapter 6).

There is evidence that frequent and prolonged visiting of their own children by parents does not have any significant effect on infection rates. However, it is useful to have a written policy for parents backed up by information leaflets stating that 'parents should consult the ward sister if they have any infection, however trivial, so as to protect other children within the unit whose resistance to infection is poor'. Similar provisos apply to visiting by siblings, but it is advisable to bar children with minor respiratory infections, as these may be prodromal signs of measles or other communicable diseases. Parents should notify staff if a visitor to the hospital develops a transmissible infection within 7 days of visiting, or a patient within the week of discharge. This enables susceptible contacts to be traced. Gowns or plastic aprons should be worn by parents nursing children with gastroenteritis, and handwashing facilities must be available to them, together with instructions on how to avoid acquiring the infection. Visiting of children with dangerous infections, such as diphtheria, poliomyelitis and (for the first 48 hours) meningococcal meningitis should be restricted to parents, and preferably those who are immune, when this is possible. Visitors of infectious patients should avoid contact with other patients. Crockery and cutlery need only be domestically clean, but washing in a machine at 70–80°C (158–176°F) is preferable, and is essential on isolation wards.

For the treatment of incubators, suction equipment, thermometers and other equipment, see Chapter 6.

TOILET ARRANGEMENTS

Because of the common occurrence of intestinal infections in children, special precautions are necessary for toilet areas and bed-pan handling. The toilet areas require a high standard of domestic cleanliness, especially the toilet seat, which should be washed at least daily, and more frequently if this is necessary. Spraying the toilet seat and cistern handle with 70 per cent alcohol or cleaning with hypochlorite solution (and rinsing) after each patient is useful during outbreaks of viral gastroenteritis, but attention to handwashing and use of paper towels is of greater importance. A steam or hot-water supply capable of destroying vegetative forms of bacteria should be fitted to bed-pan washers (see Chapter 6).

LAUNDRY

Disposable napkins ('nappies' or diapers) are standard practice in developed countries and are preferable from an infection control viewpoint. If reusable napkins are used, they should be sealed in plastic or alginate bags for transport, and the bags may be labelled with the words 'used napkins', depending on the laundry policy (see Chapter 7).

PERSONNEL

Communicable diseases may be acquired from patients by staff if they are not immune, and may then in turn be passed on to patients and visitors. One of the most important of these is rubella. Staff of both sexes should be screened for immunity to rubella and be immunized if they are non-immune, because of the number of pregnant women who visit children in hospital. The acquisition of salmonella and shigella by nursing staff can have disastrous consequences, and most outbreaks of infection in hospital owing to these organisms have been associated with the infection among the nursing staff. Herpes simplex infection in attendants may produce a variety of lesions and may cause severe infections in children. Staff with herpetic lesions should not handle babies.

RECORD-KEEPING

A list of patients with infection admitted to the ward or acquired in the ward is useful in the investigation of spread of infection. The infections which are most usefully recorded are those due to shigellae, rotavirus and other gastrointestinal pathogens, methicillin-resistant *S. aureus* (MRSA), group A streptococci, RSV and the common infectious diseases (particularly chickenpox).

Burns

Michael J Weinbren

INTRODUCTION

Information for staff in hospitals without a burns unit

Significant burns require the specialist care provided by a burns unit. As the numbers of dedicated units are relatively small, most microbiologists/Infection Control Teams do not have the experience of dealing with this patient group on a day-to-day basis. Staff in hospitals without a burns unit should be aware that the admission of a burn patient (new or old) should be viewed as a potential source of resistant organisms and precautions to minimize the spread of infection taken as appropriate. Equally should a burn patient be managed in a non-specialist centre initially, it is good practice to inform the burns unit of any relevant microbiology prior to transfer.

OVERVIEW OF THE BURNS PROCESS

The thermal injury producing a burn usually renders the burn surface free of bacteria. Unless managed appropriately, in the extensive burn, there can be an almost relentless progression from an initially 'sterile' surface through to heavy colonization and finally invasive infection. The burn wound consists of protein-rich necrotic tissue (the eschar) providing an ideal culture medium for micro-organisms (Church *et al.*, 2006). Compared with a surgical wound, it is more complex and should be regarded as a three-dimensional structure within which the eschar may provide a nidus for the proliferation of organisms. The avascular nature of the eschar not only hinders the delivery of systemic antibiotics and most topical agents to the infection site, but is thought to be important in maintaining the systemic inflammatory response that occurs in burn patients. The large numbers of organisms that may be present in the burn wound readily predispose to cross-infection. Altered drug pharmacokinetics, poor penetration of agents into the wound together with a high bacterial load can lead to the selection of resistant strains during treatment. Transfer of burn patients from abroad is not unusual and may lead to the import of organisms with unusual resistance patterns/mechanisms. This may become more common with global conflict. Shortly after the new burns unit opened at Queen Mary's University Hospital, Roehampton in 1985, a patient was transferred from abroad with a strain of *Pseudomonas* that was sensitive only to amakacin and carbapenems. The strain persisted in the unit until it closed almost 15 years later.

MANAGEMENT OF THE BURN PATIENT

In addition to the local effects of the burn, there are systemic changes (that may be profound), the intensity of which varies with the size of the burn and over time. Some of the more important steps in the management of burns are:

- emergency medical treatment;
- fluid resuscitation;
- treatment of inhalation injury – lung damage poses a significant and serious risk from pulmonary infection;
- nutritional support (modulation of the hypermetabolic response to trauma);
- burn wound care.

Although burn mortality has decreased in recent years, infection remains a leading cause of death. The primary focus of this section is to give an overview of burn management with particular reference to infection and cross-infection. Ayliffe, Lawrence and Lowbury are significant contributors to the understanding of burn microbiology/infection control, and the *Journal of Hospital Infection* supplement covering a symposium on burns remains a useful source of information (Ayliffe and Lawrence, 1985). Lowbury (1992) proposed the concept of a first and second line of defence in preventing infection in the burn patient. The first line, to prevent the patient acquiring organisms, consists of antisepsis, primary excision and grafting of the burn and asepsis. The second line is formed from methods of preventing organisms that have reached the wound from invading the tissues and bloodstream. This includes systemic antibiotics, general supportive measures and active and passive immunization. Prophylaxis against tetanus is recommended for significant burns. The early hopes of a *Pseudomonas* vaccine/immunoglobulin have not wholly materialized (Tredget *et al.*, 2004).

THE BURN PATIENT

The burn patient population is over-represented by extremes of age and those with predisposing conditions such as diabetes or mental health disorders. The susceptibility of the burn patient to infection is compounded by the diffuse effects of the burn on the immune system. This ranges from the obvious and immediate loss of skin, an important part of the innate immune system, to widespread depression of the adaptive immune system (Greenfield and McManus, 1997). Thus, the large burn is truly immunocompromised and the risk of infection is further added to by the requirement for invasive devices such as intravenous cannulae and endotracheal intubation.

CLASSIFICATION OF BURNS

Burns may be classified into scald, flame or flash, contact (with hot or cold surfaces), radiation chemical and electrical. These are further sub-classified into size (percentage area burn) and depth of burn. The depth of the burn is important. Partial thickness burns, which include superficial dermal and deep dermal burns, have the capacity to heal spontaneously from undamaged epidermal appendages. With full thickness burns only small deep burns will heal spontaneously.

MANAGEMENTS OF THE BURN

The burn wound can be managed essentially in one of three ways – the exposure method, the closed method and early tangential excision. With the exposure method, the burn is left to dry forming an environment which is inhospitable to Gram-negative bacteria but favours the growth of Gram-positive organisms. In the closed method, a dressing along with a topical antiseptic is applied to the burn. When these two methods are used for the management of full-thickness burns, grafting is usually delayed until spontaneous separation of the eschar unless infection intervenes. However, full-thickness burns should, where possible, be managed by early tangential excision. Following the burn, the patient is stabilized and topical antiseptics are applied to the burn wound to prevent/minimize early bacterial contamination. Excision of the burn wound can then take place as early as 24–48 hours post injury. Removal of the necrotic eschar reduces both the risk from infection and the systemic inflammatory response mediated by the tissue. With large burns, successive operations are required as there is a limit to the area that can be operated on at any one time. Wound closure is achieved through either autologous skin grafts, human homograft skin, cultured skin or biosynthetic skin substitutes. Early tangential excision is demanding on resources and not all patients are suitable for this method of treatment.

MICROBIOLOGICAL SURVEILLANCE

Routine microbiological surveillance is an essential component of management, the results providing information used to guide topical and systemic antibiotic therapy (reserved for when the patient becomes infected) as well as an indication of cross-contamination within the unit.

The burn wound can be heavily contaminated with a mixture of organisms. The use of selective media, for example, staphylococcal/streptococcal or *Pseudomonas* selective agars, produces higher isolation rates of the respective organisms that would otherwise be missed in mixed culture.

The burn raw area is sampled either using a swab or by taking a biopsy (Church *et al.*, 2006). Surface swabs offer the advantage of being easy to take and relatively cheap to process. Biopsy specimens can be processed in two ways – quantitative microbiological cultures are performed, high counts having a better correlation with infection. Histology is also performed and may show invasion of healthy tissues by micro-organisms consistent with infection.

SPECIFIC ORGANISMS

Contamination of the burn wound is almost inevitable. Organisms gaining access to the raw area may come either from the patient's own flora or as a result of cross-contamination. While colonization of the burn wound is common, only a small percentage go on to become infected. The diagnosis of infection can be difficult as the systemic inflammatory response arising from the burn process may mimic signs of sepsis. The range of organisms that can colonize/infect the burn patient include bacteria, fungi and viruses. Anaerobes in general are not of importance apart from certain specific instances (i.e. electrical or deep burns where there may be necrotic muscle). Gram-positive organisms tend to colonize the burn initially with Gram-negative organisms usually following later.

Beta-haemolytic streptococci

Streptococcus pyogenes would appear to be less common and less virulent than in the past; however, it may still cause severe infection and the failure of skin grafts. Although universally susceptible to penicillin, it is recommended in burn patients that a β-lactamase-stable penicillin such as flucloxacillin be used in treatment. The basis for this recommendation is that *Staphylococcus aureus*, invariably also present in the burn wound, liberates β-lactamases into the tissues, thereby indirectly protecting nearby *Streptococcus pyogenes* from the penicillin. It is customary to treat β-haemolytic streptococci (BHS) irrespective of the patient's condition because of the potential to spread to other patients and cause disease. Other BHS have been associated with infection and destruction of skin grafts.

Staphylococcus aureus

This is the commonest organism to colonize raw areas possibly arising from the depths of sweat glands/hair follicles where it may survive a more superficial burn. *S. aureus* may produce invasive infection or disease owing to the production of toxins. Some units have reported cases of toxic shock syndrome, particularly in paediatric burns.

There has been debate over the pathogenicity of methicillin-resistant *S. aureus* (MRSA) in burn patients (Shannon *et al.*, 1997). Reardon *et al.* (1998) retrospectively compared patients with MRSA and MRSA free controls. Although this study lacked statistical power, they suggested that methicillin resistance *per se* is not associated with increased morbidity or mortality in burns patients.

Pseudomonas aeruginosa

In a survey of 176 burn care centres in North America in 1994, *Pseudomonas* was considered the most serious cause of life-threatening infection in the thermally injured patient (Shankowsky *et al.*, 1994). The ready emergence of resistant strains and the use of hydrotherapy in burn patients have aided this organism in establishing itself within burns units. For further information, readers are referred to the comprehensive review by Tredget *et al.* (2004).

Acinetobacter

In recent years, this organism has emerged as a significant pathogen in intensive care units and burns units (Hèritier *et al.*, 2005). Strains can be highly resistant to antibiotics including carbapenems which previously had been the drugs of choice. For highly resistant strains, colistin, ampicillin/sulbactam or the new tetracycline derivative tigecycline should be considered following the results of sensitivity testing.

PROPHYLAXIS/TREATMENT OF INFECTIONS

Topical agents

These are applied to the raw area and should be used from the outset prior to bacterial contamination of the wound in order to be effective. Most do not penetrate into the necrotic tissue and their effectiveness may also be limited through neutralization by organic matter. Topical antibiotics have been used, but while some claim these to be the most effective, resistance emerges rapidly and therefore their use should be prohibited in most instances. Care has to be exercised as systemic toxicity may arise from absorption through the burn wound raw area: application of a neomycin-containing spray has been reported to cause deafness in children (Clarke, 1992).

The following agents are commonly used: silver sulphadiazine (flamazine)/caerium silver sulphadiazine, silver nitrate and mafenide acetate. The latter agent is of note as it is one of the few compounds that penetrate the burn wound eschar. Side effects include pain on application and metabolic acidosis owing to it being a carbonic anhydrase inhibitor.

Systemic antibiotics

Prophylaxis

Prophylactic use of penicillin at the time of admission was commonplace in the past to prevent serious streptococcal infection. With a reduction in incidence of such infections, this has been largely abandoned. However, in the event of an outbreak, widespread administration of a β-lactamase-stable penicillin (or an alternative for those allergic to penicillin) may be indicated.

It is common practice to administer systemic antibiotics at the time of burn wound manipulation owing to the association of this procedure with transient bacteraemia. This practice has been questioned, in particular the need for peri-operative antibiotic therapy in patients with burns involving less than 40 per cent of the total body surface area during the first 10 days post burn (Mozingo et al., 1997). The choice of antibiotic should be based on the results of routine surveillance cultures.

Treatment of infection

When a patient develops clinical signs of infection, an examination should be performed to identify the source and should include raw burn areas, the respiratory system and old and new vascular access sites. Specimens should be taken for culture and the patient started on antibiotics, which would be guided by the results of routine surveillance cultures and knowledge of the sensitivity patterns of organisms commonly found on the unit. Surgery may be an important adjunct to treatment depending on the site of infection (see below).

The pharmacokinetics of antibiotics are extremely variable in this patient group, with some patients requiring significantly higher than the standard recommended dose in order to achieve therapeutic levels (Weinbren, 1999). Owing to the significant and often unpredictable handling of drugs by burn patients, measuring first-dose pharmacokinetics of aminoglycosides is advocated in order that the dose may be individualized to the patient. For other drugs, such as β-lactams, where levels are not routinely measured, achieving a therapeutic level can be difficult especially where the minimum inhibitory concentration of the organism is close to the breakpoint.

Suppurative thrombophlebitis is a serious infectious complication that occurs with increased frequency in burn patients (Gillespie et al., 2000). It may be difficult to diagnose but it is important to do so, as surgical removal of the infected vessel, where possible, is an integral part of treatment.

CROSS-INFECTION/INFECTION CONTROL

Burns units represent a significant infection control challenge. Prevention of cross-infection requires the culmination of a number of factors: well-trained and motivated staff, good aseptic practices, good staffing levels and surgical practices, and design of the unit. It has been stated that the most efficient infection control measure introduced in burn care over the last decades is the early surgical excision of the burn wound and eschar followed by wound coverage (Herndon and Spies, 2001). This procedure significantly decreases the risk of colonization of the wound and the associated contamination of the environment and, therefore, risk of spread to other patients.

Acquisition rates for hospital-associated organisms would appear to vary widely between different units. While there are many variables such as size of burns unit, age of patient, and size and depth of burn, it would appear that, in some large units, cross-contamination of burns can be minimal. Hodle *et al.* (2006) conducted a survey of infection-control practices in US burns units. Their findings showed that 'although all units practice some form of infection-control, the lack of standardized guidelines makes it difficult for units to identify and use the best practices.' The use of national surveillance systems either for specific organisms or selected patient groups in other specialties has helped in allowing individual units or hospitals compare their performance and reduce rates of infection. Whether this is practicable or useful for burns where there are a large number of variables remains to be seen.

In line with infection control practices in any arena, good aseptic technique including handwashing is important in the burns unit. New burn patients admitted to a unit are usually isolated until their condition has improved sufficiently and the risk from infection is thought to be minimal, at which time they can be managed in an open part of the unit. All burns admitted from other centres (irrespective of age of burn), especially from abroad, should be isolated until the results of surveillance cultures are known.

The use of bacteria-controlled nursing units (BCNUs) has been advocated by some (Weber *et al.*, 2002). A BCNU is a laminar airflow unit surrounded by plastic walls, providing patient isolation and enabling control of the patient environment. Airflow is through high-efficiency particulate air filters located at the top of the units. BCNU side wards are entered by staff donning plastic aprons, shoulder-length gauntlets and examination gloves.

Mattresses and the use of hydrotherapy are recognized as significant sources of cross-infection within units. Small breaks in the mattress cover may allow contaminated secretions to gain access to the inner parts of the mattress. Unless inspected closely, the breach can be missed and, when the next patient is placed on the mattress, the compression from their weight causes the secretions to be liberated leading to cross-contamination. Hydrotherapy is used for cleaning the burn wound and aiding the removal of dressings. Saline baths have been used to immerse the large burn. Burns units that avoid hydrotherapy as well as maintaining high levels of reverse isolation in lamina flow units are stated to have very low rates of cross-contamination with multi-drug resistant organisms (Weber *et al.*, 2002). In general, saline baths and the associated platform used for lowering the patient into the water are difficult to clean. As with other areas outside of burns, greater consideration of infection control requirements needs to be incorporated into the design of equipment.

DESIGN OF A BURNS UNIT

The principles of design of burns units was reported on by a working group of the British Burn Association and Hospital Infection Society in 1991. This provides a good foundation for anyone building a new unit. In order to minimize the spread of organisms between burn patients and other groups of hospital patients, it is recommended that burns units should be self-contained, being able to provide the same level of care as an intensive care unit (ICU) – ability to ventilate and give renal support – to the large burn within the unit. The unit should also house its own dedicated operating theatre and equipment. Where this has not been the case, there are reports of ongoing outbreaks between the burn ward and general ITU patients (Thompson *et al.*, 2002; Bayat *et al.*, 2003). The problems of the large burn being initially 'bacteria free' requiring protective isolation followed by source isolation once colonized/infected is discussed and various options provided. The internal design of rooms, including storage of equipment, has become increasingly important with the emergence of *Acinetobacter* species as a pathogen both inside and outside of burns units. Although Gram-negative, it possesses characteristics of Gram-positive organisms, such as the ability to survive in the dry environment. Large numbers of horizontal surfaces in rooms that are difficult to clean predispose to survival of the organism and cross-infection when the next patient is admitted to the room.

Burns units require the support of specialist staff (anaesthetics, paediatric, physiotherapy, dietetics, infection control, etc.) and other services especially pathology including blood transfusion and microbiology. Thus a burns unit needs to be located where it has ready access to such services.

Renal

Muhammad Raza and Alison Hames

INTRODUCTION

Renal replacement therapy (RRT), haemodialysis (HD) and peritoneal dialysis (PD) constitutes a set of expensive and complex medical interventions. At the end of 2005, there were 41 776 patients on RRT in the UK. Of these, 71 per cent of patients were started on HD while 26.5 per cent were started on PD (Tsakiris *et al.*, 1996). Patients on RRT are at higher risk of acquiring infections owing to the immune suppression associated with altered homeostasis in renal failure, and also its management via repeated access to the blood or the peritoneal cavity. Furthermore, a proportion of these patients proceed to receive organ transplants with associated immunosuppressive therapy. Principles of infection control described elsewhere for general clinical areas are also applicable to renal units, while the issues related to kidney transplantation are considered in the section on 'Transplant'. In this section, considerations relating to bacterial and viral infections associated with RRT will be discussed.

CHARACTERISTICS OF PATIENTS ON RENAL REPLACEMENT THERAPY

These patients are particularly prone to bacterial and viral infections, ranking as the second most frequent cause of mortality and morbidity after cardiovascular disease (UK Renal Registry, 2006). Several predisposing factors have been described, which are listed below.

- repeated exposure of blood or peritoneal cavity to carry out RRT;
- immune dysregulation in these patients, resulting in defects in both cellular and humoral immunity. (These defects not only predispose patients to infections but also render them more likely to suffer with severe manifestations of infection. In addition, interventions (e.g. vaccination) are relatively ineffective.) The following factors have been described as responsible for an abnormal immune response:
  - uraemia
  - deranged metabolism of immunologically active proteins
  - RRT
  - chronic exposure to foreign bodies
- malnutrition
- chronic anaemia and repeated blood transfusions.

Haemodialysis

Haemodialysis involves blood from the patient pumping through a system of semi-permeable membranes, the dialyser unit, which brings the blood in contact with a specially prepared fluid, the dialysate, running on the other side of the membrane. Diffusion across the membrane results in the plasma chemicals moving towards the dialysate. Apart from the dialyser unit, the dialysis machine comprises blood pumps and pressure monitors, an air trap and air detector, a proportionating unit, a heparin pump and a blood leak detector. For a flow of 200–500 mL/min of the blood, about double the volume of dialysate runs in a countercurrent direction. The proportionating unit is employed to prepare the dialysate by mixing solute concentrates with specially purified water.

For adequate flow of blood for haemodialysis, the following methods for access to blood are employed: temporary access venous catheters, tunnelled catheters, arteriovenous fistulae or arteriovenous grafts. Access-associated infections are considered later (see 'Bacterial infections' below).

Equipment and supplies

Dialysis membranes are not impermeable to micro-organisms, therefore a supply of pure water is required. Water used in dialysis in the UK should contain not more than 10 colony-forming units (CFUs)/mL and 0.06 IU of endotoxin/mL of water. The water should be tested by analysing a sample from the outlet of the water treatment plant and other points where high bacterial load is suspected (R. James, Dialysis Unit, Barts and The London NHS Trust, London, UK). Water samples in 100 mL volumes should be tested, which should include culture for defined indicator bacteria (e.g. *Pseudomonas*). Several disinfection cycles plus an additional ultraviolet disinfection may be necessary to achieve these levels. A regular monthly bacteriological testing on the quality of water is mandatory (Vorbeck-Meister *et al.*, 1999).

Machines should be disinfected either chemically or by heat between patients; the entire dialysis circuit should be replaced after use for patients with known bloodborne viruses (BBVs).

A stationary medication cart or dedicated medication area should be used to prepare injectable medications. There are reports of outbreaks of hepatitis B virus (HBV) infection due to use of multi-dose vials in the medication (Alter *et al.*, 1983). Ideally, the medication should be prepared in a dedicated central area away from the treatment area. Clean supplies should be stored separately from the patient area and should not be returned to the store, so that blood contamination in the patient area can be avoided (Centers for Disease Control and Prevention; CDC). CDC also recommends that the containers used to collect priming solution from venous tubing from individual patients should be discarded or cleaned thoroughly between the patients.

BACTERIAL INFECTIONS

Methicillin-resistant *Staphylococcus aureus* screening and decolonization

Infections with MRSA and vancomycin-resistant enterococci (VRE) present a particular challenge. While outbreaks of VRE can be mainly controlled by antibiotic stewardship and infection control, high MRSA colonization rates and a high prevalence of infections amongst colonized patients pose a more significant problem. The Department of Health (DoH) in England recommends that all patients on dialysis should be screened for MRSA on admission to the programme and then at regular intervals, determined by local practice in the light of national guidance, and also prior to creation of vascular or peritoneal access. The DoH (2006) guidance, *Safer practice in renal medicine*, advises local surveillance programmes for the carriage of MRSA from nose, groin, wounds and skin breaks, sputum and catheter urine if applicable and, depending on local preferences, throat. Colonized patients should be isolated according to standard principles, offered topical decolonization treatment in an attempt to eradicate the infection, then re-screened to assess clearance. Re-screening should then be performed on a regular basis.

MRSA bacteraemias should be regarded as adverse incidents and investigated using root cause analyses. Each renal unit should have its own antimicrobial prescribing protocol to avoid the unnecessary or inappropriate use of antibiotics. The Renal Association recommends screening also for *Staphylococcus aureus* carriage on a 3-monthly basis and eliminating carriage with either a defined course or with regular topical use of mupirocin.

Haemodialysis vascular access-associated infections

In 2000, the National Audit Office estimated the additional cost of an episode of bloodstream infection to be £6209. Numerous studies report high rates of catheter-associated bloodstream infections (e.g. 5.2/1000 catheter-days; Brun-Buisson *et al.*, 2004), indicating a significant financial burden.

Types of catheter

The infection rate using temporary catheters as opposed to permanent catheters (tunnelled or cuffed central venous catheters) is significantly higher; however, it is significantly lower with native arteriovenous (AV) fistula (George *et al.*, 2006). Surveillance studies from the USA, Canada and Italy (Taylor *et al.*, 2002; Tokars *et al.*, 2002; Quarello *et al.*, 2006) showed that compared with AV fistula, the risk of bacteremia was around 30 times greater with a non-cuffed temporary catheters and around 20 times greater with a tunnelled cuffed catheter used for haemodialysis. While the proportion of haemodialysis patients using fistulae is 90 per cent in Italy and 67 per cent in the USA (Taylor *et al.*, 2002), it was only around 29 per cent in the UK in 2004 (UK Renal Registry, 2006). This practice reflects the relatively high access-related infection rate in the UK, being 0.08 per patient compared with 0.01 in Italy (Rayner, 2004).

A native AV fistula is therefore the access of choice in HD patients, followed by a prosthetic graft when a native AV fistula is surgically not possible. However, there are conditions that necessitate the use of catheters rather than the

AV fistula (e.g. high-output cardiac failure, ischaemic heart disease, steal syndrome and infection with BBVs). Fully implantable subcutaneous catheters have been shown to perform better compared with tunnelled cuffed catheters (Quarello *et al.*, 2006).

General issues related to vascular catheters, catheter care, vascular catheter-related infections and various management strategies are discussed in Chapter 13.

Arteriovenous fistula care

As described earlier, AV fistulae pose a far lower infection risk compared with catheters. The fistulae should be used once they are mature and should be able to permit blood flow greater than the pump rate (Beathard *et al.*, 1999). Thorough skin preparation of over a large area of the arm should be performed prior to accessing the fistula. Needle placement should avoid the previous point of insertion as this poses a higher risk of introducing organisms from this wound into the bloodstream. When placed, the needle should then be secured to avoid trauma.

PERITONEAL DIALYSIS

In 2005, there were 150 000 patients worldwide on PD representing around 15 per cent of the chronic dialysis patients (Thodis *et al.*, 2005). In this method the peritoneal membrane is used instead of a dialysis machine. A soft catheter positioned in the pelvic peritoneum and placed in a tunnel through the abdominal wall is employed to deliver and drain dialysate. The dialysate remains in the peritoneal cavity except at the times of exchange in continuous peritoneal dialysis (CAPD) or for short periods of active dialysis in intermittent peritoneal dialysis (IPD). Considerations of infections associated with peritoneal dialysis catheter and care of the catheter are discussed in the section on catheter care (p. **346**).

Infections associated with peritoneal dialysis

A squamous epithelial layer covers the newly inserted catheter from the exit site to the peripheral cuff, enclosed by a layer of collagen fibres. This arrangement can be damaged if extreme tension is applied to the cuff or if a badly draining sinus leads to infection as far as the peripheral cuff. Early infection in this case is only rarely treatable and withdrawal of the infected catheter is usually necessary for healing. The peripheral cuff should be placed as far from the skin as possible. Neither exit-site location (i.e. with respect to the belt-line) nor patient gender appear to be significantly associated with infection. Compared with an upward pointing exit site, downward pointing exit sites exhibit lower infection rates probably due to the effect of gravity (Thodis *et al.*, 2005). There are conflicting reports on the use of antibiotic prophylaxis at the time of catheter insertion.

Catheter design has evolved over the years to minimize the risk of infection of the exit site and the tunnel leading to peritonitis. Double-cuff Tenkhoff catheters are most widely used for PD, and they are shown to be associated with significantly fewer infections compared with single-cuff catheters. The difference in infection rates between standard Tenkhoff and curled catheters, and straight and swan-neck catheters were not significant in most studies (Thodis *et al.*, 2005). In paediatric populations, single-cuff catheters were associated with lower rate of infections compared with double-cuff (Macchini *et al.*, 2006).

An Italian cooperative PD study group presented data on a 10-year survey and found 69 per cent of PD catheters were still working at 4 years. The overall peritonitis rate in their study was 0.7 episodes per patient per year, of which 11 per cent were associated with exit-site infections. Over time, prevalence of infection decreased with *S. epidermidis* and increased with *S. aureus*, while it remained unchanged for other types of pathogens (Lupo *et al.*, 1994).

Catheter care

Exit sites should be kept covered and dry, and movement should be minimized until the site is healed and a stable tract is formed around the catheter; this may take up to a week. Large volumes of dialysate fluid, particularly during the early period after catheter insertion, can cause leakage and should not be left in the peritoneal cavity, especially if the patient is very active. Intermittent dialysis is the preferable method during the early period. The catheter site should be secured, cleaned daily using aseptic technique by patients or staff during manipulation. Iodine-based solutions should be avoided owing to the damage they may cause to both synthetic material and to the granulation tissue. There is no conclusive evidence that topical application of povidone–iodine, water and soap or even the use of no cleansing agents are significantly different from each other in terms of infection risk. The exit site should be cleaned and dried immediately after it has become dirty or wet after use (Thodis *et al.*, 2005). Topical mupirocin has been shown to reduce bacterial load, the incidence of peritonitis and the need for catheter removal significantly (Thodis *et al.*, 1998).

Frequent routine visual inspections of the exit site, and manipulation if necessary, are mandatory to proper care, but should take place only after proper handwashing. When not in use, the catheter should be anchored to the skin to prevent movement. The recommended cleaning solution is 2 per cent aqueous chlorhexidine gluconate solution in 4 per cent isopropyle alcohol and an air-permeable dressing should be used to cover the site (Thodis *et al.*, 2005).

Diagnosis of peritoneal dialysis-associated infection and management

While exit-site infections are mainly caused by S. *aureus*, both coagulase-negative staphylococci and S. *aureus* are commonly involved in peritonitis along with less common organisms: streptococci, coliforms, *Pseudomonas* and yeasts. *Pseudomonas* site infections in particular can spread subcutaneously. Exit-site and tunnel infections are characterized by local inflammation, whereas peritonitis may be diagnosed by abdominal pain and cloudy effluent, and by a peritoneal fluid leucocyte count of more than 0.1×10^9/L with more than 50 per cent neutrophils and with or without the presence of organisms on microscopy or on culture.

Intraperitoneal antibiotics should be started immediately before culture results are known and rationalized thereafter. Recurrent peritonitis is associated with an increased likelihood of treatment failure and may necessitate catheter withdrawal.

BLOODBORNE VIRUSES

Screening

The prevalence of human immunodeficiency virus (HIV) among HD patients has not changed during the past years and remained around 1.5 per cent in various centres. Incidence of HBV and hepatitis C virus (HCV) has declined over the years; however, there are reports of new cases resulting from transmission in the dialysis centres owing to inadequate infection control practices (Finelli *et al.*, 2002).

All patients who are waiting to go for dialysis and those receiving dialysis should be screened for HIV antibodies, HBV surface antigen (HBsAg) and HCV antibody, followed by a 1–3-monthly screening for HBV and HCV, and for HIV based upon a risk assessment (e.g. following foreign travel). Annual HIV testing may be a reasonable routine in many units. Patients displaying adequate antibody titres to HBV should be screened annually and considered for a booster dose if levels are low. Staff members should also be tested for HBV.

Patients with bloodborne viruses

Patients with HBV, HCV or HIV should ideally be nursed in separate rooms. Patients with HBV should have dedicated dialysis machines with disposable dialysers. Patients with HCV and HIV may use machines in general use provided they are thoroughly disinfected and the dialysis circuit adequately decontaminated between patients. In all cases, staff should wear appropriate personal protective gear when manipulating catheters and used lines should be disposed of in appropriate double-bagged clinical waste bags. Patients with a BBV should not have AV fistulae formed.

Infection prevention

Measures to prevent infections are needed for both individual patients and the environment where patients receive dialysis. There are numerous opportunities for transmission of infectious agents either directly from person to person or indirectly via contaminated devices and environmental surfaces. Nursing staff should ideally care exclusively for either infected or non-infected patients during any particular shift, and those caring for HBV-infected patients should have demonstrated immunity to HBV.

Following a new case of HBV, patients sharing the same session or machine with inadequate immunity should be screened weekly for 3 months, given a booster vaccine and, in those with no immunity, given hepatitis B immunoglobulin (HBIG). Following a new case of HCV, RNA detection should be used to screen contacts.

Application of standard infection control measure such as use of personal protective equipment, management of spills, avoidance of needlestick injuries and eye splashes, and the handling of blood specimens are dealt with elsewhere.

VACCINATION

Increased susceptibility to infections and a more severe and persistent course in chronic dialysis patients has been attributed to immunodeficiency amongst other factors in these patients. Responses to vaccines and the immune response following natural infection is also impaired in terms of a lower rate of vaccine response, lower resultant antibody titres, and a rapid decline of titres over time. Modifications might be needed in vaccination schedules plus frequent screening for immunity in these patients. All patients should receive routine vaccines, sometimes at higher doses than in the normal population. In contrast to some other immunocompromised groups, patients on dialysis can receive live attenuated vaccines, with the exception of live polio vaccine (Rangel et al., 2000).

Hepatitis B virus vaccine in three doses at 40 µg/dose should be offered to patients in the early course of their illness. Compared with around 90 per cent seroconversion rates in immunocompetent adults, only 50–75 per cent of dialysis patients develop protective response to this vaccine. The Advisory Committee on Immunization Practices (ACIP) in the USA and the UK DoH recommend a full repeat course, if the response to the first course is inadequate. These authorities also recommend testing of antibody levels 1–2 months after completion of the course and annually thereafter. Those with a marginal response may benefit from a single booster dose or yearly booster doses depending on their antibody titres. Those who fail to respond should be offered HBIG following significant exposure.

Chronic HD patients should also be offered pneumococcal and influenza vaccines.

PATIENT EDUCATION

The importance of patient education and training in prevention of infection is reflected in the higher rate of infection in the first than later years. Patients should be educated to care for the exit site and should learn to recognize the signs and symptoms of exit-site infection and peritonitis. There should be clear guidelines informing the patients how to deal with an episode of infection, including reporting to the renal unit. A leaflet containing instructions about self-cleanliness, bathing (avoid tub bathing) and care of the exit site should be given to patients and periodic refresher training should be provided. Facilities for counselling, vaccination and prophylaxis before travelling abroad should be available. After an episode of infection, retraining on the use of the catheter is mandatory. Both patient and family members should be trained in access site care and aseptic manipulation techniques. Root cause analysis should be used for each episode of infection.

SUMMARY

While the availability of dialysis has promoted the health of RRT-dependent patients enormously and resulted in prolongation of life, the intervention has presented an array of complex challenges to nephrologists, nursing staff and microbiologists, with infections being one of the most important. Prevention of infections in this group of patients requires team work, active development of policies and their meticulous application on a day-to-day basis. Frequent auditing and review of the policies and procedures, with application of root cause analysis to individual untoward infectious incidents are essential in continuous development of the service.

Critical care units

Michael A Cooper

The patients housed on critical care units are extremely vulnerable to health-care-associated infection. Many factors contribute to this: they commonly have several breaches of their anatomical barriers, such as peripheral and central intravenous catheters, urinary catheters, endotracheal tubes or a tracheostomy, plus surgical drains; they may be immunosuppressed from malnutrition, underlying disease, drugs, such as steroids, or secondary to multi-organ failure;

and they require frequent handling by staff, because of sedation and the need for physiotherapy, pressure area care and the care of lines, catheters etc. Additionally, critical care units have a high level of antimicrobial usage, often with broad-spectrum agents and antibiotic combinations that change the ecology of the patients' and the environmental flora in favour of multi-resistant organisms. Lapses in ideal infection control technique allow the spread of these multi-resistant organisms from patient to patient via the hands of healthcare personnel or, occasionally, fomites. The pressure of work within such units, especially during emergency situations, results in breaches of infection control protocols despite the best efforts of the infection prevention team (ICT) to ensure these are in place and the necessary training has occurred. It follows that adequate staffing, especially with trained nursing staff, is absolutely fundamental to the prevention of healthcare-associated infection on critical care areas (Halwani *et al.*, 2006).

DESIGN OF THE UNIT

There is an array of additional equipment that has to be available at each bed space on critical care units to monitor and provide support for patients in multi-organ failure. The space between beds has to be adequate not only to house this equipment but also to allow full access to the patient from all directions. This is not just for reasons of infection prevention and control, although it certainly is extremely difficult to decontaminate the environment and equipment properly around a cluttered bed space. As a minimum, all bed spaces must have an area of at least 25.5 m^2 with an unobstructed corridor space of at least 2.5 m beyond the working space. From an infection prevention viewpoint, the ideal would be for every bed space to be housed in a single room, but this is usually impractical. Therefore, a compromise has to be agreed over the ratio of single-bedded rooms in the total bed numbers: Health Building Note 57 *Facilities for critical care* (NHS Estates, 2005b) suggests half of the total beds should be in single rooms. Mechanical ventilation must ensure air movement is from clean to dirty areas and allow adequate airflow into areas that only have mechanical extract ventilation, via transfer grilles in doors or walls. Fresh air should be tempered and filtered (minimum of 99 per cent filtration to a particle diameter of 5 μm in clinical areas) before being distributed via high-level outlets via a low-velocity system. If highly infectious patients are to be housed in an area, a minimum of 15 air changes per hour is required but, for most patients, six air changes per hour are sufficient. Dirty areas, such as toilets, require a separate extract system. Air intakes and exhaust systems must be placed to avoid the re-circulation of air and minimize the effects of back pressure from strong winds. Isolation rooms should have ventilation that provides both source and protective isolation; this requires a balanced supply and exhaust system. An alternative is to have switchable positive/negative pressure ventilation, but such systems are generally not advisable, as there is a risk that the correct mode for a particular patient may not be used. Single rooms should have a gowning lobby, which requires a high balanced air change rate to act as a functional airlock. This is easier to achieve if the lobby is designed to be as small as possible, though a hand wash-basin is essential in every side-room lobby (NHS Estates, 2005b).

There must be adequate storage space for equipment, such as ventilators and haemofiltration units, disposables and linen. Dirty utility rooms or sluices should only be as large as required for their primary purpose; there is a huge temptation for equipment and supplies to be stored in these non-clean areas if there is any excess space. These 'dirty' areas should be situated away from any food preparation or 'clean' clinical areas. If waste is not to be transported from the areas immediately, the waste storage area should have easy access to the route by which waste is taken away from the unit. This should not involve transporting waste through clean or patient areas. Waste storage must be of adequate size to allow for segregation into the appropriate waste streams. Floors and walls should be of easily cleanable materials and finishes which can withstand repeated applications of strong disinfectants. There is little evidence to suggest that antibacterial paints and finishes have any advantage over other readily cleanable materials. Floors must be of a material sufficiently durable to withstand the heavy traffic inevitable in a critical care area while also being slip resistant for obvious safety reasons. Where the floor meets walls and other vertical surfaces, there should be a smooth junction with the floor material covering the lower 15 cm of the wall to allow for easy cleaning and prevent the build-up of dust and dirt. All joints in the floor must be heat sealed. Walls must be washable and durable. Counter tops must be constructed of a non-porous durable material able to withstand repeated applications of strong disinfectants. Protective seals must be intact; inspection as part of regular environmental audits is probably the optimal method of ensuring they are maintained to a suitable standard. Ceilings must be appropriate for their location. In clinical areas, they must be cleanable and, in single-room areas, sealed to avoid the ingress of potentially contaminated air from dead spaces. Ceiling tiles designed to reduce noise are not suitable for clinical areas but may be used in corridors, waiting areas, etc. (O'Connell and Humphreys, 2000).

PREVENTION OF INFECTION

Rules about hand decontamination and the removal of white coats and jackets worn around the rest of the hospital should be strictly enforced on entry to the unit. All staff must feel empowered to challenge breaches of these rules. Alcohol hand gel must be placed at the entry points to the unit and by every bed space. Hand wash-basins should also be adjacent to, or within easy reach of, every bed space. It is not necessary to have an individual hand wash-basin for every bed space as there is a risk of *Legionella* and other infections associated with infrequently used water outlets. All water outlets must be run daily to minimize the potential for *Legionella* to multiply within the pipework and outlet.

Within the unit, strict adherence to local infection prevention policies must be observed at all times by all staff and visitors. This includes those staff who are based on the unit as well as those who visit it as part of their duties around the hospital, such as clinicians, radiographers and physiotherapists. Hand hygiene between patients is of paramount importance, and audits of hand-hygiene practice must be regularly undertaken to ensure compliance with the policy is being maintained. Staff based on the unit must challenge poor practice and breaches of guidelines on the unit.

Environmental cleanliness is also important, as many of the multi-resistant organisms that are commonly responsible for healthcare-associated infection on critical care units, such as MRSA and *Acinetobacter* spp, can survive for prolonged periods on floors and other surfaces. Cleaning schedules must be devised that ensure all areas are cleaned thoroughly and regularly, and compliance with the schedules monitored. Audits of the environment should be undertaken on a regular basis; both the domestic and ward staff should participate in these, and the results monitored by the Director of Infection Prevention and Control (DIPC) or other members of the ICT. Education of domestic staff is fundamental to ensuring that environmental cleaning is carried out in an appropriate manner, as domestics who do not understand the principles of how organisms can spread between staff, patients and the environment will not necessarily carry out their duties in a manner that minimizes the risks, and surfaces that appear to be physically clean may still be colonized with potential pathogens. Periodic environmental swabbing for adenosine triphosphate (ATP) activity can be a useful adjunct to visual assessment of the cleanliness of the environment in critical areas (Lewis *et al.*, 2008). It is impossible to adequately clean cluttered areas, so all equipment not in use must be stored away from the immediate patient area. Any equipment essential to the care of the patient or that which has to be stored in the patient areas must be cleaned regularly; guidelines on what items of medical equipment, if any, domestics can clean and what can be cleaned only by nursing staff or other specialist staff, such as medical physicists, must be in place. Likewise, the domestics must be clear about which items of equipment they can move to clean around, which they can not, and how these latter places are to be cleaned, or areas of the ward could go undisturbed for a considerable length of time (Schabrun and Chipchase, 2006).

PREVENTION OF NOSOCOMIAL AND VENTILATOR-ASSOCIATED PNEUMONIA

Patients who require mechanical ventilation are much more likely to develop pneumonia than those who are able to breathe spontaneously. Ventilator-associated pneumonia (VAP) is a major cause of morbidity and mortality in critical care patients. Education programmes in infection prevention, including hand hygiene and the use of personal protective equipment, as part of induction and mandatory updates, can reduce the rates of many healthcare-associated infections, including VAP and such programmes are an essential part of any infection control strategy. It is also essential that there is an adequate number of nursing staff, of an appropriate grade, who have received adequate training on the care of the ventilated patient.

The tracheal cuff pressure should be maintained such that it minimizes the risk of tracheal damage, but also does not allow the aspiration of pharyngeal contents. Subglottic secretions should be drained. Oral antiseptics (e.g. chlorhexidine) should be included as part of the oral hygiene regimen for all patients who are intubated and receiving mechanical ventilation (Gastmeier and Geffers, 2007). Reduction of gastric acid secretion increases the risks of VAP. Therefore, if possible, acid suppression therapy should not be used. If the patient is only at low to moderate risk of stress ulceration, sucralfate should be used in preference to other gastric ulcer prophylactic regimes.

There is evidence that the semi-recumbent position is associated with a lower risk of VAP, so this position is preferred unless it is contraindicated (National Institute for Health and Clinical Excellence, 2008). Oral, rather than nasal, intubation has a lower risk of VAP. Screening the environment or patients routinely for the causative organisms of VAP is of no benefit. The elderly and other groups at risk should be immunized against influenza virus and the pneumococcus, but this needs to be as part of a community-wide immunization programme and is not something that can be addressed by the critical care staff.

Clinical care and weaning protocols have been shown to reduce the incidence of VAP and these should be in place and compliance with them audited regularly. Care bundles, such as the 'Saving Lives' VAP high-impact intervention can also help reduce the incidence of VAP (see http://www.clean-safe-care.nhs.uk/toolfiles/25_SL_HII_5_v2.pdf).

All ventilator equipment must be maintained, cleaned and decontaminated following the manufacturers' instructions. New ventilator circuit tubing should be provided for each patient, but there is no evidence that changing this more frequently than every 7 days reduces the incidence of VAP, unless the circuit becomes physically soiled or damaged. Condensate should be drained periodically and healthcare workers should wear appropriate masks and visors when opening a closed breathing circuit to protect themselves from contamination. The use of heat moisture exchangers lowers the rate of VAP in patients who require mechanical ventilation for more than 7 days and are safe to use as long as the manufacturers' instructions are followed and the patient is not at risk of airways obstruction. These should be changed according to the manufacturers' instructions or if they become contaminated. Nebulizers should be for single-patient use only, and disinfected and cleaned with sterile water between uses. If they form part of the ventilator circuit, they must be single use. Filters should be used to protect the ventilator circuit, but they do not directly influence the rate of VAP. Suction equipment needs to be changed only weekly, unless it becomes contaminated or damaged, in which case it should be changed immediately. The anaesthetic machine should not be a source of infection as long as filters are used, the heat and moisture exchanger, and anaesthetic machine valve are changed between patients, and the ventilator tubing is changed weekly. If a machine is used on an infected patient, the filter and tubing must be replaced before that machine is used on another patient.

There is no difference between open or closed suctioning in terms of the rates of VAP, but closed suctioning decreases the chances of aerosolization of secretions and, therefore, reduces the exposure of staff and other patients to potential pathogens. Special consideration needs to be given to immunosuppressed patients, who may be at increased risk of acquiring an invasive aspergillus infection unless the air in the unit it suitably filtered. Even then, if building or demolition work is taking place nearby, there may still be an increased risk, and consideration should be made to nursing such patients in rooms with high-efficiency particle/particulate filtered air and using antifungal prophylaxis. Selective decontamination of the digestive tract (SDD) has been shown to be effective in preventing VAP and cost-effective overall. There is no evidence that SDD contributes to the acquisition of multi-resistant organisms, but the use of regimens that include cephalosporins or fluoroquinolones may produce increased morbidity and mortality associated with *Clostridium difficile* infection, and should be used with caution in hospitals where C. *difficile* is endemic (Masterton *et al.*, 2008).

MANAGEMENT OF LINES

Almost all patients on critical care units require intravascular catheters (often multiple) for the administration of fluids, nutrition and drugs and for monitoring physiological parameters. Such lines are potential sources of sepsis to the patient, as they breach the skin at their insertion site and also allow direct access to the bloodstream for organisms. Consequently, intravascular catheters must be inserted only if they are necessary. It is important that the correct type of line is used and that it is inserted using the correct technique, in an appropriate environment and in the most appropriate anatomical site. The insertion site must also be maintained properly; and lines must be removed when indicated (i.e. as soon as the line is no longer required or if there is any evidence of infection). Lines should also be removed if they have been in place for the maximum period stated by the manufacturers; in the case of short peripheral venous lines, they should not be left *in situ* beyond 72 h.

Education, including hand-hygiene education, for all staff involved in the insertion and use of intravascular lines, is crucial to minimize the risk of line-associated sepsis. Compliance with the local hand-hygiene guidelines should be audited and the results of these audits fed back to the DIPC or other ICT members.

Central lines should be inserted using maximum sterile barrier precautions, with sterile gloves, cap, mask, gown and a large sterile drape. With these precautions in place, it probably makes little difference if the procedure takes place in an operating theatre or on the unit itself. Before line insertion, hands must be decontaminated. The skin at the insertion site must be cleaned and disinfected using an appropriate disinfectant (e.g. 2 per cent chlorhexidine in either alcoholic solution) prior to insertion. The antiseptic must remain on the insertion site for an appropriate length of time before inserting the catheter; alcoholic solutions must be allowed to dry. Antimicrobial ointment or organic solvents (e.g. acetone or ether) should not be applied to the insertion site prior to insertion. Either a gauze or transparent semi-permeable dressing should be used. A gauze dressing is preferable if the insertion site is oozing, otherwise a transparent dressing allows better visualization of the insertion site and requires less frequent changes. Aseptic technique must be used when accessing the catheter. The giving sets should be changed every 72 h (Pratt *et al.*, 2007).

SPECIFIC PROBLEMS

Methicillin-resistant *Staphylococcus aureus*

Methicillin-resistant *Staphylococcus aureus* (MRSA) has become endemic in many critical care units. Its ability to survive for prolonged periods on inanimate surfaces and its ready transmission from the hands of healthcare workers (contaminated either from infected or colonized patients, or the environment) has made it a common cause of line-associated, urinary tract, respiratory tract and other nosocomial infections. Properly applied control strategies can be successful in reducing the impact of MRSA. Meticulous environmental decontamination, strict adherence to hand-hygiene practices, isolation of known positive patients and admission plus regular (at least weekly) screening of all patients on the unit can reduce the prevalence and impact of MRSA (Cepadia *et al.*, 2005). Rapid (same-day) screening using molecular techniques has been shown to have a greater impact on the transmission and carriage rate of MRSA when compared with traditional culture techniques (Cunningham *et al.*, 2007). Decolonization should be attempted on MRSA carriers, but this is often less successful with this patient group because the application of skin disinfectants is more problematic with non-ambulant patients. Evidence-based line, ventilator, wound and urinary tract care also help reduce clinical infections with all nosocomial pathogens, including MRSA (Raineri *et al.*, 2007).

Acinetobacter

Multi-resistant strains of *Acinetobacter*, particularly *A. baumanii*, are another common cause of critical care-acquired infections, particularly VAP and bacteraemia. This organism is well adapted for survival in the environment and thorough decontamination of all equipment, the bed space and all other clinical areas is an essential component of dealing with outbreaks with this organism. The isolation of all patients transferred from other hospitals, especially from abroad, until it has been established that they are not carrying multi-resistant organisms, such as acinetobacters, is recommended good practice. The overuse of broad-spectrum antibacterials must also be discouraged to reduce the selective pressure for multi-resistant organisms. All antibacterial therapy must be reviewed on a daily basis by the critical care team, which should include a microbiologist and/or an antibiotic pharmacist. Patients found to be colonized with multi-resistant acinetobacters should be isolated if at all possible (Pimental *et al.*, 2005). Skin carriage can be reduced or eliminated with a daily regimen of 4 per cent chlorhexidine body washes (Boer *et al.*, 2007).

Glycopeptide-resistant enterococci

These organisms can arise from the endogenous flora of patients, but the selective pressure created by the overuse of glycopeptides, particularly vancomycin, along with antibacterials with little or no activity against the enterococci, such as the cephalosporins and fluoroquinolones, provide favourable conditions for these organisms to proliferate. Like *Acinetobacter*, they are very well adapted for survival on inanimate objects and readily contaminate the environment, which can lead to persistence of the organism on the unit (Lund *et al.*, 2002). Unlike MRSA, decolonization of colonized patients is not possible because the organism is carried in the gastro-intestinal tract. Manipulation of the antimicrobials used on the unit can remove the survival advantage of glycopeptide-resistant enterococci and reduce the carriage rate among patients. Screening for carriage in outbreak situations, along with the isolation of carriers can prevent further spread of the organism. Thorough environmental cleaning is also essential to prevent recurrent outbreaks (Cookson *et al.*, 2006; Hayden *et al.*, 2006; Lucet *et al.*, 2007).

Stenotrophomonas maltophilia

Although often considered a low-grade pathogen, this has become an important nosocomial pathogen on critical care units. Its intrinsic resistance to many antibiotics, including the carbapenems, makes its presence more common on units where antibiotic use is high, particularly where carbapenems are used extensively (Meyer *et al.*, 2007). Again, environmental contamination seems to play an important role in transmission between patients. VAP and line-associated infections are its most common clinical manifestation.

Pseudomonas aeruginosa

Despite the availability of various antipseudomonal antibiotics, this remains an important pathogen on critical care units. Tap water can be the source of this organism and its elimination from the plumbing system can be very difficult. Sink drains will commonly grow *P. aetuginosa*; the environment and equipment can then become contaminated through splash-back if the taps are fitted immediately above the drain (Bert *et al.*, 1998; Trautmann *et al.*, 2005). Urinary and respiratory tract infections are the usual clinical manifestations and care in the management of the airway in patients on ventilators is vital in controlling this organism.

Obstetrics and gynaecology

Richard PD Cooke and Julie Hughes

OBSTETRICS

Introduction

Maternity services have received considerable public attention in recent years. National publications that have set out good practice for maternity services include *The National Service Framework for Children, Young People and Maternity Services* (Department of Health, 2004) and the National Institute for Health and Clinical Excellence (NICE, 2001) *Guidelines for Maternity Services 2001*. In addition, there have been two reports from the Confidential Enquiry into Maternal and Child Health (CEMACH; 1997–99, 2000–02): *Why Mothers Die 1997–1999* and *Why Mothers Die 2000–2002*. In the UK, the risk of women dying from a pregnancy-related cause is extremely small and has reduced over the years. During the period 2000–2002, 391 maternal deaths were reported, giving an incidence of 11.4 deaths per 100 000 maternities (CEMACH, 2000–02).

Throughout these reports, infection prevention and control practices are often mentioned only briefly, probably because many policies and procedures are considered common to other specialities. Other issues are often given greater prominence. These include lack of effective systems and processes for the management of risk in maternity services, poor clinical leadership and poor interprofessional and intraprofessional relationships, excessive reliance on the use of locum and agency staff, poor planning in relation to the refurbishment or development of maternity services, and failure or lack of equipment.

Nevertheless, specific infection control prevention and policies are needed in obstetrics, since both pregnant women and their unborn children are more susceptible to infection despite the fact that they usually have no underlying medical pathology. Using the National Service Framework template, these can be conveniently divided into three key areas: pre-birth, birth and post-birth care for mothers and their babies (Department of Health, 2004).

Pre-birth care

Patient antenatal screening

Congenital infections acquired in pregnancy can be the cause of multi-system fetal disease resulting in permanent damage. This can be avoided by identification of at-risk mothers who can receive appropriate prophylaxis or early treatment particularly during delivery or the post-natal period. Hence screening for HBV, HIV, rubella and syphilis is recommended at the first antenatal appointment (NICE, 2003).

Cytomegalovirus (CMV) infection is a common concern in pregnancy, in view of its association with fetal malformation and the fact that infection is usually not apparent. It is excreted in urine, saliva, breast milk and cervical secretions, and can be transmitted from mother to baby *in utero*, during delivery and in the post-natal period. However, avoiding occupational exposure to infected urine and saliva (e.g. from young children) has not been proven to prevent infection in susceptible pregnant women. Therefore, general advice should be to encourage universal infection control precautions, particularly handwashing, after exposure to body fluids.

Screening for parvovirus B19 immunity is currently not recommended. Approximately 50 per cent of the antenatal population in the UK will be immune to B19. Although most commonly associated with 'slapped cheek syndrome' (Fifth disease), maternal infection during the first 20 weeks of pregnancy can result in increased fetal loss, fetal anaemia and subsequent cardiac failure (hydrops fetalis) (Miller *et al.*, 1998). This can be reversed by intrauterine blood transfusion. Parvovirus is transmitted via contact with infected respiratory secretions and is probably most communicable before the onset of the rash. The incubation period is usually between 4 and 20 days. Prevention and control relies on patient information to avoid exposure and early reporting in the event of contact with an exanthematous rash (see Health Protection Agency [HPA] guidelines; Morgan-Capner and Crowcroft, 2002).

Similarly, there is no recommendation for toxoplasmosis screening in pregnancy (NICE, 2003). Prevention and control relies on general advice to pregnant women concerning the need to avoid cleaning cat litter trays, wearing gloves for gardening and washing hands thoroughly after handling raw meat.

In the non-immune patient, chickenpox in pregnancy may increase the risk for congenital varicella syndrome by 0.5 to 1.5 per cent above the baseline risk for major malformation (Tan and Koren, 2006). Third-trimester infection may lead to maternal pneumonia, which can be life threatening if not treated appropriately.

Screening for varicella-zoster virus (VZV) IgG antibody is not recommended at antenatal booking, since about 95 per cent of adults patients born in the UK are immune to chickenpox. However, all laboratory sera should be stored for up to 2 years. Hence, in the event of exposure to VZV in pregnancy, the patient's stored antenatal blood should be tested for VZV antibody if there is not a positive history of chickenpox. VZV immunoglobulin (VZIG) is recommended for all VZV antibody-negative contacts exposed at any stage of pregnancy providing VZIG can be given within 10 days from contact. VZIG should be re-administered if a second exposure occurs after a further 3 weeks (Salisbury *et al.*, 2006; HPA, 2006).

Up to 30 per cent of pregnant women are colonized with Group B streptococcus (GBS) in the vagina and/or rectum. As early-onset GBS disease is the commonest cause for severe infection in newborn infants in developed countries, the Royal College of Obstetricians (RCOG, 2003) has published specific guidelines on the prevention of GBS. These guidelines provide a clinical risk-based approach to prevention and do not recommend routine screening for antenatal GBS carriage.

Similarly, screening for listeriosis is not recommended (NICE, 2003). General advice for prevention includes eating meats and dairy products only when properly cooked, avoiding non-pasteurized dairy products and washing vegetables thoroughly.

With a fall in the use of the combined vaccine for measles, mumps and rubella (MMR), reported cases of measles and mumps are on the increase. There remains no recommendation for routine antenatal measles immunity screening in pregnancy. However, human normal immunoglobulin (HNIG) should be considered for pregnant women if they have been in contact with a confirmed case or if their contact is associated with a local outbreak (HPA, 2006). HNIG may attenuate the infection in the mother but there is no evidence that it prevents fetal loss. If possible, an assessment of antibody status should be undertaken before HNIG is administered. HNIG is not recommended for post-exposure protection to mumps, since there is no evidence that it is effective.

Urinary tract infection in pregnancy increases the risk of premature delivery and post-partum infection. Hence, all pregnant women should be screened for asymptomatic bacteruria early in pregnancy (NICE, 2003).

Although syphilis is a rare condition, screening for this disease continues to be offered in early pregnancy owing to the benefits of treatment for both the mother and fetus (NICE, 2003).

Staff screening

In obstetrics, protection of healthcare workers (HCWs) against rubella and measles is especially important in the context of their ability to transmit these infections to pregnant patients. Satisfactory evidence of protection includes documentation of having received two doses of MMR vaccine or a positive antibody test for measles and rubella. Staff born before 1970 are likely to have acquired natural immunity. MMR vaccine should be offered to such individuals on request or if they are considered to be of high risk of exposure (Salisbury *et al.*, 2006).

Hepatitis B virus immunization and screening for bloodborne viruses in staff undergoing exposure-prone procedures has been dealt with in Chapter 9. It is particularly important that HCWs in obstetrics know their responsiveness to HBV vaccination, as this is a high-risk specialty for BBV cross-infection. At least one occupational exposure with blood or amniotic fluid is thought to occur in about 39 per cent of vaginal deliveries and in 50 per cent of caesarean sections (Popejoy and Fry, 1991; Panillo *et al.*, 1992). Midwives sustain the greatest number of exposures, followed by obstetricians.

In view of the potentially devastating consequences of VZV infection in pregnancy, it is important to ensure that HCWs have either documented evidence of a past history of chickenpox/shingles, immunity or are offered varicella vaccination (Varivax or Varilrix; Breuer, 2005). Although 95 per cent of adult patients born in the UK and hospital staff are immune to chickenpox, only 75–85 per cent of adults who have grown up in tropical countries such as the Philippines, the Indian subcontinent and the West Indies are immune. Hospitals with greater numbers of staff (or patients) from these areas are at increased risk of nosocomial VZV outbreaks. HCWs with a definite history of VZV infection can be considered immune, otherwise antibody testing is recommended. As a history of chickenpox is a less reliable predictor of immunity in individuals born and raised overseas, routine immunity testing should be considered in this group. Varicella vaccine should be offered to non-immune HCWs. Though a two-dose vaccination schedule in adults provides about 75 per cent protection, post-vaccination serology testing is not recommended unless HCWs are dealing with highly vulnerable patients (e.g. neonatal intensive care units; Salisbury *et al.*, 2006). Occupational health departments should seek advice for HCWs who fail to seroconvert (see HPA guidance). Vaccinated HCWs, or those with a definite history of VZV infection, with a significant exposure to VZV should be considered protected and allowed to continue working. However, they should be advised to report to their occupational health department if they develop fever or rash. Unvaccinated HCWs without a definite history of VZV infection and a significant exposure to VZV should be either excluded from contact with high-risk patients (e.g. maternity or neonatal units) from 8 to 21 days after exposure or be advised to report to their occupational health department before having patient contact, if they feel unwell or develop a fever or rash (Salisbury *et al.*, 2006).

Occupational health screening policies for maternity units should follow national guidelines on MRSA (Coia *et al.*, 2006) and tuberculosis control (National Collaborating Centre for Chronic Conditions, 2006). They should also emphasize the importance of early HCW self-reporting if herpetic whitlow or septic lesions are suspected, to minimize herpes simplex virus (HSV) and Group A streptococcus (GAS) transmission.

Maternity unit design

The labour ward is an archetypal 'high-risk area', where high-level emergency care may be needed at any time of the day or night throughout the year. Obstetric units can vary greatly in design, ranging from birthing centres for low-risk deliveries to standard labour and delivery units, including operating theatres for caesarean sections. However, basic design needs will be similar to other clinical areas, namely conveniently placed alcohol hand rubs, sinks for hand disinfection, easily cleaned surfaces and suitable isolation facilities for patients with airborne infectious diseases (e.g. chickenpox or tuberculosis).

The British Association of Perinatal Medicine (BAPM, 1998) has published obstetric standards for the provision of perinatal care. Guidance on staffing, facilities and organization for obstetric units is divided into three levels of care:

- Level 1 for general practitioner or midwifery units within or adjacent to a consultant obstetric unit;
- Level 2 for district general hospitals with a short-term intensive care capability; and
- Level 3 for intensive care tertiary referral units.

Detailed planning advice on maternity departments is also available from Health Building Note 21 prepared by NHS Estates (1996). The American College of Obstetricians and Gynaecologists (2002) has also outlined basic standards for obstetric facilities that may be applicable to UK units.

The BAPM has also produced guidance on neonatal unit (NNU) design and emphasizes the importance of building new NNUs as close as possible to the labour suite (Laing *et al.*, 2004). Ideally the NNU should be immediately adjacent to the labour suite and on the same floor. Handwashing sinks should be large enough to avoid splashing, with one large sink for every three infants in the unit. Incubators should never be more than 6 m away from a hand washbasin. The NNU should be air conditioned throughout with a minimum of six air changes per hour plus at least 90 per cent efficient filtration of ventilation air. Temperature and humidity control is also of vital importance (air temperature between 22 and 26°C, relative humidity 30–60 per cent). If it is planned to clean all NNU equipment outside the NNU, then a small equipment store area is adequate. However, if cleaning of equipment is 'in house', then the need for adequate space should be carefully addressed. A clean utility area of at least 20 m² should be included in the NNU design to ensure that clean materials do not pass through the dirty utility area. The dirty utility area is needed for cleaning soiled items such as cots, incubators, humidifiers and basins. This room should have a negative air pressure facility. A cleaner's room of 10 m² is considered suitable for domestic staff to store their cleaning equipment. Every NNU should have a milk kitchen for refrigeration and freezing of expressed breast milk. Where this is strongly encouraged, four refrigerators and two large freezers are essential. A designated milk expression room of at least 8 m^2 is also required for mothers.

Birth

General considerations

Pregnant women should be at low risk of nosocomial infection owing to their short hospital stay and by minimizing the use of invasive devices and procedures. Frequent vaginal examinations, rectal examinations and intrauterine monitoring and caesarean section increase the risk of chorioamnionitis or post-partum endometrial infection. The risk of urinary tract infection will be increased by caesarean section, forceps or vacuum extraction, epidural anaesthesia and urinary catheterization. The use of fetal scalp electrodes should be kept to the minimum and should be avoided in women with HSV, HBV or HIV infection. Shaving increases the risk of wound infection and should be avoided. For instance, shaving of perineal hair does not reduce rates of infection post episiotomy. Antibiotic use needs to be judicious and should focus on the prevention/treatment of GBS infection, wound infection, post-caesarean section, endometritis, chorioamnionitis and urinary tract infection. Single-dose antibiotic prophylaxis is recommended for caesarean section surgery following clamping of the umbilical cord (NICE, 2004). Such issues highlight the importance of establishing clear infection control policies in obstetric units, staff training, strict adherence to aseptic techniques and operator skills.

Universal infection control precautions

Semmelweis' original observations on the value of good handwashing with an antibacterial agent have remained the cornerstone of both good obstetric and general infection control practice. The universal application of good hand hygiene practice is therefore of critical importance. Obstetric procedures result in a high risk of exposure to the obstetric team of blood and body fluids during deliveries. A patient may have BBV disease at the time of delivery even if antenatal screening during the first trimester was undertaken. Hence appropriate protective equipment should always be worn, including gloves, long-sleeved impervious gowns, shoe covers, surgical masks and eye protection. Obstetricians should also be aware of glove perforation which occurs commonly and is often unrecognized (Serrano et al., 1991).

Other key universal infection control precautions for staff include the routine covering of cuts and abrasions with an occlusive waterproof dressing, safe handling and disposal of sharps, management of blood and body-fluid spillages, segregation of contaminated linen, and the decontamination of reusable devices and equipment by a sterile services department.

The HIV-positive patient

Vertical transmission of HIV can be reduced to <2 per cent by a combination of high uptake of antenatal HIV screening, provision of antiretroviral therapy to mothers from early in the second trimester, delivery of the baby electively by planned caesarean section or safe vaginal delivery, administration of anti-retroviral therapy during delivery (if the mother is not optimally suppressed), antiretroviral prophylaxis to the baby and avoidance of breast feeding. Evidence for these interventions is available from the British HIV Association (2005) guidelines on HIV in pregnancy.

Prevention of mother-to-child transmission of maternal infections by caesarean section

NICE guidelines were published on this issue in 2004. Apart from HIV infection, women with primary genital HSV infection occurring in the third trimester should be offered planned caesarean section. Mother-to-child transmission of HBV can be reduced if the baby receives immunoglobulin and vaccination as appropriate, and caesarean section is not usually indicated. Also caesarean section has not been shown to reduce the risk of vertical transmission of HCV.

Birthing pools

Water birth is popular, with more than half of all NHS obstetric units having installed a birthing pool. Although there is a lack of prospective studies concerning maternal or neonatal outcomes in similar groups of women delivering in water or conventionally, water birth is not considered to be more risky than conventional labour (Nikodem, 1998; Gilbert and Tookey, 1999).

Pool design and maintenance are essential elements in minimizing infection risks. Problems have been reported in pools with combined entry/exit hoses, which are not plumbed in and allow for stagnant water (George and Hobbs, 1990). Infection control policies should be available and focus on legionella precautions, decontamination after use (preferably use of detergent and then a chlorine-releasing disinfectant), HBV vaccination of staff and universal infection control precautions with the provision of personal protective equipment to minimize mucous membrane contamination and post-natal surveillance (Kingsley et al., 1999).

Post-birth care

Mothers

Good perineal surgical site and breast care are essential in the post-partum period for the prevention of wound infections and mastitis. Surgical site infection (SSI) following caesarean section is the second most common infectious complication after urinary tract infection in obstetrics. SSI can occur in up to 11 per cent of caesarean sections, including incision and organ space infections, and are associated with significant morbidity and socio-economic consequences (Johnson *et al.*, 2006). Surveillance programmes, which provide surgeon-specific SSI rates, have been shown to be effective in reducing infection rates. Methodology can be problematic as many SSIs may only be detected post discharge, reflecting the short length of stay associated with this procedure.

Post-partum endometritis from *Streptococcus pyogenes* has been considered the classic obstetric infection but with good infection control practices is now uncommon. Such infections may occur in previously colonized mothers or may be acquired by cross-infection from HCWs, other patients or colonized infants. If *S. pyogenes* infection is diagnosed, the patient should be isolated because of the risk of airborne spread, and early epidemiological investigation should be undertaken by the infection control team. Outbreaks of *Staphylococcus aureus* infections, in particular MRSA, occasionally occur and should be managed with standard outbreak control measures.

Transmission of infection through breast milk can occur in HIV and human T-lymphocytic virus type I and II seropositive mothers. Breast feeding should therefore be avoided. There are no such contraindications concerning CMV, HBV, HCV or HSV infection (Brady, 2006). However, babies of HBV carriers should be offered vaccination (± immunoglobulin). Mothers should refrain from breast feeding until any herpetic breast lesions have resolved.

Baby

Prevention and control of neonatal infection are discussed earlier in this chapter (p. 333).

GYNAECOLOGY

In the absence of specific infection control guidelines for gynaecology, prevention and control of infection should follow the key principles outlined in earlier chapters. For women requiring induced abortion, UK guidelines recommend routine antibiotic prophylaxis or genital tract screening and treatment of positive cases to avoid post-abortion infection morbidity with *Chlamydia trachomatis* following instrumentation (RCOG, 2004).

Endoscopy in gynaecology (colposcopy, hysteroscopy, laparoscopy and cystoscopy) is a rapidly expanding service. Existing guidelines for the decontamination of medical devices, from the Medicines and Healthcare Products Regulatory agency, should be followed (Medical Devices Agency, 2002; Medicines and Healthcare Products Regulatory Agency, 2004). Decontamination of transvaginal probes widely used in the investigation of infertility remains problematic. Although disposable probe covers are used during an examination, the probe then should be cleaned and disinfected after use. However, specific guidance on the choice of disinfectant used should be sought from the specific probe manufacturer.

Transplants

Manjusha Narayanan and Kate Gould

Transplantation involves the transfer of tissues, cells or organs from an individual and grafting into another area of the same individual or in another individual. All such procedures carry risk of infection, but those pertaining to the use of immunosuppression, broadly divided into solid organ transplants (SOTs) and haematopoietic stem cell transplants (HSCTs), will be discussed in this section.

SOLID ORGAN TRANSPLANTS

Between 2005 and 2006, 2794 patients received organs for transplantation in the UK, 2195 from brainstem dead or non-heart-beating donors, and 599 from a living (related or non-related) donor (Transplant activity in the UK, 2005–6). Organ transplantation is usually the last resort for patients with end-stage organ failure.

The use of immunosuppressive agents in transplant patients inhibits the immune system from rejecting the new organ and therefore plays a significant role in improving patient survival. Unfortunately these agents also complicate the infectious disease process by inhibiting inflammatory responses to microbial invasion, and make the recipient more prone to infections.

The level and duration of immunosuppression required is dependent on the type of organ transplanted. The choice and dose of immunosuppressive agent depends on whether it is being given for potent 'induction' therapy in the immediate peri-transplant period, when the risk of rejection is highest, or for long-life 'maintenance' therapy, usually with reduced doses of drugs. In the event of an episode of rejection, more potent immunosuppressants are used, thereby greatly increasing the risk of infection. Most rejection episodes occur in the first 3 months after transplantation.

Modern immunosuppressive therapy follows a concept of 'steroid-sparing' therapy with various combinations of drugs, such as azathioprine, mycophenolate mofetil, the calcineuron inhibitors (ciclosporin and tacrolimus), rapamycin (sirolimus), and polyclonal and monoclonal antilymphocyte antibodies to achieve a balanced state of immunosuppression.

HAEMATOPOIETIC STEM CELL TRANSPLANTS

Haematopoietic stem cell transplant is indicated to treat haematological malignancies, such as chronic myeloid leukaemia, acute leukaemia, myelodysplasia, non-Hodgkin's lymphoma, Hodgkin's disease, multiple myeloma and some high-risk solid tumours, such as Ewing's sarcoma. Non-malignant conditions where HSCT is indicated arise out of bone marrow failure, such as aplastic anaemia, haemoglobinopathies and metabolic storage disorders. Haematopoietic stem cells for transplant are sourced from bone marrow or peripheral blood stem cells mobilized from bone marrow, using granulocyte colony-stimulating factor or stem cells derived from umbilical cord. Stem cells were obtained from bone marrow by direct puncture, but more recently, the harvesting of cells from other sources has led to the use of the term 'haematopoietic stem cell transplant'. The donor may be autologous (self) or allogeneic: identical twin, related and human leukocyte antigen (HLA) matched, related but HLA mismatched, or unrelated – HLA matched or mismatched. Umbilical cord blood can also be used for stem cell transplants (Cant *et al.*, 2007).

The patient's own marrow is ablated by chemotherapy, or a combination of chemotherapy and total body irradiation prior to transplant. Cryopreserved harvested cells from donor are infused into the patient. The intensity of conditioning used depends on the underlying disorder and is considered on an individual basis. The immunosuppressive effects of chemotherapy and radiotherapy reduces the risk of graft rejection and graft versus host disease (GVHD). Additional immunosuppression may be required if alternative donors are used and this is provided by serotherapy in the form of antithymocyte globulin (polyclonal antibody) directed against T lymphocytes or Alemtuzumab (family of monoclonal antibodies) directed against B and T lymphocytes and monocytes.

Post-HSCT immunosuppression is provided by a combination of different drugs, such as cyclosporine, methotrexate, tacrolimus (FK 506), corticosteroids and mycophenolate mofetil. The resulting immunosuppression can make way for opportunistic bacterial, fungal, viral or parasitic infections.

SPECIAL PROBLEMS

Infection-related problems in transplant recipients can be exacerbated by their underlying morbidity, and are related to disease management, for example hospitalization for the transplant procedure, related intensive care interventions and immunosuppression. Community-acquired infections should also be considered following discharge from hospital.

The recognition and diagnosis of infection in this group of patients is a challenge as clinical symptoms and signs may be subtle or modified compared with a non-transplant patient. Treatment strategies may be delayed as a result thereby compromising survival outcomes. It is therefore imperative to implement optimum measures to prevent infections and have the best possible multi-disciplinary approach to recognize and treat infections as early as possible. The measures taken by transplant centres to prevent nosocomial infections will vary according to availability of resources and local risk assessment (Murphy and Gould, 1999).

DESIGN OF UNITS

There are no specifications available for structural designs for SOT or HSCT units. Designing of units is therefore based on a combination of general principles of hospital infection control (room ventilation, construction and renovation, isolation and barrier precautions), the degree of immunosuppression (HSCT patients are generally more immunosuppressed than SOT patients, and allogeneic HSCT patients are more susceptible to infections than autologous HSCT patients) and the resources available locally. No two centres are environmentally identical and local experiences in management of these patients will have a bearing on the working of the units. Guidelines for the prevention of opportunistic infections in HSCT (Dykewicz and Kaplan, 2000) are detailed and can be adapted to local needs in conjunction with isolation facilities conforming to Department of Health standards (HBN4; NHS Estates, 2005a).

Haematopoietic stem cell transplants patients should be nursed in single rooms (with or without anterooms) at positive pressure, when compared with any adjoining lobby/hallway, toilets or anterooms. They should have clean environments, be clutter free and have the highest hygiene standards. The use of high-efficiency particulate air (HEPA) filters and air change of >12/h is essential for allogeneic HSCT and may be desirable for autologous HSCT if they have prolonged neutropenia. The use of laminar air flow (LAF) is optional as the value of routine LAF rooms for all HSCT recipients is doubtful. LAF has been demonstrated to protect patients from aspergillosis outbreak during hospital construction. Provision of facilities (e.g. correct placement of hand washbasins, hand gels or toilets for visitors) while designing or renovating should involve dialogue between the transplant team, infection control team, and the representative of estates and facilities department.

However, HEPA filtration alone is not a foolproof method of infection prevention in HSCT units. In a survey report of 23 outbreaks of infectious diseases in stem cell transplant units (13 centres), eight out of eight viral, four out of ten bacterial and three out of five fungal outbreaks occurred in HEPA-filtered rooms. Cross-infection was a major factor (except in fungal outbreak) and could have been prevented by simple measures like rapid exclusion of infected staff with viral upper respiratory tract infections and scrupulous handwashing or isolation of patients infected with VRE (McCann et al., 2004).

Solid organ transplant units have different approaches towards post-transplant care. Protective isolation offered no benefit over standard care in protecting cardiac allograft patients from infections and was discontinued as a routine in some units (Walsh et al., 1989). The SOT patient (usually heart, lung, liver) will require ICU support in single rooms post transplant before moving to specialty wards. It is desirable to have ICU services within a hospital where HSCT is performed and, if possible, should also include facilities for critical care outreach services. A team of specialist nurses, trained specifically in the management of SOT or HSCT specific to adult and paediatric group of patients, is essential.

SCREENING

It is immensely useful for transplant centres to have protocols in place to screen for infections prior to the transplant procedure and for close environmental and clinical surveillance following transplant for early detection and management of infections. Susceptibility of a transplant patient to infection largely depends on exposure to pathogens exogenously (which can be primary or secondary), or acquired in the donated organ or tissue.

Solid organ transplantation

The advantage of pre-transplantation screening for infections is the ability to exclude a donor or to tailor specific antimicrobial therapy following transplantation. The rates and types of infectious complications vary among different transplant centres around the world, and largely reflect the epidemiology of infectious agents in different geographic regions. For example, tuberculosis can be a major problem with transplant patients in countries where it is endemic. Pre-transplant screening of donor and recipient for tuberculosis is therefore essential in this situation.

There is a wide variety of approaches to screen for infections and this is reflected in a survey of 147 renal transplant centres in the USA (Batiuk *et al.*, 2002). Uniform screening for donors and recipients (>95 per cent) was carried out for CMV and HIV, and 91 per cent for syphilis in donors and 84 per cent in recipients. Screening for other agents was variable, e.g. varicella-zoster (donor 41 per cent, recipient 64 per cent). There was no correlation between geographical location and screening for histoplasmosis and coccidioidomycosis.

Whereas donors with active HBV or HIV infection are not used, the use of organs from HCV-seropositive donors is controversial and depends on local policies. Some centres transplant HCV-positive organs into patients who are already HCV positive.

Travel history is important to look for exposure to geographically limited endemic infections such as coccidioidomycosis (an endemic mycosis in the south-western USA and Mexico), other geographically restricted systemic mycoses, infections with *Strongyloides stercoralis* and malaria.

Recipients

For pre-transplant evaluation, in general, genitourinary tract infections, recurrent respiratory tract infections, sinusitis, active dental infections, skin and nail infections, diverticulitis and diarrhoeal disease should be diagnosed and treated in good time.

Viral infections play a significant role in increasing morbidity and mortality of transplant patients, with some variation in rates of infections depending on pathogen and the type of transplant. The herpes group of viruses – HSV, VZV, CMV, Epstein–Barr virus (EBV), human herpes virus (HHV 6 and 7) – are particularly important, as they can lie dormant in the patient's body or in the transplanted organ, and are reactivated on immunosuppression, augmentation or during GVHD. They are generally more difficult to diagnose and treat than bacterial infections and can themselves lead to further immunosuppression (particularly CMV), thereby increasing the patient's susceptibility to other infections.

In SOTs, CMV can be transmitted in the donor organ, whereas it is mainly a reactivation of latent infection in HSCTs. CMV viraemia can cause life-threatening pneumonitis and gastrointestinal symptoms, or organ-specific infection such as CMV hepatitis.

Serological screening is performed for antibodies to CMV, EBV, VZV, *Toxoplasma gondii*, hepatitis B and C, HIV 1 and 2, and *Aspergillus precipitins* for lung transplantation.

Donors

Pre-transplant evaluation for infections is necessary, as the risk of transmitting them to an immunosuppressed recipient in the transplanted organ is high, and can delay recovery by weeks. All donors should be serologically tested for HIV, hepatitis B and C, CMV, EBV, syphilis and *Toxoplasma gondii*.

Organ donors usually have had major trauma or intracranial haemorrhage, and may have been on ICUs for some time. They are usually intubated, ventilated and have intravascular access devices fitted, and are likely to be colonized or infected in various organ sites.

Appropriate specimens (e.g. blood culture, sputum or bronchoalveolar lavage as clinically indicated) should be sent for culture, and significant positive results should be relayed to the transplant centre via the transplant coordinator to guide peri-operative antibiotic therapy.

Haematopoietic stem cell transplants

Recipients

The following tests should be considered: serological tests for syphilis, toxoplasma, CMV, EBV, HIV 1 and 2, HSV, VZV, hepatitis A and C, and hepatitis B surface antigen. MRSA screen and glycopeptide-resistant enterococci/VRE screen may also be required according to local protocols. Mid-stream urine, stool cultures and screening for respiratory tract infections, including viral infections, should be taken if indicated by symptoms.

Donors

Screening for infectious diseases should be completed 30 days before the harvest of cells. It should include serological tests for syphilis and toxoplasma antibodies, and antiviral antibodies for CMV, EBV, HIV 1 and 2, human T-lymphocytic virus type I and II, HSV, VZV, measles, hepatitis A and C, and HBsAg.

For cord blood donation, serological tests are performed on the mother for syphilis, HIV 1 and 2, CMV antibodies and HBsAg. These tests are repeated 3–6 months after delivery.

CONTROL OF INFECTION

General aspects

The general principles of infection control such as handwashing, good aseptic care, standard and protective isolation, described in Chapter 13, must be applied. Certain additional precautions are given below.

Specific measures in solid organ transplants

It is essential that those involved in the care of transplant patients have a good understanding of infections, and the knowledge to prevent them. In one study from Stanford University Hospital, infection-related episodes occurred at a rate of 1.73/patient, and were the leading cause of late death more than 30 days and 1 year after transplantation surgery (Montoya *et al.*, 2001).

With improved immunosuppressive agents and prophylactic strategies, the overall incidence of infections after transplantation has decreased in recent years. Use of prophylaxis, such as trimethoprim–sulfamethoxazole has reduced the incidence of infection with *Pneumocystis jirovecii* (previously *P. carinii*), *Listeria* and *Nocardia*, and to a certain extent infections with susceptible bacteria causing urinary tract infections (UTIs). Similarly, use of antivirals and antifungals has reduced the incidence and severity of viral and fungal infections.

Care of post-SOT patients in ICUs may involve ventilatory support, intravascular devices such as central lines and pulmonary artery catheters for central venous pressure and pulmonary artery pressure, Swan–Ganz catheters for cardiac monitoring and arterial lines for monitoring of blood pressure, pacemakers for epicardial pacing in cardiac transplants, other intravenous lines for drugs and fluid replacements, and urinary catheters (Wade *et al.*, 2004).

Experience over the years has helped in formulation of a consistent timetable when different infections develop after transplantation (Patel and Paya, 1997; Fishman and Rubin, 1998). This timetable is divided into three segments: the first month, 1–6 months, and >6 months after transplantation.

In the early period, usually within the first month after surgery, infections with nosocomial bacterial pathogens and *Candida* are commonly seen, and do not differ greatly from infections seen postoperatively in other general surgical patients. Such infections include UTIs, surgical site wound infections, sepsis related to the use of intravascular devices and respiratory tract infections. Other infections in the early postoperative period may relate to a surgical procedure of a specific organ (e.g. sternotomy-associated mediastinitis in the thoracic organ recipients, infected perigraft haematomas and lymphocoeles in renal transplants, and hepatic abscess secondary to bile duct manipulations in liver transplantation).

In the period between the second and sixth month after transplant, viral infections usually predominate, and this may be in addition to infections from the early period in some patients. Viruses of the herpes group, particularly CMV, can be particularly problematic in SOT patients with their wide range of presentations and immunomodulating effect. Other opportunistic infections due to *Pneumocystis jirovecii*, *Nocardia*, *Listeria*, and reactivation of tuberculosis and fungal infections can be encountered.

After 6 months post transplant, most patients are at home and exposed to the same infections as other non-transplant patients in the general community. Some transplant patients on higher immunosuppression owing to chronic rejection, will be at additional risk and may not strictly fit into a 'timetabled' pattern of infections. In these, a higher degree of suspicion is necessary for early diagnosis and treatment (Gould, 1998).

Non-cytomegaloviral respiratory viral infections can be acquired from visitors or from healthcare workers or from other patients. In HSCT patients, both in adults and children, influenza A and B viruses, parainfluenza (serotype 3 is the most common) and respiratory syncytial virus are an important cause of nosocomial spread of community-acquired infections, which can be fatal if disease (pneumonia) occurs pre-engraftment. In one study, 23 per cent of adult lung transplant recipients had viruses other than CMV isolated (herpes, adenovirus and parainfluenza) at diagnostic bronchoscopy, which was associated with significant morbidity (Holt *et al.*, 1997).

Managing bilateral lung transplant patients (for chronic lung disease) can be very challenging, as they may be colonized pre-operatively with multi-resistant bacteria, or may be colonized and infected with nosocomial microbials if the post-transplant ICU or hospital stay is prolonged.

Some cystic fibrosis patients are colonized and infected with pathogens that are difficult to treat, such as *Burkholderia cepacia* complex, *Stenotrophomonas maltophilia*, *Alcaligenes xylosoxidans*, *Aspergillus* spp, non-tuberculous mycobacteria and respiratory viruses. Some genomovars of *B. cepacia* complex confer increased morbidity and mortality, and are more likely to cause cross-infection and outbreaks. This can therefore be a major problem in lung transplant patients and in outpatient clinics (Saiman and Siegel, 2004).

Infectious complications occur in 60–80 per cent of all liver transplant patients. UTIs are common and infections related to the surgical procedure, e.g. bile leaks or biliary strictures, can lead to formation of liver abscesses containing bacteria from the gut flora, such as anaerobes, coliforms and enterococci.

Infection with vancomycin resistant enterococcus has emerged in some transplant centres, with 1-year mortality as high as 82 per cent in the liver transplant population. Outbreaks of VRE may be associated with excessive and inappropriate use of vancomycin, thus infection with other microbial pathogens or biliary complications following liver transplant may trigger such use and therefore are risk factors for VRE infection. Cross-infection is also common if VRE infections are prevalent in units caring for transplant patients (Orloff *et al.*, 1999).

Many transplant centres use selective decontamination of the digestive tract with a combination of antibacterial and antifungal agents to prevent colonization of the oral cavity and gastrointestinal tract, and minimize risk of nosocomial infections after liver transplantation. Use of surveillance cultures and targeted infection control interventions has proved to be effective in reducing new acquisition and mortality with *Staphylococcus aureus* infections (bacteraemia and deep seated) in liver transplant recipients (Singh *et al.*, 2006). A locally agreed peri-operative surgical antibiotic prophylaxis should be used based on the local antibiotic susceptibility pattern of bacteria and local preference of antibiotics.

Nosocomial transmission of legionnaire's disease in HSCT and heart transplant patients has been reported. Hot water sources for non-pneumophilia *Legionella* species (e.g. *L. cincinnatenensis* and *L. micdadei*) were responsible for an outbreak in renal and cardiac transplant patients (Kool *et al.*, 1998; Knirsch *et al.*, 2000). Routine surveillance and use of specialist anti-*Legionella* water systems, such as chlorination, etc., may be indicated in some units. Similarly, units with a high prevalence of nosocomial aspergillosis or those close to building work may opt for regular surveillance with or without the use of prophylactic antifungal therapy. Outbreaks of infections caused by HBV have been described in cardiac transplant recipients caused by inadequate decontamination of biopsy forceps (Drescher *et al.*, 1994).

It is important to ensure that patients are up to date on all routine immunizations and potential transplant recipients receive tetanus–diphtheria updates, and pneumococcal, hepatitis A and B, and influenza vaccinations.

Specific measures in haematopoietic stem cell transplants

Recipients of HSCTs experience certain infections at different times after transplant. Immune-system recovery for HSCT recipients takes place in three phases beginning at day 0, the day of transplant: phase I, the pre-engraftment phase (<30 days after HSCT); phase II, the post-engraftment phase (30–100 days after HSCT); and phase III, the last phase (>100 days after HSCT). Prevention strategies should be based on these three phases and the following information.

Pre-transplant

Prevention and prompt treatment of infections based on local protocols are advocated (see earlier). CMV-seronegative (or unknown status) patients awaiting HSCT should be given CMV-seronegative or white-cell-depleted blood products to prevent CMV infections in their immunosuppressed state.

Post transplant

Prevention of severe oral mucositis following chemotherapy/radiation is essential to avoid superadded infection with *Candida* and HSV. Use of antifungals (azoles) and antivirals (acyclovir) prophylaxis is routinely recommended. Prompt treatment of typhilitis (neutropenic enterocolitis) due to bacterial or fungal infection of damaged intestinal mucosa is indicated after appropriate cultures of stool and blood are sent to the laboratory.

PATIENT EDUCATION

The risk of acquired infection remains following the patient's discharge from hospital after transplantation. Most centres have a comprehensive teaching package, which includes specific reference to infection risks. These patients may be re-admitted to non-specialist wards in other healthcare facilities. In such circumstances, protective isolation of the patient should be necessary only if the transplant recipient becomes neutropenic.

Operating theatres
Eric W Taylor and Peter Hoffman

THE DESIGN PROCESS

The role of the Infection Control Team

It is recommended that the Infection Control Team should take a significant role in the design of operating theatres. As stated in Department of Health guidance Health Building Note 26 (NHS Estates, 2004):

> Infection control teams should be consulted from the outset of any new-build or renovation project and should remain integral planning team members throughout. In a new-build project this means that they should be members of the team that develop the business case from its inception.

This involvement at an early stage can prevent errors occurring in the planning stage, after which they maybe costly, inconvenient or impossible to rectify.

Location within the hospital

Although the precise location has little or no relevance with regard to infection control, theatres should be located in a single unit in a hospital to enable economic use of resources and have good access from those parts of the hospital functionally related to them (e.g. SSD, stores, critical care, etc.).

Design

The design of a new theatre should allow effective working and flow though the department (NHS Estates, 2004). Matters of infection control significance are detailed as follows.

• The design should encourage staff to move around the department by the corridors and only to access theatres and other clean areas when this is necessary.
• The use of a 'dirty' corridor for disposal of waste packed in impervious bags and used instruments is unnecessary. These items should not contribute to environmental contamination and can be removed via the 'clean' corridor. The use of a separate 'service corridor' by non-theatre staff is not an infection control issue.
• Separate scrub rooms are unnecessary, but a scrubbing area in theatre should be sited so that exposed instruments are not splashed.
• There should be sufficient storage to accommodate all sterile and clean items, as well as all equipment used. Storage is one of the first areas to be scaled-down if overall reductions are required during the design process. However, this does not mean that fewer items will need storage, just that they will be stored in inappropriate areas.
• Surfaces should be easily cleanable, both in the materials used and the style of construction (e.g. coving between floors and walls in the theatre). There is no value currently perceived for 'antibacterial' surfaces in the theatre environment.

VENTILATION

Conventionally ventilated operating theatres

The ventilation of operating theatres has two main infection control functions:

• to prevent entry of contaminated air from areas around the theatre;
• to dilute airborne contamination generated inside the theatre and preparation room.

Air originating in areas containing infected and colonized patients, particularly wards, can carry pathogens. To exclude them from sensitive areas of the operating suite, air is supplied in excess to these areas such that it flows out to surrounding areas, thus preventing any inward flow of contaminated air. This ventilation is referred to as 'positive pressure'. Such pressure can be measured in pascals, but robust flow in the desired direction is more important than its precise value. Alteration of a theatre's ventilation such that air flowed outwards from it, rather than in from contaminated areas, has been associated with a reduction in infection of clean wounds from nearly 9 per cent to 1 per cent (Ellis et al., 1956). Similarly, in the area of the operating suite that may itself generate airborne contamination (the dirty utility or 'sluice'), air is mechanically extracted so as to put the room under negative pressure such that all airflow to this area is inward, preventing escape of potentially contaminated air to surrounding clean areas of the theatre suite.

The main source of airborne contamination in the operating theatre is contaminated particles dispersed from the skin of those present. Such dispersal will increase with the number of people present and the amount of movement (i.e. the patient disperses very little). This contamination, present as microcolonies on skin scales or 'squames' (usually 5–15 µm in size) can either settle in a wound or on exposed instruments that will subsequently be used in the wound; this latter route usually provides the major route of wound contamination by airborne bacteria (Whyte et al., 1982). This makes cleanliness in preparation rooms used for laying-up instruments at least as important as in operating theatres. The contamination is removed by supplying large amounts of clean air to the most sensitive areas of the suite (theatre and preparation room) and encouraging it to flow into surrounding areas, taking its entrained contamination with it. The air supplied to a new operating theatre should equate to 25 air changes per hour (i.e. air equivalent to 25 times the volume of the theatre should be supplied every hour) when it first comes into service, but should be at least around 20 air changes per hour in any older or pre-existing theatre. The air supplied to preparation rooms used for lay-up of surgical instruments should be changed at least 25 times per hour and preferably higher.

The air change rate is derived from the rate of air supply divided by the room volume (e.g. a room of $50\,m^3$ supplied with air at $200\,m^3/h$ has an air-change rate of $200 \div 50 = 4$ air changes per hour). The clean air should be supplied via filters installed in the air-handling unit. Experience has shown that the use of high efficiency particulate air (HEPA) filters is unnecessary and expensive, both to install and maintain. Conventional filters of grades F (or 'EU') 7 are adequate.

For economic reasons, operating suites can be ventilated at a reduced rate ('setback'), or the ventilation turned off, when not in use. The ventilation status should be clearly indicated in the theatre. It is not unusual for the setback or off status to be controlled by a timer but, in case of extended operating lists or faulty timers, there should be an override linked either to a movement sensor or the operating light. Normal ventilation should be resumed 15 minutes before use from setback (Hoffman *et al.*, 2002). One hour of full ventilation before use has been recommended, if the ventilation was turned completely off (Clarke *et al.*, 1985), but this allowed a very generous safety margin and 30 minutes should be adequate.

Ultraclean ventilated theatres

In ultraclean ventilated (UCV) theatres, sometimes referred to as 'laminar flow' theatres, highly filtered air descends in an organized flow from a canopy in the theatre ceiling over the centre of the theatre. This unidirectional downward flow rapidly removes contamination generated by the surgical team working within this area and resists ingress of contamination from outside, resulting in very low bacterial counts in this area. UVC theatres are commonly used for orthopaedic prosthetic surgery where, because of the amount of non-self-material implanted, the wounds are unusually susceptible to infection and the consequences of wound infection are substantial.

Other surgical facilities

Treatment rooms have no special ventilation but should have readily cleanable surfaces and good handwashing facilities. Rooms for interventional radiology (cardiac catheterization 'laboratories', etc.) are essentially facilities for surgery, and should be equipped and ventilated as operating theatres.

Commissioning and monitoring

As well as being involved in operating theatre design, the Infection Control Team should be part of the commissioning process and should be kept informed about routine monitoring. *Commissioning* (sometimes called 'validation') is a process that assesses a facility has been supplied and functions as required, and *monitoring* (sometimes called 'verification') is the ongoing assessment that the facility continues to function within acceptable limits. Infection control aspects of commissioning both conventionally ventilated and UCV operating theatres have been described fully elsewhere (Holton and Ridgway, 1993; Hoffman *et al.*, 2002).

For conventional theatres, infection control commissioning should involve an assessment of the air supply in terms of air-change rates (using data supplied by the commissioning engineers), ensuring that there are clear indications in the theatre of ventilation functioning correctly and of setback (reduced levels of flow when the theatres is not in use) status; smoke tracing should show turbulent flow in all areas of the theatre and air flowing robustly from the theatre into all surrounding areas except the preparation room where air should flow into the theatre, and the theatre should be free from obvious defects. Current guidance (HTM 03-01, Part A; Department of Health, 2007a) is that there should be ventilation that gives 25 air changes per hour in newly built theatres or in older theatres undergoing a major refurbishment.

Microbiological sampling of air supplied to the theatre, usually established by sampling the air in a clean, unoccupied theatre, should show 10 colony forming units per cubic metre (cfu/m^3) or less. Guidance on sampling methods is in Hoffman *et al.* (2002).

For UCV theatres, there should be no obvious defects and clear indication of UCV ventilation status (full or setback), and the commissioning engineers should supply data showing the unit is functioning adequately. This involves downward air-velocity measurements at multiple points under the UCV canopy, particle challenging of the filters in the canopy to show they prevent passage of all particles and showing absence of ingress into the area under the canopy from the theatre periphery. Air movement between rooms in a UCV suite is unimportant but, if air flows from the preparation room into the theatre, it should not interfere with the UCV flow. There is no requirement for microbiological sampling of the air entering an ultraclean theatre.

The routine monitoring or verification of operating theatre ventilation is a matter of periodic engineering assessments: inspection every 3 months and verification annually (HTM 03-01, Part B; Department of Health, 2007b). There is no requirement for direct microbiological input. However, the Infection Control Team should be involved if defects are found that could increase the transmission of infection. The ventilation should give at least 75 per cent of the design value (i.e. that given on initial commissioning). For theatres designed to have 25 air changes per hour (these would normally be fairly new theatres); this equates to around 19 air changes per hour. For older theatres built with lower air-change rates, a similar minimal flow rate (around 20 air changes per hour), should be present. If microbiological air sampling is carried out in a working operating theatre, there should be < 180 cfu/m^3 in a conventional theatre (anywhere in the room) and < 10 cfu/m^3 in an ultraclean theatre (within 300 mm of the wound). Such sampling can be useful as an educational tool to demonstrate the effects of poor theatre discipline, but is not normally performed otherwise.

THE OPERATING SUITE AND EQUIPMENT

Cleaning

Items in contact with the intact skin of a patient (supports, pulse oximeters, etc.) should be cleaned between patients, followed by disinfection if a patient is known or suspected to be infected or colonized with infectious micro-organisms. The more remote inanimate environment of a theatre suite is not closely concerned with infection control. Floors should be cleaned with detergent after each session. There is no point in attempts to protect the theatre floor by use of sticky mats by the entrance; the floor is of minimal relevance and such mats soon become overloaded.

Spills of blood or body fluid should be cleared immediately (see Chapter 6). The tradition of wall washing once or twice a year is for aesthetic reasons and not infection control.

Theatre equipment

Equipment used in theatres should be cleaned, disinfected or sterilized according to the risk it poses (see Chapter 6). If contamination can be prevented, for example, by use of filters in anaesthetic machine tubing (Rathgeber *et al.*, 1997) or between suction collection bottle and vacuum source, this greatly reduces the need for difficult decontamination. Laryngoscope blades should be reprocessed via a sterile supply department (SSD). Laryngoscope handles also acquire patient-derived contamination, both as micro-organisms and blood (Ballin *et al.*, 1999); these can either be reprocessed via the SSD or receive a local thorough clean followed by an alcohol wipe. Alternatively, single use may be used.

'Dirty' or infectious cases

If the air-change rate is adequate (see earlier), any airborne contaminants will be effectively removed in the time between cases. If extra time is needed to disinfect items that have been in contact with the patient (see earlier), then an infectious patient could be last on the list. Similarly, assuming good theatre discipline, there is no reason why different surgical specialties should not have sequential use of the same theatre. It is important that infection control precautions should also apply to the recovery area.

Theatre staff

The nursing, medical and support staff in the operating theatre provide the greatest source of airborne and other forms of exogenous bacterial contamination. Dispersal of skin particles (or 'squames') carrying bacteria into the atmosphere is inevitable and control of this form of wound contamination is the principal benefit of theatre ventilation. It has been traditional for all members of staff entering the operating theatre complex to change into freshly laundered theatre suits and special theatre footwear. It should have low linting properties, be antistatic and cost effective. Some theatre clothing claims to reduce the release of the wearer's skin particles into the theatre environment by means of fine-mesh fabrics that 'filter out' such particles. If this claim is to be effective, then the neck, wrists, waist and ankles of such clothing must be elasticized so as to prevent unfiltered release.

Headgear

It is traditional, but probably unnecessary, for most members of the operating theatre staff to wear headgear. There is little evidence that wearing headgear reduces bacterial contamination in the operating theatre (Humphreys *et al.*, 1991b). The scrub team should wear disposable hats that enclose all loose hair.

Masks

Facemasks were introduced by Mikulicz in Breslau in 1897 as a means of preventing droplets from the nose and mouth of the operating team being shed into the patients wound. They are now commonly worn by all operating theatre staff, and often by ward staff for routine wound dressings, midwives for delivery, etc. There is no study to show that wearing facemasks reduces the incidence of infection, and the principal benefit from their use is in preventing blood droplets from the patient entering the mouth and nostrils of the operating team. In a study of 3088 operations in which the operating team were masked for 1537 operations and wore no mask for 1551 operations, Tunevall (1991) reported that infection occurred after 4.7 per cent of the operations where the team were masked and 3.5 per cent of the operations in which the team wore no mask. There was no difference on the species of organisms isolated from infections that did occur. While there is no evidence on which to base the statement, it would seem sensible for bearded members of the scrub team to be masked with their beard fully enclosed within the mask. There is no indication for non-scrubbed members of the operating department staff to wear masks. This includes the anaesthetists.

Footwear

It is traditional for the staff entering the operating theatre complex to change into special clean footwear. Humphreys *et al.* (1991a) showed no change in the bacterial count of the operating theatre floor when staff wore their outdoor shoes into the operating theatre, and donning a pair of plastic overshoes made no difference. The practice of donning overshoes does, however, risk transferring bacteria from the staff member's shoes to their hands. Overshoes are not necessary for visitors, parents, etc. entering the theatre complex and anaesthetic room, but staff entering the operating theatre itself should probably wear theatre shoes. Wellington boots are appropriate for situations in which blood or other bodily fluids are likely to be spilled excessively. Theatre shoes/boots should be cleaned regularly, and whenever they are contaminated by blood or body fluids. They do not need to be sterilized.

Patients' beds in theatre

There is no reason why a patient's bed should not be wheeled into the operating theatre, and the patient then be transferred directly from it to the operating table and back again at the end of the operation. However, the ward sheets and blankets should be changed for freshly laundered ones immediately before transfer to theatre.

Jewellery and false fingernails

The scrub team should remove all jewellery except wedding rings. Glove perforation is more common at the base of the left fourth finger when wedding rings are worn (Nicolai *et al.*, 1997). The glove material is traumatized between the wedding ring and the instruments. There is some low-level evidence that false fingernails predispose to contamination and can prevent adequate decontamination (Pratt *et al.*, 2007). For many reasons, including infection control, it seems reasonable that false fingernails should not be worn by the surgical team.

Surgical scrub

Pre-operative cleaning of the hands is considered an essential part of the preparation of the scrub team for an operation. While the benefit of this has never been proven, to conduct such a trial would no longer be considered ethical. Current guidelines would suggest that the initial scrub of the day should be with a soft single-use brush to remove debris from beneath the fingernails, but that the use of chlorhexidine or a similar agent such as povidone-iodine or triclosan for 2 minutes is adequate. Thereafter, between cases, the use of the scrubbing brush is not necessary. There is currently a debate as to whether it is sufficient to use alcoholic solutions for subsequent operations. Although studies have been based on bacterial counts, and chlorhexidine would appear to be preferable, no study has indicated benefit in terms of the incidence of post-operative wound infection.

'Scrub' gowns

After scrubbing, the operating team should don sterile operating ('scrub') gowns. The gown should form a barrier between patient and surgeon yet be comfortable and breathable. The material should be impervious to water to prevent wicking of blood through the fabric, sufficiently robust to prevent tearing and, if not single use, capable of withstanding repeated washing and autoclaving. Some gowns are now available made from non-woven material and designed for single use. They are, however, more expensive.

Gloves

It is now considered obligatory for the scrub team to wear sterile gloves, but this practice is of unproven value in reducing the incidence of surgical site infection (SSI) and similarly with protection of the surgeon from bloodborne viruses, but their use as standard seems prudent. Double gloving has been advocated to prevent spread of viral infections from patient to surgeon and extra thickness gloves have also been produced for this purpose.

It has become traditional to replace a glove that becomes perforated during the course of an operation. However, Dodds *et al.* (1988), in a study of 582 surgical gloves, found 74 (12.7 per cent) were perforated at the end of the operation, but that perforation did not influence the bacterial count on the surgeons hands or the outside of the glove. The authors concluded that glove perforation was of no clinical significance to the patient. In order to minimize the contamination caused during the changing of a glove, it is probably preferable simply to don a second glove over the perforated first glove.

Wearing cover-gowns when leaving theatre

It is occasionally necessary for theatre staff to leave the operating theatre complex briefly to attend to patients in the recovery room or elsewhere. This applies particularly to the anaesthetists. There is no evidence that donning a cover-gown reduces the incidence of SSI, but whether staff should change their theatre garb after visiting wards, going to the toilet, etc. remains a local decision.

THE PATIENT

Microbiological studies would suggest that the most common source of wound contamination is from the patient's own bacteria (i.e. the contamination is endogenous). Each patient, indeed each human being, carries in the order of 10^{14} bacteria, of some 500 different species, on or in their body, and it is this magnitude of bacterial load that is brought into the operating theatre with each patient. Taking steps to prevent the patient's own bacteria gaining access to, and contaminating, the surgical site is, therefore, at least as important as the rituals we pursue to prevent exogenous contamination in the operating theatre.

Hypothermia

There is evidence (Melling *et al.*, 2001) that patients with peri-operative hypothermia (a body core temperature of less than 36°C) are more likely to develop post-operative infection. Patients who have a low body core temperature or are likely to develop one should be actively warmed, usually with a forced-air warming device, where warm air is blown into a special blanket under the patient. Other forms of patient warming devices exist. This recommendation is supported by NICE.

Pre-operative shower

One of the most common sources of endogenous contamination is the skin. Hayek *et al.* (1987), in a study of 2015 patients, suggested that pre-operative showers with chlorhexidine led to a lower incidence of SSI by comparison with showers with bar soap or placebo. Lynch *et al.* (1992) studied 3482 patients having three pre-operative showers with chlorhexidine and were unable to show a significant benefit. Ostrander *et al.* (2005) compared three types of skin preparation in 125 patients: 2 per cent chlorhexidine led to a lower toenail, web-space and control-site culture positivity in comparison with 3 per cent chloroxylenol or 0.7 per cent iodine in alcohol. They presumed that this would lead to a reduced incidence of SSI but the results did not show this benefit. This study echoed that of Garibaldi *et al.* (1988) who showed that chlorhexidine led to a lower incidence of skin colonization than povidone–iodine or bar soap, but could show no benefit in terms of the incidence of SSI. In summary, there would appear to be no benefit from whole-body showering or washing of the surgical incision site before the patient is brought to the operating theatre.

Hats

There is no evidence that gathering the patient's hair into a theatre hat has any influence on the incidence of SSI.

Clothes

It has been traditional to divest a patient of their own clothing and put them into theatre gowns before entering the operating theatre. Clearly this has application in major limb, thoracic or abdominal surgery, but there is no evidence that this reduces the incidence of SSI. For more minor operations, such as cataract operations, the patient can be taken into the theatre fully clothed without detriment.

Jewellery

There is no reason to remove patients' jewellery other than for security and electrical reasons. This is particularly important when diathermy is to be used when it is important to ensure that jewellery is not in contact with metal fittings on the operating theatre table, etc., which could lead to serious and significant burns to the patient.

Shaving

In the past, it was usual to shave the operation site on the day before operation. However, this practice was called into question by Seropian and Reynolds (1971) who, in their study of 406 clean wound operations, showed a 5.6 per cent incidence of SSI when the patient was shaved compared with 0.6 per cent SSI when the patient was not shaved or hair was removed with a depilatory cream. Shaving causes microscopic trauma to the surface of the skin converting the operation site from a clean surface to an infected site.

Use of a shaving brush simply exacerbates the problems. Oie and Kamiya (1992) examined 24 brushes used for shaving. They found 18 to be contaminated with *Pseudomonas aeruginosa*, *Xanthomonas maltophilia* and *Candida* and the mean bacterial skin count increased from 4×10^3 to 4.6×10^5 cfu/cm^2. They concluded that shaving brushes should not be used.

In a review of 20 clinical studies on the effects of shaving, Kjonniksen *et al.* (2002) concluded that pre-operative hair removal is unnecessary. If it has to be removed, hair should be removed using depilatory cream or electric clippers; shaving should not be performed. Unless hair is going to cause a technical problem during the procedure, there is no reason to shave the patient; the hair can be disinfected as least as adequately as the skin which bears it.

Other forms of patient preparation

Preparation of the stomach

Occasionally it is considered necessary to attempt to deflate the stomach. A stomach full of gas may obstruct the view when performing laparoscopic surgery to the gall bladder or oesophageal hiatus, and gastric outlet obstruction caused by gastric ulcer, pyloric hypertrophy or ulceration, duodenal ulcer or antral malignancy can render the stomach full of fluid and food residue. Bacterial overgrowth can occur in the presence of food residue in the stomach or if the acid secretion of the stomach is reduced by drug therapy. It has also been traditional to pass a nasogastric tube in an attempt to keep the stomach empty post-operatively after major colonic or small bowel surgery, but this is no longer considered appropriate. Nasogastric tubes can be the cause of sinusitis, laryngitis, pneumonia and oesophageal perforation. They can be misplaced into the trachea, cause acid reflux and aspiration into the lungs. They should be used as infrequently as possible.

Pre-operative mechanical bowel preparation

Until recently, pre-operative mechanical bowel preparation (MBP) was considered an important part of the preparation of a patient about to undergo elective colorectal surgery. Controversy existed as to whether pre-operative oral antibiotics to reduce the bacterial load in the colon added benefit, but more recent work has suggested that the bowel preparation itself led to a higher incidence of post-operative wounds and other SSIs. Guenaga *et al.* (2005) conducted a systematic review of the Cochrane database and published a meta-analysis of nine studies (1592 patients) showing a significantly lower incidence of an anastomotic leak and a lower incidence of SSI, with no bowel preparation compared with mechanical bowel preparation.

Pre-operative administration of non-absorbable antibiotics (neomycin and erythromycin base) has been shown to reduce the incidence of SSI in elective colorectal surgery when combined with pre-operative MBP (Nichols *et al.*, 1973), but no study has yet been published to show whether oral antibiotics confer the same benefit when there is no MBP.

The operating theatre

Skin preparation

A disinfectant compatible with skin should be used on the area of the surgical incision. It is probably more effective when that microbicide is in alcoholic solution, which has a significant additional disinfectant effect and whose evaporation will leave a layer of the microbicide on the skin to continue working after surgery. When alcoholic solutions are used, the alcohol should be allowed to evaporate completely before the operation commences and particularly before diathermy is used. Explosions of alcohol vapour have been reported and burns to patients have occurred where pooled alcohol has ignited.

Only aqueous-based disinfectants should be used on mucous membranes. A cream containing 1 per cent chlorhexidine can be used in urological or obstetric practice.

Drapes

It is traditional to drape the patient's body, exposing only the area of incision. The drapes should provide sterile cover over a wider area of the body than the incision site and it is important that, when they are placed on the body, a waterproof sheet is placed to prevent bacterial strikethrough, which would lead to contamination of the instruments and subsequently the wound. Disposable, waterproof materials are now available for draping the patient. These are more expensive than reusable materials but have the advantage of a lower wetting ability, reducing bacterial strikethrough.

Wound guards/adhesive drapes

Protective adhesive plastic drapes placed across the wound have been advocated to prevent skin bacteria coming into contact with the wound. Similarly plastic sheeting attached to a flexible ring, which is placed inside the abdominal cavity, has been devised with the intention of preventing contamination of the wound edges by gut bacteria. Whilst these devices have theoretical advantages, they have not proven to be beneficial in reducing the incidence of SSI in clinical trials.

More recently, a plastic solution, which can be painted on to the wound with the same objective, has been brought on to the market. Clinical trials of efficacy are awaited.

Wound dressings

It is common practice to cover the wound with an absorbent wound dressing at the end of the operation. Again there is a lack of clinical evidence that these dressings prevent SSI and, in 1989, Chrintz *et al.* (1989) showed no difference in the incidence of SSI when the wound was dressed (*n* = 633 patients) or left exposed (*n* = 569 patients).

Antibiotic prophylaxis

See Chapter 8.

Management of HIV- or hepatitis B-infected patients

See Chapter 9.

REFERENCES

Allen KD, Ridgway EJ and Parsons LA (1994) Hexachlorophane powder and neonatal infection. *Journal of Hospital Infection* **27**, 29.

Alter MJ, Ahtone J and Maynard JE (1983) Hepatitis B virus transmission associated with a multiple-dose vial in a hemodialysis unit. *Annals of Internal Medicine* **99**, 330.

Ayliffe GAJ and Lawrence JC (eds) (1985) Symposium on infection control in burns. *Journal of Hospital Infection* **6**(Suppl B), 3.

Ballin MS, McCluskey A, Maxwell S and Spillsbury S (1999) Contamination of laryngoscopes. *Anaesthesia* **54**, 1115.

Batiuk TD, Bodziak KA and Goldman M (2002) Infectious disease prophylaxis in renal transplant patients: a survey of US transplant centres. *Clinical Transplantation* **16**, 1.

Bayat A, Shaaban H, Dodgson A and Dunn KW (2003) Implications for Burns Unit design following outbreak of multi-resistant *Acinetobacter* infection in the ICU and Burns Unit. *Burns* **29**, 303.

Beathard GA, Settle SM, Shields MW (1999) Salvage of the nonfunctioning arteriovenous fistula. *American Journal of Kidney Disease* **33**, 910.

Bert F, Maubec E, Bruneau B, Berry P and Lambert-Zechovsky N (1998) Multiresistant *Pseudomonas aeruginosa* outbreak associated with contaminated tap water in a neurosurgical intensive care unit. *Journal of Hospital Infection* **39**, 53.

Boer A, Gilad J Porat N *et al.* (2007) Impact of 4% chlorhexidine whole-body washing on multidrug-resistant *Acinetobacter baumannii* skin colonisation among patients in a medical intensive care unit. *Journal of Hospital Infection* **67**, 149.

Brady MT (2005) Healthcare-associated infections in the neonatal intensive care unit. *American Journal of Infection Control* **33**, 268.

Breuer J (2005) Varicella vaccination for healthcare workers. *BMJ* **330,** 433.

British Association of Perinatal Medicine (1998) *Obstetric standards for the provision of perinatal care.* Available online at: http://www.bapm.org.

British HIV Association (2005) *Guidelines for the management of HIV infection in pregnant women and the prevention of mother-to-child transmission of HIV.* Available online at: http://www.bhiva.org.

Brun-Buisson C, Doyon F, Sollet JP, Cochard JF, Cohen Y and Nitenberg G (2004) Prevention of intravascular catheter-related infection with newer chlorhexidine-silver sulfadiazine-coated catheters: a randomized controlled trial. *Intensive Care Medicine* **30,** 837.

Cant A, Galloway A and Jackson G (eds, 2007) *Practical haematopoietic stem cell transplantation.* Oxford: Blackwell Publishing Ltd, 2.

Cepadia JA, Whitehouse T, Cooper B *et al.* (2005) Isolation of patients in single rooms or cohorts to reduce spread of MRSA in intensive care units: prospective two-centre study. *Lancet* **365,** 295.

Chrintz H, Vibits H, Harreby JS *et al.* (1989) Discontinuing postoperative wound dressings. *Ugeskrift for Laeger* **151,** 2667.

Church D, Elsayed S, Reid O, Winston B and Lindsay R. (2006) Burn wound infections. *Clinical Microbiology Reviews* **19,** 403.

Clarke JA (1992) *A colour atlas of burn injuries.* London: Chapman and Hall Medical.

Clarke RP, Reed PJ, Seal DV and Stephenson ML (1985) Ventilation conditions and air-borne bacteria and particles in operating theatres: proposed safe economies. *Journal of Hygiene, Cambridge* **95,** 325.

Coia JE, Duckworth GJ, Edwards DI *et al.* (2006) Guidelines for the control and prevention of meticillin-resistant *Staphylococcus aureus* (MRSA) in healthcare facilities. *Journal of Hospital Infection* **63**(Suppl 1), 1.

Confidential Enquiry into Maternal and Child Health (2000–02) *Why mothers die 2000–2002.* Available online at: http://www.cemach.org.uk.

Confidential Enquiry into Maternity and Child Health (1997–99) *Why mothers die 1997–1999.* Available online at: http://www.cemach.org.uk.

Cook D, Randolph A, Kernerman P *et al.* (1997) Central venous catheter replacement strategies: a systematic review of the literature. *Critical Care Medicine* **25,** 1417.

Cookson BD, Macrae MB, Barrett SP *et al.* (2006) Guidelines for the control of glycopeptide-resistant enterococci in hospitals. *Journal of Hospital Infection* **62,** 6.

Craven DE and Steger KA (1989) Nosocomial pneumonia in the intubated patient. In Weber DJ and Rutala WA (eds) *Nosocomial infections: new issues and strategies for prevention. Infectious Disease Clinics of North America.* Philadelphia: WB Saunders, 843.

Crossley K, Landesman B and Zaske D (1979) An outbreak of infection caused by epidemic strains resistant to methicillin and aminoglycosides. Two epidemiologic slides. *Journal of Infectious Diseases* **139,** 280.

Cunningham R, Jenks P, Northwood J, Wallis M, Ferguson S and Hunt S (2007) Effect on MRSA transmission of rapid PCR testing of patients admitted to critical care. *Journal of Hospital Infection* **65,** 24.

Department of Health (2004) *The national service framework for children, young people and maternity services.* London: Department of Health.

Department of Health (2006) *Safer practice in renal medicine.* Available online at:

http://www.dh.gov.uk/en/Publichealth/Healthprotection/Healthcareacquiredinfection/ Healthcareacquiredgeneralinformation/Thedeliveryprogrammetoreducehealthcare associatedinfectionsHCAIincludingMRSA/index.htm.

Department of Health (2007a) Health Technical Memorandum 03-01. *Specialised ventilation for healthcare premises. Part A: design and validation*. Department of Health, Estates and Facilities Division. London: The Stationery Office.

Department of Health (2007b) Health Technical Memorandum 03-01. *Specialised ventilation for healthcare premises. Part B: Operational management and performance verification*. Department of Health, Estates and Facilities Division. London: The Stationery Office.

Dodds RD, Guy PJ, Peacock AM *et al.* (1988) Surgical glove perforation. *British Journal of Surgery* **75**, 966.

Drescher J, Wagner D, Haverich A *et al.* (1994) Nosocomial hepatitis B virus infections in cardiac transplant recipients transmitted during transvenous endomyocardial biopsy. *Journal of Hospital Infection* **26**, 81.

Dykewicz CA, Kaplan JE, Centers for Disease Control and Prevention (2000) Guidelines for preventing opportunistic infections among haematopoietic stem cell transplant recipients. *Morbidity and Mortality Weekly Report* **49**(RR10), 1.

Ellis G, Ross JP, Shooter RA, Ellis G, Taylor GW (1956) Postoperative wound infection. *Surgery, Gynecology and Obstetrics* **103**, 257.

Finelli L, Miller JT, Tokars JI, Alter MJ, Arduino MJ (2005) National surveillance of dialysis-associated diseases in the United States, 2002. *Seminars in Dialysis* **18**:52.

Fishman JA and Rubin RH (1998) Medical progress: infections in organ transplant recipients. *New England Journal of Medicine* **338**, 1741.

Ford-Jones EL, Mindorff CM, Langley JM *et al.* (1986) Epidemiologic study of 4684 hospital acquired infections in pediatric patients. *Pediatric Infectious Diseases*, **8**, 668.

Gantz NM and Godofsky EW (1996) Nosocomial central nervous system infections. In Mayhall CG (ed.) *Hospital epidemiology and infection control*. Baltimore, MD: Williams & Wilkins, 246.

Garibaldi RA, Skolnick D, Lerer T *et al.* (1988) The impact of preoperative skin disinfection on preventing intraoperative wound contamination. *Infection Control and Hospital Epidemiology* **9**, 109.

Gastmeier P and Geffers C (2007) Prevention of ventilator-associated pneumonia: analysis of studies published since 2004. *Journal of Hospital Infection* **67**, 1.

George A, Tokars JI, Clutterbuck EJ, Bamford KB, Pusey C and Holmes AH (2006) Reducing dialysis associated bacteraemia, and recommendations for surveillance in the United Kingdom: prospective study. *BMJ* **332**, 1435.

George R and Hobbs P (1990) Bacteria in birthing tubs. *Nursing Times* **86**(14), 14.

Gilbert RE and Tookey PA (1999) Perinatal mortality and morbidity among babies delivered in water: surveillance study and postal survey. *BMJ* **319**, 483.

Gillespie P, Siddiqui H and Clarke J (2000) Cannula related suppurative thrombophlebitis in the burned patient. *Burns* **26**, 200.

Gould K (1998) Microbiological aspects of heart and heart-lung transplantation. In: Schofield PM, Corris P (eds) *Management of heart and lung transplant patients*. London: BMJ Publishing Group, 85.

Greenfield E and McManus A (1997) Infectious complications – prevention and strategies for their control. *Burn Management* **32**, 297.

Grohskopf LA, Sinkowitz-Cochran RL, Garrett DO *et al.* (2002) A national point-prevalence survey of pediatric intensive care unit-acquired infections in the United States. *Journal of Pediatrics* **140**, 432.

Guenaga KF, Matos D, Castro AA *et al.* (2005) Mechanical bowel preparation for elective colorectal surgery. *Cochrane Database Systematic Review* **25**, CD001544.

Halwani M, Solaymani-Dodaran M, Grundmann H, Coupland C and Slack R (2006) Cross-transmission of nosocomial pathogens in an adult intensive care unit: incidence and risk factors. *Journal of Hospital Infection* **63**, 39.

Hayden MK, Bonten MJ, Blom DW *et al.* (2006) Reduction in acquisition of vancomycin-resistant Enterococcus after enforcement of routine environmental cleaning measures. *Clinical Infectious Diseases* **42**, 1552.

Hayek LJ, Emerson JM and Gardner AMN (1987) A placebo-controlled trial of the effect of two preoperative baths or showers with chlorhexidine detergent on postoperative wound infection rates. *Journal of Hospital Infection* **10**, 165.

Hayes-Lattin B, Leis JF and Maziarz RT (2005) Isolation in the allogeneic transplant environment: how protective is it? *Bone Marrow Transplantation* **36**, 373.

Health Protection Agency (2006) *Immunoglobulin handbook 2006.* Available online at: http://www.hpa.org.uk.

Health Protection Agency (2008) Management of vesicular rash (varicella/herpes zoster) in pregnancy. Available online at: http://www.hpa.org.uk/web/HPAweb&HPAwebStandard/HPAweb_C/1195733798289 (accessed 15 October 2008).

Hèritier C, Dubouix A, Poirel L, Marty N and Nordmann P (2005) A nosocomial outbreak of *Acinetobacter baumannii* isolates expressing the carbapenem hydrolysing oxacillinase OXA-58. *Journal of Antimicrobial Chemotherapy* **55**, 115.

Herndon DN and Spies M (2001) Modern burn care. *Seminars in Paediatric Surgery* **10**, 28.

Hodle AE, Richter KP and Thompson RM (2006) Infection control practices in US Burn units. *Journal of Burn Care Research* **27**, 142.

Hoffman PN, Williams J, Stacey A *et al.* (2002) Microbiological commissioning and monitoring of operating theatre suites. *Journal of Hospital Infection* **52**, 1.

Holt ND, Gould FK, Taylor CE *et al.* (1997) Incidence and significance of non-cytomegalovirus viral respiratory infection after adult lung transplantation. *Journal of Heart Lung Transplantation* **16**, 416.

Holton J and Ridgway GL (1993) Commissioning operating theatres. *Journal of Hospital Infection* **23**, 153.

Humphreys H, Marshall RJ, Ricketts VE *et al.* (1991a) Theatre over-shoes do not reduce operating theatre floor bacterial counts. *Journal of Hospital Infection* **17**, 117.

Humphreys H, Russell AJ, Marshall RJ *et al.* (1991b) The effect of surgical theatre head-gear on air bacterial counts. *Journal of Hospital Infection* **19**, 175.

Johnson A, Young D and Reilly J (2006) Caesarean section surgical site infection surveillance. *Journal of Hospital Infection* **64**, 30.

Kingsley A, Hutter S, Green N, Speirs G (1999) Waterbirths: regional audit of infection control practices. *Journal of Hospital Infection* **41**, 155.

Kjonniksen I, Andersen BM, Sondenaa VG and Segadal L (2002) Preoperative hair removal – a systematic literature review. *Association of Operating Room Nurses Journal* **75**, 928, 940.

Knirsch CA, Jakob K, Schoonmaker D, Kiehlbauch JA, *et al.* (2000) An outbreak of *Legionella micdadei* pneumonia in transplant patients: evaluation, molecular epidemiology, and control. *American Journal of Medicine* **108**, 290.

Kool JL, Fiore AE, Kioski CM *et al.* (1998) More than 10 years of unrecognized nosocomial transmission of legionnaires' disease among transplant patients. *Infection Control and Hospital Epidemiology* **19**, 898.

Laing I, Ducker A, Leaf A and Newmarch P (2004) *Designing a neonatal unit. Report for the British Association of Perinatal Medicine.* Available online at: http://www.bapm.org.

Leclair JM, Freeman J, Sullivan DB *et al.* (1987) Prevention of nosocomial RSV infections through compliance with glove and gown isolation precautions. *New England Journal of Medicine* **317**; 329.

Lewis T, Griffith C, Gallo M and Weinbren M (2008) A modified ATP benchmark for evaluating the cleaning of some hospital environmental surfaces. *Journal of Hospital Infection* **69**, 156.

Lowbury EJL (1992) Special problems in hospital antisepsis. In: Russell AD, Hugo WB and Ayliffe GAJ (eds) *Principles and practice of this infection, preservation and sterilisation*, 2nd edn. Oxford: Blackwell Scientific Publications, 310.

Lucet J-C, Armand-Lefevre L, Laurichess J-J *et al.* (2007) Rapid control of an outbreak of vancomycin-resistant enterococci in a French University hospital. *Journal of Hospital Infection* **67**, 42.

Lund B, Agvald-Ohman C, Hultberg A *et al.* (2002) Frequent transmission of enterococcal strains between mechanically ventilated patients treated at an intensive care unit. *Journal of Clinical Microbiology* **40**, 2084.

Lupo A, Tarchini R, Carcarini G *et al.* (1994) Long-term outcome in continuous ambulatory peritoneal dialysis: a 10-year-survey by the Italian Cooperative Peritoneal Dialysis Study Group. *American Journal of Kidney Disease* **24**, 826.

Lynch W, Davey PG, Malek M *et al.* (1992) Cost-effectiveness analysis of the use of chlorhexidine detergent in preoperative whole-body disinfection in wound infection prophylaxis. *Journal of Hospital Infection* **21**, 179.

Macchini F, Valade A, Ardissino G *et al.* (2006) Chronic peritoneal dialysis in children: catheter related complications. A single centre experience. *Pediatric Surgery International* **22**, 524.

Masterton RG, Galloway A, French G *et al.* (2008) Guidelines for the management of hospital-acquired pneumonia in the UK: Report of the working party on hospital-acquired pneumonia of the British Society for Antimicrobial Chemotherapy. *Journal of Antimicrobial Chemotherapy* **62**, 5.

McCann S, Byrne JL, Rovira M *et al.* (2004) Outbreaks of infectious diseases in stem cell transplant units: a silent cause of death for patients and transplant programmes. *Bone Marrow Transplantation* **33**, 519.

Medical Devices Agency (2002) *Decontamination of endoscopes.* Device Bulletin DB 2002 (05). London: Department of Health.

Medicines and Healthcare Products Regulatory Agency (2004) *Flexible and rigid endoscopes.* Medical Device Alert, MDA 2004/028. London: Department of Health.

Melling AC, Ali B, Scott EM and Leaper DJ (2001) Effects of preoperative warming on the incidence of wound infection after clean surgery: a randomised controlled trial. *Lancet* **358**, 876.

Meyer E, Schwab F, Gastmeier P, Rueden H, Daschner FD and Jonas D (2007) *Stenotrophomonas maltophilia* and antibiotic use in German intensive care units: data from Project SARI (Surveillance of Antimicrobial Use and Antimicrobial Resistance in German Intensive Care Units). *Journal of Hospital Infection* **64**, 238.

Miller E, Fairley CK, Cohen BJ and Sang C (1998) Intermediate and long-term outcome of human parvovirus B19 infection in pregnancy. *British Journal of Obstetrics and Gynaecology* **105**, 174.

Montoya JG, Giraldo LF, Efron B *et al.* (2001) Infectious complications among 620 consecutive heart transplant patients at Stanford University Medical Center. *Clinical Infectious Disease* **33**, 629.

Morgan-Capner P and Crowcroft NS (2002) Guidelines on the management of, and exposure to, rash illness in pregnancy (including consideration of relevant antibody screening programmes in pregnancy). *Communicable Disease and Public Health* **5**, 59.

Mozingo W, McManus, Kim SH and Pruitt BA Jr (1997) Incidence of bacteraemia after burn wound manipulation in the early post burn period. *Journal of Trauma Injury Infection and Critical Care* **42**, 1006.

Murphy OM and Gould FK (1999) Prevention of nosocomial infection in solid organ transplantation. *Journal of Hospital Infection* **42**, 177.

National Collaborating Centre for Chronic Conditions (2006) *Clinical diagnosis and management of tuberculosis and measures for its prevention and control.* London: Royal College of Physicians.

National Institute for Health and Clinical Excellence (2001) *Guidelines for maternity Services.* Available online at: http://www.nice.org.uk

National Institute for Health and Clinical Excellence (2003) *Clinical Guideline 6: Antenatal care – routine care for the healthy pregnant women.* Available online at: http://www.nice.org.uk.

National Institute for Health and Clinical Excellence (2004) *Clinical guideline 13: Caesarean section.* Available online at: http://www.nice.org.uk.

National Institute for Health and Clinical Excellence (2008) Patient safety guidance PSG002: *Technical patient safety solutions for ventilator-associated pneumonia in adults.* Available online at: http://www.nice.org.uk.

NHS Estates (1996) *Maternity department health building notes (21).* London: HMSO.

NHS Estates (2004) Health Building Note 26: *Facilities for surgical procedures,* Vol. 1. London: The Stationery Office.

NHS Estates (2005a) HBN 4: *In-patient accommodation: options for choice Supplement 1: Isolation facilities in acute settings.* London: The Stationery Office.

NHS Estates (2005b) Health Building Note 57: *Facilities for critical care.* London: The Stationery Office.

Nichols RL, Broido P and Condon RE (1973) Effect of preoperative neomycin–erythromycin intestinal preparation on the incidence of infectious complications following colon surgery. *Annals of Surgery* **178**, 453.

Nicolai P, Aldam CH and Allen PW (1997) Increased awareness of glove perforation in major joint replacement. A prospective, randomised study of Regent Biogel Reveal gloves. *Journal of Bone and Joint Surgery, British* **79,** 371.

Nikodem VC (1998) Immersion in water during pregnancy, labour and birth. In: *Cochrane Collaboration. Cochrane Library,* Issue 3. Oxford: Update Software.

O'Connell NH and Humphreys H (2000) Intensive care unit design and environmental factors in the acquisition of infection. *Journal of Hospital Infection* **45,** 255.

Oie S and Kamiya A (1992) Microbial contamination of brushes used for preoperative shaving. *Journal of Hospital Infection* **21,** 103.

Orloff SL, Busch AMH, Olyaei AJ *et al.* (1999) Vancomycin-resistant *Enterococcus* in liver transplant patients. *American Journal of Surgery* **177,** 418.

Ostrander RV, Botte MJ and Brage ME (2005) Efficacy of surgical preparation solutions in foot and ankle surgery. *Journal of Bone and Joint Surgery (American)* **87,** 980.

Panililio AL, Welch BA, Bell DM *et al.* (1992) Blood and amniotic fluid contact sustained by obstetric personnel during deliveries. *American Journal of Obstetrics* **167,** 703.

Patel R, Paya CV (1997) Infections in solid organ transplant recipient. *Clinical Microbiological Reviews* **10,** 86.

Pimental JD, Low J, Styles K, Harris OC, Hughes A and Athan E (2005) Control of an outbreak of multi-drug-resistant *Acinetobacter baumannii* in an intensive care unit and a surgical ward. *Journal of Hospital Infection* **59,** 249.

Popejoy SL and Fry DE (1991) Blood contact and exposure in the operating room. *Surgery, Gynaecology and Obstetrics* **172,** 480.

Pratt PJ, Pellowe CM, Wilson JA *et al.* (2007) epic 2: National evidence-based guidelines for preventing healthcare-associated infections in NHS hospitals in England. *Journal of Hospital Infection* **65**(Suppl), S1.

Quarello F, Forneris G, Borca M and Pozzato M (2006) Do central venous catheters have advantages over arteriovenous fistulas or grafts? *Journal of Nephrology* **19,** 265.

Raineri E, Crema L, De Sivestri A *et al.* (2007) Meticillin-resistant *Staphylococcus aureus* control in an intensive care unit: a 10 year analysis. *Journal of Hospital Infection* **67,** 308.

Rangel MC, Coronado VG, Euler GL, Strikas RA (2000) Vaccine recommendations for patients on chronic dialysis. The Advisory Committee on Immunization Practices and the American Academy of Pediatrics. Semin Dial.;13(2):101-7.

Rathgeber J, Kietzmann D, Mergeryan H, Hub R, Zuchner K and Kettler D (1997) Prevention of patient bacterial contamination of anaesthesia-circle-systems: a clinical study of the contamination risk and performance of different heat and moisture exchangers with electret filter (HMEF). *European Journal of Anaesthesiology* **14,** 368.

Raymond J and Aujard Y (2000) Nosocomial infections in pediatric patients: a European, multicenter prospective study. *Infection Control and Hospital Epidemiology* **21,** 260.

Rayner HC, Pisoni RL, Bommer J, Canaud B, Hecking E, Locatelli F, et al. (2004) Mortality and hospitalization in haemodialysis patients in five European countries: results from the dialysis outcomes and practice patterns study (DOPPS). *Nephrology, Dialysis, Transplantation* **19,** 108.

Reardon CM, Brown TP, Stephenson AJ and Freedlander E (1998) Methicillin resistant *Staphylococcus aureus* in burns patients – why all the fuss? *Burns* **24,** 393.

Royal College of Obstetricians and Gynaecologists (2003) *Green top guide guideline number 36: prevention of early onset neonatal group B streptococcal disease.* London: RCOG Press.

Royal College of Obstetricians and Gynaecologists (2004) *Evidence-based clinical guideline no. 7: the care of women requesting induced abortion.* London: RCOG Press.

Royal College of Physicians, American Academy of Pediatrics and American College of Obstetricians and Gynecologists (2002) *Guidelines for perinatal care*, 5th edn. Washington, DC: American College of Obstetricians and Gynecologists, 17.

Saiman L and Siegel J (2004) Infection control in cystic fibrosis. *Clinical Microbiological Reviews* **17**, 57.

Salisbury DM, Ramsay M, Noakes K (eds; 2006) *Immunisation against infectious diseases.* London: HMSO.

Schabrun S and Chipchase L (2006) Healthcare equipment as a source of nosocomial infection: a systematic review. *Journal of Hospital Infection* **63**, 239.

Serody JS and Shea TC (1997) Prevention of infections in bone marrow transplant recipients. *Infectious Disease Clinics of North America* **11**, 459.

Seropian R and Reynolds BM (1971) Wound infections after preoperative depilatory versus razor preparation. *American Journal of Surgery* **121**, 251.

Serrano CW, Wright JW and Newton ER (1991) Surgical glove perforation in obstetrics. *Obstetrics and Gynecology* **77**, 525.

Shankowsky HJ, Callioux LS and Tredget EE (1994) North Americans survey of hydrotherapy in modern burn care. *Journal of Burn Care and Rehabilitation* **15**, 43.

Shannon T, Edgar RP, Villarreal C, Herndon DN, Phillips LG and Heggers J (1997) Much ado about nothing: methicillin resistant *Staphylococcus aureus.* *Journal of Burn Care and Rehabilitation* **18**, 326.

Singh N, Squier C, Wannstedt C, Keyes L, Wagener MM and Cacciarelli TV (2006) Impact of an aggressive infection control strategy on endemic Staphylococcus aureus infection in liver transplant recipients. *Infection Control and Hospital Epidemiology* **27**, 122.

Tan MP and Koren G (2006) Chickenpox in pregnancy: revisited. *Reproductive Toxicology* **21**, 410.

Taylor G, Gravel D, Johnston L, Embil J, Holton D, Paton S, Canadian Hospital Epidemiology Committee (2002) Canadian nosocomial infection surveillance program. Prospective surveillance for primary bloodstream infections occurring in Canadian hemodialysis units. *Infection Control and Hospital Epidemiology* **23**, 716.

Thodis E, Bhaskaran S, Pasadakis P, Bargman JM, Vas SI, Oreopoulos DG (1998). Decrease in *Staphylococcus aureus* exit-site infections and peritonitis in CAPD patients by local application of mupirocin ointment at the catheter exit site. *Peritoneal Dialysis International* **18**: 261.

Thodis E, Passadakis P, Lyrantzopooulos N, Panagoutsos S, Vargemezis V and Oreopoulos D (2005) Peritoneal catheters and related infections. *International Urology and Nephrology* **37**, 379.

Thodis E, Passadakis P, Panagoutsos S, Bacharaki D, Euthimiadou A and Vargemezis V (2000) The effectiveness of mupirocin preventing *Staphylococcus aureus* in catheter-related infections in peritoneal dialysis. *Advances in Peritoneal Dialysis* **16**, 257.

Thompson JT, Meredith JW and Molnar JA (2002) The effect of burn nursing units on burn wound infections. *Journal of Burn Care and Rehabilitation* **23**, 281.

Tokars JI, Miller ER and Stein G (2002) New national surveillance system for haemodialysis-associated infections: initial results. *American Journal of Infection Control* **30**, 288.

Trautmann M, Lepper PM, Haller M. (2005) Ecology of *Pseudomonas aeruginosa* in the intensive care unit and the evolving role of water outlets as a reservoir of the organism. *American Journal of Infection Control* **33**: S41.

Tredget EE, Shanaowsky HA, Rennie R., Burrell R and Logsetty S (2004) Pseudomonas infections in the thermally injured patient. *Burns* **30**, 3.

Tsakiris D, Simpson HK, Jones EH *et al.* (1996) Report on management of renal failure in Europe, XXVI, 1995. Rare diseases in renal replacement therapy in the ERA-EDTA Registry. *Nephrology, Dialysis, Transplantation* **11**(Suppl 7), 4.

Tunevall TG (1991) Postoperative wound infections and surgical face masks: a controlled study. *World Journal of Surgery* **15**, 383.

UK Renal Registry (2006) *The Renal Association, UK Renal Registry, the 9th annual report, December 2006.* Available online at: http://www.renalreg.com/Report%202006/Cover_Frame2.htm.

Vorbeck-Meister I, Sommer R, Vorbeck F and Horl WH (1999) Quality of water used for haemodialysis: bacteriological and chemical parameters. *Nephrology, Dialysis, Transplantation* **14**, 666.

Wade CR, Reith KK, Sikora JH and Augustine SM (2004) Postoperative nursing care of the cardiac transplant recipient. *Critical Care Nursing Quarterly* **27**, 17.

Walsh TR, Guttendorf J, Dummer S *et al.* (1989) The value of protective isolation procedures in cardiac allograft recipients. *Annals of Thoracic Surgery* **47**, 539.

Weber JM, Sheridan RL, Schultz JG, Tomkins RG and Ryan CM (2002) Effectiveness of bacteria controlled nursing units in preventing cross colonisation with resistant bacteria in severely burned children. *Infection Control and Hospital Epidemiology* **23**, 549.

Weinbren MJ (1999) Pharmacokinetics of antibiotics in burn patients. *Journal of Antimicrobial Chemotherapy* **44**, 319.

Welliver RC and McLaughlin S (1984) Unique epidemiology of nosocomial infection in a children's hospital. *American Journal of Diseases in Childhood* **138**, 131.

Whyte W, Hodgson R and Tinkler J (1982) The importance of airborne bacterial contamination of wounds. *Journal of Hospital Infection* **3**, 123.

Working party report – principles of design of burns units: report of a working group of the British Burn Association and Hospital Infection Society (1991) *Journal of Hospital Infection* **19**, 63.

15 PREVENTION OF INFECTION IN ALLIED HEALTH AND SERVICE DEPARTMENTS

Christina Bradley, Rebecca Evans, Adam Fraise, Conor Jamieson, Said Noorazar, Christine Perry, Andrew J Smith, Avril Weaver

Radiology

Rebecca Evans

The aim of this section is to provide healthcare professionals working within imaging departments with a practical overview of the principles of infection prevention and control, and should be used in conjunction with other associated professional and national guidelines.

The prevention and control of healthcare-acquired infections (HCAI) should be paramount to all clinical practice. Healthcare-associated infections not only place an increased financial burden on healthcare organizations, but also have an associated morbidity and mortality (Plowman *et al.*, 1999; National Audit Office, 2000; Department of Health, 2003). While it is recognized that not all HCAI are preventable, the application and adherence to infection control policies, procedures and guidelines will facilitate a reduction in the level of HCAI.

Radiography, whether diagnostic or therapeutic, offers a diverse and complex service involving the assessment, diagnosis and treatment of abnormalities/disease – including interventional techniques (e.g. angiograms, intravenous urograms) – with a proportion of patients having identified risk factors such as immunocompromise/immunosuppression or incubation of a communicable infection (e.g. pulmonary tuberculosis, bloodborne viruses and enteric infections).

Infection prevention and control should be incorporated as part of all education and training programmes (e.g. pre- and post-registration, induction/mandatory training packages, new procedures and protocols) and should include instruction on:

- the correct methods of hand decontamination, hand hygiene and aseptic technique, and the use of intravascular devices;
- the use of personal protective equipment (PPE);
- the management of sharps/clinical/hazardous waste and decontamination of the equipment and environment.

Reducing the risk of cross-infection is largely dependent on the susceptibility of the patient, the procedures undertaken, the complexity of the equipment used and the environment in which the patient is seen. Departments should have clearly defined operational policies that identify the risk and action to be taken to minimize the risk of patients acquiring a HCAI. Risk assessments should form an integral part of the management and care of any procedure undertaken and should include:

- complexity of procedure being undertaken;
- clinical condition of the patient;
- any associated risk factors (such as immunocompromise/immunosuppression, infections, e.g. pulmonary tuberculosis, infective diarrhoea);
- environment – is the environment fit for purpose? can procedures be undertaken safely?
- equipment used and decontamination methods required;
- facilities available to decontaminate equipment;
- contamination risk (e.g. transmission of micro-organisms, solutions, dressings, environment, equipment);
- use and availability of PPE;
- type of waste generated and facilities available to collect, store and dispose of waste.

MODE OF TRANSMISSION

How micro-organisms are transmitted will influence risk factors in relation to the procedures being undertaken and methods required to minimize cross-infection (Table 15.1). Micro-organisms are primarily transmitted by four routes: airborne; contact; blood/body fluids; and enteric. Practices required to reduce transmission will be dependent upon the mode of spread.

Prior to undertaking any procedures, risk assessments should identify any other factors which may increase or alter the mode of transmission (e.g. risk of

Table 15.1 Transmission of micro-organisms

Route of transmission	Examples of micro-organisms
Blood and body fluids	Hepatitis B, C HIV
Faecal/oral (enteric)	*Salmonella* spp *Shigella* spp *Campylobacter* spp
Airborne	Pulmonary tuberculosis MRSA (if dispersing)
Contact	Multi-resistant Gram-negative organisms Fungi (e.g. *Candida* spp, *Tricophyton* spp)

HIV, human immunodeficiency virus; MRSA, methicillin-resistant *Staphylococcus aureus*.

aerosol or splash injury from using, decontaminating or disposing of equipment).

LOCATION/ENVIRONMENT

The optimum environment is one which allows treatments to be undertaken with the minimum risk of cross-infection. Determining the suitability of the environment/location will depend upon the functionality of the department and should include an assessment of the complexity of proposed procedures, associated patient risk factors and the ability of the environment to allow the practitioner to undertake defined procedures or treatments with minimum risk.

When new builds or upgrades are being considered, it is essential that operational policies clearly identify the complexity and diversity of procedures being undertaken, decontamination processes anticipated, equipment/facilities required and storage needs to ensure the design complements the functionality of the service requirements. As part of any new build/upgrade, consideration should be given to the availability of isolation facilities especially in waiting/recovery areas for patients with known or suspected communicable infections (e.g. pulmonary tuberculosis).

It is recognized that specific procedures will need to be undertaken in designated rooms to accommodate the type, size and complexity of equipment used (e.g. magnetic resonance imaging, computerized tomography, angioplasties, barium studies, ultrasound, radiotherapy). As these procedures may involve invasive techniques and contact with blood or body fluids, it is essential that the design incorporates support facilities in close proximity to facilitate best practice. Such facilities may include:

- sluice (to contain sluice hopper, macerator, general and hand-wash sink);
- clinical room;
- designated waste storage;
- linen storage;
- sufficient storage for sterile equipment and supplies;
- domestic cleaning facilities.

PREVENTING/REDUCING THE RISK OF CROSS-INFECTION

Outlined below are key principles for the prevention and control of cross-infection. These guidelines should be used in conjunction with local infection control guidelines.

Identification of patients

Early identification of susceptible patients and patients with known or suspected communicable infections facilitates better management of patient case loads and reduces the risk of cross-infection. Ideally, this should be incorporated as part of the referral process whether via hospital or general practitioner. Identification of patients can either be electronically through Patient Administration Systems or manually. To maintain patient confidentiality, it is more practical to identify risk by mode of transmissions as outlined above as opposed to diagnosis, for example hepatitis B and C, or human immunodeficiency virus (HIV) identified as blood/body-fluid risk.

Scheduling of patients

- Scheduling of patients should be based on clinical need and risk of infectivity, with those with the lowest risk of infectivity reviewed first (e.g. immunocompromised/immunosuppressed), and patients with infected wounds/lesions or communicable diseases reviewed last. Where this cannot be achieved owing to clinical need, risk assessments should identify the best action taken to minimize the risk.
- For waiting areas, consideration should be given to reducing the waiting time (back to wards or awaiting transport into the community) for patients with communicable diseases.
- Practitioners should check the origin of the patient with the person in charge of the ward to ascertain if there are other risk factors (e.g. outbreaks of diarrhoea and/or vomiting). If so, consideration should be given to rescheduling appointments if clinically safe.

Hand hygiene

Good compliance with hand decontamination is the single most effective action that can be taken to prevent the spread of infection. Hand decontamination should be carried out:

- between all patient contact;
- following any task where contact with body fluids has taken place;
- prior to performing an aseptic technique;
- following contact with any contaminated or potentially contaminated equipment.

Wrist watches and stoned rings should not be worn in clinical areas or when undertaking clinical procedures.

Alcohol hand rubs/gels are recommended for use on physically clean hands and should be available at key locations within departments (e.g. imaging workstations, procedure trolleys).

Clinical practices

When any clinical invasive procedure is undertaken, the principles of asepsis should be maintained to reduce the risk of cross-infection.

Intravascular device insertion

The following guidelines apply for the insertion of intravascular devices (Infection Control Nurses Association, 2001; Pratt *et al.*, 2001; Royal College of Nursing, 2005):

- Any intravascular device insertion should comply with national guidelines.
- Aseptic technique should be used for all intravascular device insertion.
- Maximum sterile barrier precautions should be implemented for central venous catheter insertion.
- Peripheral cannulae should be inserted in an optimal area that can be clearly visualized during use.
- Prior to line insertion, the skin should be decontaminated with an antimicrobial solution (e.g. 2 per cent alcoholic/chlorhexine).
- Invasive devices should be secured with an appropriate sterile dressing in accordance with local and national guidelines.
- Any access ports should be disinfected prior to use with an appropriate antimicrobial solution.
- Regular observation of the intravascular device should be carried out to identify signs of complications (e.g. phlebitis/infection).
- Intravascular device insertion details (including date and time of insertion) should be documented.

Use of personal protective equipment

Personal protective equipment should be readily available within each department for use as appropriate. Staff should be trained and understand the correct use and application of PPE. Where chemical or hazardous substances are used compliance with legislation is essential (Health and Safety Executive, 1974, 1992, 1999a, b).

Personal protective equipment should be used to protect both the practitioner and patient from any potential risk of cross-infection.

The type of PPE worn should be based on a risk assessment of:

- the proposed risk of transmission of any potential organisms;
- the patient's status (e.g. infectivity and susceptibility to infection);
- the procedure being undertaken;
- the type of equipment used (Box 15.1).

Visiting wards/departments

When entering wards, staff should ascertain whether the patients they are to visit have known or suspected communicable infections. They should also

---

Box 15.1 Types of personal protective equipment

GLOVES

- Are only effective if worn properly
- Are not substitutes for hand decontamination
- Should be fit for purpose (local policy should be consulted)
- Should be worn when in contact with blood, body fluids, chemicals or chemotherapeutic agents

PLASTIC APRONS

- Provide a barrier to prevent the transfer of micro-organisms from a practitioner's uniform and clothing to the patient and vice versa

Aprons and gloves should be worn when in contact with a patient with a known or suspected communicable infection or infected wounds, and should be single use only.

MASKS

- The principal function of facemasks is to reduce the risk of airborne contamination
- If a patient in isolation with known or suspected multi-drug resistant tuberculosis is being treated, masks conforming with national recommendations must be worn.

GOGGLES/VISORS

- Eye protection should be worn when there is a risk of splash or aerosol is likely

---

ensure that the correct PPE is available for use and that facilities are in place to decontaminate equipment effectively.

Outbreaks of communicable infections

During outbreaks and/or ward closures (e.g. owing to diarrhoea and/or vomiting) consideration should be given to scheduling cases to minimize the risk of cross-infection. Radiography staff working in an affected area should, where practical, avoid working in non-infected areas.

Blood and body fluids

- Care should be taken when handling all blood and body fluids.
- Appropriate PPE should be worn when in contact with and cleaning up blood/bodily fluids:
  - gloves and aprons should be worn when in contact with blood/body fluids;
  - goggles/face visors should be used if there is a risk of splashing.

- Solidifying agents, such as gels, should be used to contain blood and body fluid spills.
- Blood/body fluids should be removed and the area/surface decontaminated in accordance with local decontamination policy.
- Equipment used to clean up spillages must be decontaminated following use.

Safe management of sharps and clinical/hazardous waste

- All sharps and clinical or hazardous waste should be handled in accordance with relevant waste regulations (NHS Estates, 1995; Department of Health, 1997; Department of Health, 2006).
- Sharps should be disposed of at the point of use (where practical) into an approved container, which must comply with national standards (e.g. UK – BS7320).
- There should be systems in place for the storage, collection, transportation and disposal of waste.
- Waste bins should be operated by foot to reduce the risk of hand contamination.

Safe handling of linen

- Clean and dirty linen should be segregated in a designated area.
- Infected linen should be handled according to the local infection control policy.

Equipment

- When purchasing equipment, consideration should be given to the use of disposable, single-use items where practical. Where single-use items are used, it is essential that equipment is disposed of and transported in accordance with waste regulations.
- Items of equipment not designated as single use but which have contact with the patient must be capable of being decontaminated between use. Equipment can be divided into high-, intermediate- and low-risk categories depending on the purpose of its use (Table 15.2; Spaulding, 1972).
- It is essential that risk assessments are undertaken to determine the suitability of equipment to be decontaminated. Cleaning, disinfection and sterilization are all processes that remove or destroy micro-organisms. The method chosen to decontaminate equipment will depend on the facilities available, the decontamination process required, the complexity of the equipment (e.g. lumens, size, sharps), the ability of the equipment to withstand the decontamination process (e.g. chemical or steam disinfection) and the infection risk associated with the equipment/medical device.

Table 15.2 Risk categories of equipment

Risk category	Description	Example
High	Items that are invasive or have close contact with a break in the skin or mucous membrane	Invasive instruments Lines, guide wires
Intermediate	Items in contact with blood/bodily fluids, mucous membrane	Scissors
Low	Equipment in contact with intact skin	Trolleys, beds, imaging tables

- Prior to purchasing any equipment, it is the responsibility of the user to ensure that the equipment can be adequately decontaminated. Within any department, there should be a programme for cleaning and maintaining all items of equipment, based on local and national policy.
- Where practical, equipment designated as reusable should be processed in a sterile services department to ensure adequate decontamination and compliance to national guidelines. If local decontamination is used, it is essential that consideration is given to dedicated decontamination facilities and systems need to be in place to ensure the effectiveness of the decontamination processes.
- Care must be taken to reduce an inoculation accident when any instruments/sharps are handled.
- There should be a maintenance programme in place and a monitoring system to ensure that each load achieves the correct temperature. Instruments with lumens should be processed only in a vacuum autoclave, which should comply with national guidelines (Medical Devices Agency, 1998, 2001).
- As part of any cleaning programme where solutions or disinfectants are used, consideration should be given to the following:
  - surfaces must be able to withstand cleaning with detergent and water and disinfectants (e.g. chlorine-releasing agents, 70 per cent alcohol);
  - no patients or staff are put at risk where disinfectants are used;
  - the appropriate PPE is available for use;
  - products used comply with national policy, Control of Substances Hazardous to Health Regulations (Health and Safety Executive, 1999a) and health and safety legislation.

Details of the specific equipment used in the radiology department and methods for its decontamination are given in Table 15.3.

Table 15.3 Specific equipment used in the radiology department

Examples of types of equipment	Method of decontamination	Comments
Blankets/sheets	Launder or use disposable	Single patient use
Diagnostic scopes	Non-heat tolerant – chemical disinfection	Ensure decontamination process is compatible with manufacturer's guidelines
Examination couches, chairs, tables, dressing trolleys and work surfaces	General use – detergent and water[a]	Disposable roll should be used between patients
Foam supports	Disposable, laundered or decontaminated with detergent and water[a]	Covers should have washable or disposable waterproof covers
Imaging equipment e.g. MRI/CT scanner, ultrasound	As per manufacturer's guidelines	Ensure compatibility with detergents and disinfectants used
Imaging tables	General use – detergent and water[a]	Ensure compatibility of detergents/disinfectants with manufacturer's guidelines
Instruments (e.g. scissors, scalpel handles)	Single use If reusable – autoclave[b]	Care should be taken to prevent an inoculation accident
Patient gowns	Launder or disposable	Single patient use only
Portable imaging equipment	As per manufacturer's guidelines	Should be stored clean Equipment should be covered where practical
Probes (e.g. vaginal, rectal)	As per manufacturer's guidelines	Ensure all crevices and lumens can be decontaminated The use of sheath may be advocated[c]
Sharps	Single use	Dispose into an approved sharps container Dispose at point of use
Suction tubing	Disposable	Dispose as clinical waste
Toys	Detergent and water[a]	All toys should be washable There should be a cleaning programme in place for cleaning any toys used
Tubing/lines	Single use	Dispose as clinical waste Sharps into an approved sharps container
Ultrasonic gels	As per manufacturer's guidelines	Nozzles must not touch the patient's skin Containers should not be topped up

[a]Cleaning should be followed by disinfection with a chlorine-releasing agent (1000 ppm) or an alcohol-impregnated wipe if used on a patient with a known or suspected infection.
[b]Where autoclave/bench-top sterilizers are used, only instruments designed to be autoclaved should be processed. Organic matter should be removed prior to autoclaving. The use of an ultrasonic washer is preferred. Where instruments require manual cleaning, a risk assessment should be undertaken to ensure that the equipment can be cleaned effectively and safely (Medical Devices Agency, 1998, 2002).
[c]Sheaths should not be used as an alternative to decontaminating probes.
CT, computerized tomography; MRI, magnetic resonance imaging.

Physiotherapy and occupational therapy

Christine Perry

Therapy staff are involved in the treatment of patients in acute hospital settings, outpatient facilities and patients' own homes. Therapists treating patients in acute ward settings come across many patients who are suspected or known to be infected or colonized with pathogenic and antimicrobial-resistant organisms. As their role requires them to treat patients in many different areas, it is vital that they understand and apply infection control principles in practice. Physiotherapy departments can treat both inpatients and outpatients; therefore, it is important to be aware of the infection transmission potential resulting from mixing patients from many different ward areas and care settings, and to manage risks accordingly. Therapy staff also undertake home visits with hospital inpatients, and need to apply infection control principles during transportation and in the patient's own home.

While reports of infection associated with physiotherapy and occupational therapy activities are rare, patient contacts within a physiotherapy department have been implicated in hospital-wide dissemination of methicillin-resistant *Staphylococcus aureus* (MRSA; Rimland, 1985). Equipment used in physiotherapy departments has been implicated in infection outbreaks, for example, *Pseudomonas aeruginosa* associated with a hydrotherapy pool (Sclech *et al.*, 1986). Therapeutic ultrasound equipment has been found to be contaminated with potentially pathogenic organisms including *Stenotrophomonas maltophilia* and *Acinetobacter baumanii* (Schabrun *et al.*, 2006). Physiotherapy staff are also actively involved in the care and treatment of patients with chronic disease, such as cystic fibrosis, where prevention of transmission of organisms including *Burkholderia cepacia* is important (Cystic Fibrosis Trust, 2002). Patient contacts in the occupational therapy department also have the potential for transfer of organisms between patients from different ward and department areas. In addition, specific activities in these departments (e.g. food preparation) require infection control consideration.

Physiotherapy and occupational therapy staff require knowledge and understanding of standard infection control precautions, specific disease precautions and decontamination of equipment in order to practise safely. Therapy staff also undertake invasive-type procedures, including wound dressings and injections, requiring them to be competent in aseptic technique. Therapists who are involved in food preparation activities should have, as a minimum, a basic understanding of food hygiene principles. Education and training in these areas will be provided to registered therapy staff during pre-registration training. Assistant practitioner and helper roles are becoming more commonplace amongst therapy disciplines. As these staff have direct patient contact, they require education and training in infection prevention and control to the same level as nursing or health care assistants.

PREVENTION OF INFECTION

Therapy departments should be designed with reference to infection control considerations, allowing patient segregation and ease of cleaning, and with facilities for decontamination of equipment. Units where wound dressings will be part of patient management should include appropriate facilities, which may include a preparation area, dressing area and disposal facilities. Units that undertake injection therapy should identify a clean area in which medications can be prepared aseptically. Hand decontamination facilities will be required, which can be achieved through the availability of a combination of sinks for handwashing and alcohol hand gel. Food preparation areas should be designed to enable compliance with food safety principles, including segregation of raw and cooked food, hand hygiene, pest control and high standards of cleanliness.

Standard precautions, as described for general wards and departments, should be applied to all patient contacts for therapy purposes, whether patients are inpatients or outpatients (Pratt *et al.*, 2007). Physiotherapy staff may need to wear masks or respirators when carrying out certain procedures on patients with respiratory infections. They should be trained in the use of respirators and included in programmes for fit testing of respirators. Ward staff and general practitioners should ensure that therapists are informed of any additional specific infection prevention requirements at the point of referral to one of the services. In some circumstances, patients' rehabilitation needs may over-ride infection control needs (Pike and McLean, 2002); a risk assessment should be undertaken, in consultation with the Infection Control Team, to ensure precautions meet individual patient needs but do not compromise the safety of other patients. Outpatient sessions may need to be planned to maintain segregation of certain patient groups; in particular, cystic fibrosis patients who are colonized with *Burkholderia cepacia* must not attend treatment sessions at the same time as patients who are not colonized (Cystic Fibrosis Trust, 2004).

Restriction on therapy staff movement and activities is an essential part of hospital outbreak management. Where wards or departments are closed (e.g. during norovirus) outbreaks, patients should not attend physiotherapy and occupational therapy departments, if such attendances are avoidable. Only essential therapy visits should take place on closed wards and departments, avoiding activities with patients who have symptoms of the outbreak infection. One therapist should be allocated to the closed ward area and, wherever possible, this therapist should not undertake any therapy activities in other wards or departments. If this is not possible, the closed ward should only be visited when all other visits are completed. During major outbreaks of infection (e.g. in an influenza outbreak), there may be a need to establish small local rehabilitation facilities within closed ward areas and to undertake rehabilitation consultations by phone or email to maintain therapy activity during periods of prolonged outbreak activity (Pa *et al.*, 2004).

Therapists undertaking home visits should apply principles of infection prevention and control relevant to community settings (National Institute for Clinical Excellence, 2003), ensuring access to hand decontamination facilities and protective clothing where appropriate. If therapists are transporting patients home in their own or lease cars, it is prudent to ensure patients are free from symptoms of enteric infection.

EQUIPMENT

Equipment used in therapy procedures has the potential to act as a vector for transmitting infection. Treatment couches should be covered with paper or cleaned between each patient use. Bedding should be changed at least daily and after use on an infected patient. Gym equipment should also be cleaned on a regular basis. Contamination of therapy equipment may be reduced by ensuring patients wear day clothing and shoes wherever possible. Principles for decontamination are described elsewhere and manufacturers' decontamination instructions should always be obtained and followed. Therapeutic ultrasound equipment has potential for infection transmission through either contamination of the transducer head or the ultrasound gel (Schabrun *et al.*, 2006). Transducer heads should be adequately decontaminated between each patient use; 70 per cent alcohol wipes are quick and effective measure, provided compatibility is assured. Gels should be stored and handled in a manner that reduces the risk of contamination, avoiding decanting from large to small bottles. Electromyography equipment should also be decontaminated in accordance with manufacturers' instructions. Electrode probes that are to be used internally in the vagina and anus should either be disposable or be decontaminated by heat rather than chemicals. Autoclavable products are available and should be preferred, with autoclaving in an accredited sterile services department between each use. Putty that is used in hand physiotherapy could also be a potential vector for infection transmission and patients should decontaminate their hands before and after using this material. Furthermore, it is preferable to avoid use in patients who have unhealed wounds on their hands. If it is necessary for a patient with a wound to use putty, then the wound should be covered with a waterproof impermeable dressing or, alternatively, a glove may be worn. Splinting baths contain heated water, which could promote bacterial growth. The water in these baths should be drained at least daily and left empty overnight; the reservoir should be decontaminated regularly. Ice-making machines must be regularly disinfected as they have been associated with outbreaks of infection caused by *Mycobacterium* spp. Hands should not be used for obtaining ice; a scoop that is regularly decontaminated should be used.

Walking and dressing aids should be decontaminated between each patient use; they will also require cleaning during use if individual patients utilize them for an extended period of time. Where hospital therapy units loan equipment for patients to use in their own home, the contamination of these items should be in line with principles for decontamination in community loan equipment stores (Medicine and Healthcare Products Regulatory Agency, 2003). This will include:

• transporting of used items separate from clean items;
• assuming used equipment is contaminated and handling it accordingly;
• documenting the decontamination status of equipment;
• storing decontaminated equipment correctly to prevent recontamination and to protect from dust.

HYDROTHERAPY POOLS

Hydrotherapy and spa pools have been associated with outbreaks of *Pseudomonas aeruginosa*, *Legionella* spp and enteroviruses. Dermatophyte infections of the feet can also be acquired from the surrounding poolside area. Therapeutic pools require strict infection prevention management as the higher temperatures at which they operate can affect the ongoing activity of disinfectants. Patients using these pools are likely to be more susceptible to infection than the general population and, in the case of hospital inpatients, are at greater risk of having been in contact with antimicrobial-resistant organisms. To avoid cases and outbreaks of infection, good management of pools is essential (Public Health Laboratory Service, 1999). A named senior physiotherapist should be responsible for the overall daily management of the pool. They should be trained in hydrotherapy and pool management, and operate under the direction of a superintendent physiotherapist with appropriate knowledge. The senior physiotherapist ensures that daily records are maintained and that regular maintenance activities occur. A named hospital engineer should have delegated responsibility for pool pumping equipment and filtering mechanisms. A hydrotherapy pool management group should be established, consisting of the senior physiotherapist, a hospital engineer, a management representative and a microbiologist. Twice-yearly, formal, minuted meetings should be held to review pool records and address unresolved issues. Where infection outbreaks are suspected or occur, the local Consultant in Communicable Disease Control may need to be involved.

The pool design should allow for continuous circulation of water that eliminates dead spots. The circulation system should also allow for the injection of reagents for disinfection and pH adjustment, obtaining samples for microbiological monitoring and back-washing of filters. The choice of filter will depend on the number and types of bathers that are likely to use the pool. The disinfectant injection site should be located immediately before the filters.

Circulation and disinfection should be a continuous process 24 hours a day for 365 days each year. The time taken for the equivalent volume of pool water to be circulated through the filters should be not less than 1 hour and not more than 1.5 hours. The patient and staff changing areas should be designed for easy cleaning and should be furnished using easily cleaned materials. Some areas may require regular disinfection, which should be taken into account during planning and building. Separate showering, changing and toilet facilities should be provided for patients and staff.

A protocol should be established for exclusion of certain patients if there is thought to be an unacceptable infection risk (e.g. patients with infected wounds that cannot be covered). Patients should be encouraged to evacuate their bladders and bowels before using the pool and should wear a clean swimming costume. All patients should shower before using the pool. Physiotherapy staff with skin conditions, such as eczema or psoriasis, may experience a worsening of these conditions owing to the chemicals in the water. An individual assessment of the severity of these conditions should be made to ensure staff are not placed at increased risk of pool-associated infections. Standard precautions should be applied to patient contact outside of the pool with hand hygiene and protective clothing being adopted as appropriate (e.g. when emptying urine catheter bags). The poolside area should be cleaned daily with pool water when the pool is not in use. Regular decontamination with a disinfectant may be employed but compatibility with the disinfectant used in the pool should be ensured. Equipment such as flotation aids and manual handling equipment should be regularly cleaned according to an agreed schedule.

An agreed programme of monitoring should be in place. At the beginning and end of each pool session, the temperature and pH value should be measured. The pool pH should be within the range 7.2–7.8. At these times, the residual free disinfectant level should be measured. Between morning and afternoon sessions the free and total disinfectant level should be determined. A visual inspection of the pool water for colour and clarity should be undertaken at the start of a working day and appropriate action taken if the pool water appears cloudy, dirty or green, or if there is obvious slime on tiles or fittings. A programme for bacteriological monitoring of the pool should be agreed and it is suggested that samples of pool water be examined twice weekly (Public Health Laboratory Service, 1999). Samples should be incubated at 37°C for 24 hours and the total bacterial count reported as colony-forming units (CFU) per volume of pool water. In addition, the presence or absence of *Pseudomonas aeruginosa* (expressed as CFU per 100 mL) should be reported. The presence of *P. aeruginosa* or overall colony counts of >100 CFU/mL requires urgent action and consideration of taking the pool out of use. To maintain pool water, quality back-washing of filters, where the flow of water through the filters is reversed, should take place regularly to ensure filters do not become clogged with debris. This should be recorded, as should other events, including pool emptying and inspection, pool closures, health complaints from staff and patients, and faecal contamination of the pool. When faecal contamination occurs, the pool should be closed to bathers. If the contamination is with a formed stool, the amount of residual disinfectant should be rapidly increased (hyperchlorination/shock-dosing) and the pool should remain closed until normal disinfectant levels are re-established. If the contamination is with a loose stool, then the pool should be closed, emptied and hosed down. Shock-dosing of disinfectant should take place, together with back-washing of filters and followed by three full-turnaround circulations of pool water. The pool should not be returned to use until normal disinfectant levels have been re-established.

Whirlpool or spa pools have been associated with additional microbiological hazards, including *Legionella* spp, *Mycobacterium* spp, amoebae, hepatitis A and *Cryptosporidium*. Guidance on pool design, hygiene, water quality and monitoring is available, and should be followed (Health and Safety Executive and Health Protection Agency, 2006).

MONITORING OF PRACTICE

Regular audit of practice within the physiotherapy and occupational therapy departments will ensure infection prevention and control practices comply with best practice. Audit tools developed by the Infection Control Nurses Association (2004) can be used for this purpose. In particular, the audit tool for management of patient equipment (specialist areas) covers physiotherapy and occupational therapy equipment. Occupational therapy kitchens can be audited using the ward/departmental kitchen tool.

Pharmacy

Conor Jamieson and Said Noorazar

A hospital pharmacy department can have different functions and specializations. Aside from the traditional role, which focuses on the supply of medicinal products to inpatients, outpatients and other departments, pharmacy departments may also manufacture medicinal products, such as radiopharmaceuticals, cytotoxic drugs and total parenteral nutrition in aseptic conditions, and undertake quality control/quality assurance activities. The pharmacy department may also have one or more satellite units that provide medicinal products for specialist areas, such as ophthalmology or dermatology centres. The fundamental principles of stock control, good manufacturing practice, quality control and appropriate storage and handling will be similar in all areas to minimize the risk of contamination of medicinal products.

The manufacture of pharmaceutical products is regulated throughout most of the world. In the UK, the Medicines and Healthcare products Regulatory

Agency (MHRA) regulates the manufacture of pharmaceuticals ensuring efficacy, quality and safety of pharmaceutical and other healthcare products. In Europe, the European Medicines Agency is a decentralized body of the European Union, which protects and promotes public and animal health through the evaluation and supervision of medicines for human and animal health. The USA was one of the first countries in the world to have comprehensive regulatory control of the quality of medicines. The Pure Food and Drugs Act of 1906 in the USA is regarded as the first attempt to prevent adulteration of drugs and to put an end to manufacturing conditions lacking sanitary precautions. The Food and Drug Administration regulates the pharmaceutical manufacturing in the USA and all manufacturers must register with this organization. Most other countries have similar organizations to regulate and supervise the manufacture of pharmaceuticals.

Some manufacturing departments in National Health Service hospital pharmacies are engaged in batch manufacturing of sterile and non-sterile pharmaceuticals under a manufacturing licence, allowing the products to be used nationwide. These products do not have a product licence (marketing authorization) number and are known as 'specials'. The MHRA has issued guidelines on the supply of unlicensed medicinal products (Anon., 2005).

However, there is often a need to obtain medicinal products without a product licence. These products could be parenteral nutrition individualized to a specific patient, cytotoxic infusions prepared for an oncology clinic, bulk preparation of a drug as a sterile eye drop or simply dilution of a proprietary ointment to one of a lower strength for a patient.

Creams, ointments and oral mixtures may be prepared extemporaneously in a general dispensary. These products are not supplied sterile, as they will be ingested or be applied to non-sterile surfaces such as the skin. However, steps should be taken to minimize the inoculation of large numbers of microorganisms into the product. High standards of hygiene are required (e.g. surface disinfection of mortars, pestles, glass tiles, spatulas and associated equipment is recommended prior to preparation of the product). Seventy per cent denatured ethyl alcohol is often used for this purpose. These products should be prepared in an appropriate environment, where potential pathogens are unlikely to be found. These products will have a short shelf-life owing to the lack of antimicrobial preservation. Worksheets recording details of ingredients used, expiry dates, method of preparation and shelf-life assigned to the product should be maintained and stored for certain number of years.

STERILE PRODUCTS

Thirty years ago, the Breckenridge report was issued, concluding that 'the addition of drugs to intravenous infusion fluid is an aseptic pharmaceutical procedure, which should ideally be carried out in appropriate environmental conditions under the direct control of a pharmacist' (Breckenridge, 1976). Pharmacy departments are involved in a range of aseptic preparation services, providing sterile medicinal products to wards and departments for individually named patients. However, many activities that should be performed in an aseptic pharmaceutical environment in accordance with the Breckenridge report are performed on the ward. Aseptic preparations undertaken by pharmacy departments' aseptic manufacturing units may include the provision of a centralized intravenous additive (CIVA) service, preparation of total parenteral nutrition (TPN), cytotoxic infusions and radiopharmaceuticals. A CIVA service reduces the risk of microbial contamination of infusion products to a minimum by preparing sterile infusions and products in a ready-to-administer form by pharmacy staff. Pharmaceutical laminar flow cabinets (LFC) and isolators situated in purpose-built clean rooms are used to prepare the products. Non-hazardous products, such as TPN are prepared in vertical LFCs or positive pressure isolators, while cytotoxic products and radiopharmaceuticals are prepared in a safety cabinet with vertical laminar flow or in negative pressure isolators (see later). As these products must be prepared under direct supervision of a pharmacist for individually named patients, a manufacturing licence is often not required.

CONTAMINATION OF ASEPTICALLY PREPARED MEDICINAL PRODUCTS

Whether prepared in a controlled environment, such as a pharmaceutical isolator, or an uncontrolled open environment such as a ward, contamination of medicinal products can occur. Risk assessment should be carried out on all sterile medicinal products to determine the risk of contamination of a product based on its physicochemical properties and formulation, the numbers of such products being prepared on a daily basis, the staff preparing the product, the extent of preparation involved, the location where preparation takes place and the level of training provided to the member of staff. An assessment of risk regarding the clinical situation of the patient receiving the aseptically prepared product should also be made. Risks can then be stratified and preparation should be carried out in an environment appropriate to the risk assessment.

Risk assessment on this basis will identify which sterile products should be outsourced from a licensed manufacturer, which can be prepared in-house in a controlled environment, such as an isolator, and which could be prepared on a ward, clinic or theatre.

PHARMACEUTICAL CABINETS

Most sterile pharmaceuticals are sterilized terminally by heat (steam or dry heat) or by filtration. Sometimes aseptic preparation without further sterilization is necessary, such as reconstituting a pharmaceutical powder in a vial by addition of diluent.

To process pharmaceuticals, a clean environment is required. Pharmaceutical clean rooms are equipped with air-handling units, which supply high-efficiency particulate air (HEPA) filtered into the clean room, making the room's pressure higher than its immediate surroundings. The rooms have workstations where the manipulation of pharmaceuticals can take place. Usually these workstations are either LFCs or pharmaceutical isolators (Midcalf *et al.*, 2004). The air from the room is HEPA filtered into the LFCs either from back to front (horizontal flow) or from top to the bottom (vertical flow). The flow is unidirectional and in a laminar fashion.

The air blowing horizontally from the back of the cabinet protects the pharmaceutical material prepared inside the cabinet by preventing any air entering into the cabinet through its open front. However, as the operator is stationed in front of the cabinet, he or she is vulnerable to any hazardous materials that may be handled in the cabinet. Only safe products such as TPN should be manufactured in a horizontal LFC.

The downward blown air in vertical laminar flow safety cabinets sweeps the material inside the cabinet, protecting it from contamination. This air is sucked away from the cabinet just in front of the work surface, preventing any harmful particulate matter reaching the operator. Preparation of potentially harmful pharmaceuticals, such as cytotoxics and radiopharmaceuticals, should be handled in safety cabinets (Allwood *et al.*, 2002).

Isolators are glove boxes which have their process chambers completely isolated from the surrounding environment. HEPA filtered air is introduced into the process chamber either as laminar flow or in turbulent fashion. Isolators have entry devices (hatches) attached to them. The hatches have their own HEPA filtered air supply and are equipped with two doors. One opens to the outside and the other into the process chamber. These doors have timing devices and the inner door will usually not open for at least for 2 minutes after closing the outer door. This allows time for the material being transferred inside the process chamber to be disinfected. Any product entering a pharmaceutical cabinet is wiped and sprayed several times using sterile wipes impregnated with 70 per cent isopropanol and sterile 70 per cent alcohol sprays.

The pressure inside an isolator can be higher than the room in which the device is sited (positive pressure isolators) or lower (negative pressure isolators).

Commissioning of cabinets (validation) is necessary to ensure their integrity and safety. Cabinets require regularly particle counting to make sure that the particulate matter in the HEPA filtered cabinets are within the set limits for a class A environment.

Tests are done on safety LFC to ensure that particles created inside the cabinet will not leak out to compromise the worker's safety (iodine disk test).

Similarly, the gloves of the isolators are checked on a daily basis to ensure their integrity. Isolators are leak-tested (pressure decay test) regularly to check the integrity of their bodies.

Laminar flow cabinets and isolators are cleaned regularly using sterile disinfectants to rid the cabinet of any bacteria and fungi, including their spores. Microbiological swabs and active air samplings are taken and contact plates are used to monitor the cabinets microbiologically.

During product manufacture, petri dishes with culture media are exposed inside the cabinets to monitor the microbiological status of the workstation. Operators are asked to dab their fingers on to the plates at the end of the work session for monitoring the cleanliness of their hands (the closest to the point of fill) during the work. The workers are trained in aseptic techniques and should perform several broth transfer tests annually to prove their dexterity.

Broth simulation exercises are used to validate a given aseptic procedure where, instead of the starting materials, double-strength broth and sterile distilled water will be used and the manufacturing procedure followed. The broth in the final container is incubated and checked for the lack of microbial growth if the procedure is to be validated.

QUALITY ASSURANCE

Quality assurance comprises steps taken to ensure the quality of a product and embraces all the stages of design, manufacture, distribution and storage of a pharmaceutical product. To ensure the quality of a product, good manufacturing practice requires buying the starting materials and containers from reputable suppliers and manufacturing the products in suitable facilities according to well-defined procedures (Sharp, 2000). Other requirements would include having a well-trained workforce and having the raw materials and manufactured products sampled, tested and analysed (quality control). Manufactured products should have suitable containers with proper labelling. However, quality assurance would go further, as the storage and distribution conditions should be appropriate to the product's requirements (Beaney, 2006).

SHELF-LIFE

Giving a product a shelf-life is intended to ensure that maximum product quality is maintained in the time interval between manufacture and use. For the majority of products, the general standard is that the product is not contaminated at the time of administration and contains not less than 90 per cent of the stated content of the active ingredient. This is determined by the physico-chemical stability tests on the product, and the risk of microbial contamination during reconstitution and administration. The physicochemical stability of a product can be influenced by the storage temperature, light, the pH of the product, the concentration of the drug, the formulation of the product and the final container.

Proprietary preparations, stored according to the manufacturer's recommendations, can be used until their expiry date. For products requiring refrigeration, there must be confidence that the cold chain has not been broken. If a breach does occur, an informed decision on whether to continue to use the stock should be made based on knowledge of the product's stability and its intended use. For preserved products, such as eye drops, used for inpatients within the hospital, a 2-week expiry is recommended once the product is opened. For oral mixtures, a 7–10 day expiry is usually recommended. Reconstituted injections should be administered immediately and any excess discarded. In some cases, if recommended by the manufacturer, reconstituted injections may be stored in a refrigerator (2–8°C) for up to 24 hours. The Farwell report (Farwell, 1995) allows aseptic medicinal products prepared under direct supervision of a pharmacist in an unlicensed unit to have up to 7 days of expiry, provided there is physicochemical stability evidence present.

STORAGE OF MEDICINAL PRODUCTS

Consideration must be given to the infrastructure of the pharmacy department to ensure appropriate storage conditions to avoid the degradation of medicinal products, contamination with micro-organisms or risks associated with spillage of medicinal products. Sufficient room is required to store thermolabile medicinal products at the appropriate temperature. All stock should be protected from extremes of temperature, exposure to direct sunlight and atmospheric moisture. When large quantities of bulky or heavy medicinal products are stockpiled, a full health and safety assessment should be undertaken. Systems should be in place to monitor storage conditions and expiry dates, and ensure appropriate stock rotation occurs. Storage areas should be kept clean and tidy.

Medicinal products may be stored in a variety of locations, such as the pharmacy department, a ward, a clinic or an operating theatre. Medicinal products vary in their particular storage requirements, so attention must be paid to the storage facilities at the final destination; dedicated storage areas should be assigned and maintained.

For medicinal products requiring refrigeration, a dedicated fridge must be available to store these products. This fridge must be maintained only for the storage of medicinal products; food and drinks must not be stored in this fridge. The fridge should be fitted with a thermometer, which must be monitored regularly to ensure the fridge operates within the required temperature range. Pharmacists have an important role to play in ensuring that medicines that require refrigeration and are used in wards, theatres or clinics, are stored appropriately.

TRANSPORT AND DISTRIBUTION OF MEDICINAL PRODUCTS

For medicinal products that require refrigeration, delays in transporting the products to the end-user department may result in products being stored above their recommended temperature for significant periods of time. Steps must be taken to ensure that transport occurs in a timely fashion, and the risk of temperature fluctuation is minimized. This may be achieved by using refrigerated transport, or simply using cool boxes with ice packs to maintain the required temperature.

Whatever transport medium is used, the transport containers must be fit for purpose, be appropriate to the medicinal product and must be able to contain potential spillages. Provision should be made for dealing with spillages of potentially hazardous products. Records should be kept of all medicinal products received by the pharmacy department, or prepared in-house, as well as the end-user areas to which they are distributed.

In addition to ensuring the production, storage and supply of sterile and non-sterile medicinal products, clinical pharmacists have an important role to play. This involves advising on the choice of medicines used for patients, to ensure optimal benefit to the patient is achieved. This can include advice on antibiotic choice, appropriate switch from intravenous drugs and infusions to alternative oral products and reminders to stop antibiotics when a treatment course is complete. This serves to reduce unnecessary antibiotic consumption, reduce the use of intravenous medicinal products and ensure appropriate treatment. Taken in context with other infection control measures, such activity may help to reduce the incidence of healthcare-associated infection.

Sterile services department

Adam Fraise and Christina Bradley

The function of the sterile services department (SSD) is to supply a range of sterilized or disinfected items to operating-theatres, wards and other units, and to healthcare establishments (e.g. community health centres). The manager is responsible for monitoring all decontamination processes, and for ensuring that all protocols for the handling and processing of equipment meet the required standards. Records must be kept of tests of efficacy of sterilizers and of all sterilization cycles and decontaminating processes. These records must be related to packs issued to users (Institute of Decontamination Science, 2007a, b).

The SSD is also responsible for the safe and effective processing of re-usable medical equipment, preventing any risk of transfer of infection or other risk to patients or staff. The responsibility for re-use of expensive 'high-risk', single-use items (e.g. cardiac catheters) is ultimately that of the user, with advice on processing and packaging from the Infection Control Team (ICT) and the SSD manager. This practice for 'single-use', high-risk items is rarely endorsed by government agencies in developed countries. Reprocessing of low-risk, single-use items is more often carried out if it is cost effective and the process conforms to recommended protocols, for example, the Medicines and Healthcare Products Regulatory Agency (MHRA, 2006). As the hospital and processor as well as the user may also be legally responsible for the safety of re-processing, it is advisable, particularly for single-use items, for decisions on whether an item is suitable for re-processing and what is an appropriate protocol to be taken by a re-processing committee (see Chapter 2). The advice in the UK is that items intended for single use should not be reused (MHRA, 2006)

The SSD must develop good communications with the users (i.e. medical and nursing staff), and should remain a clinical service as well as an efficient distribution and cost-effective processing unit. The manager should be a member of relevant committees (e.g. theatre users, reprocessing of single-use items and control of infection). Communication is essential with theatre staff, infection control and the estates department.

Central supply services were developed in the USA, and the first purpose-built civilian central sterile supply department in the UK was opened in Belfast in 1958. Since then there have been many developments, including the addition of independent sections or units, such as a theatre sterile supply unit and a hospital sterilization and disinfection unit (HSDU). The latter unit processes items of medical equipment (e.g. respiratory ventilators, suction pumps and respiratory circuits and infant incubators). Periodic maintenance and instrument calibration may be carried out (e.g. by medical engineers either in the unit or in an adjacent area). This should be done after decontamination and before the items are returned for use. Processing of respiratory ventilators is now infrequently required, as they are protected by filters and patient circuitry is autoclavable. Babies' incubators are usually processed in a room in the clinical area. The requirement for a specialized HSDU has therefore decreased, but it is important that staff who carry out local re-processing in other parts of the hospital have received appropriate training.

In the UK, many SSDs are being centralized to 'off-site' centres, which will provide a service to numerous trusts and hospitals, and possibly primary care facilities.

The present SSDs have rationalized their function and now obtain a large range of sterile procedure packs, dressings and single-use supplementary instruments from commercial sources.

With the introduction of consumer legislation, recent European Community Directives and the loss of crown immunity, departments should operate good manufacturing practices, which should be in accordance with existing guidelines and practices, such as those produced by the Institute of Sterile Supplies Management (1989, Institute of Decontamination Science, 2007b) and the Medical Devices Agency (1993, 1996, 1999, 2006). The European Medical

Devices Directive 93/42/EEC indicates that an SSD which supplies products to another organization (e.g. another hospital or healthcare establishment) is considered to be a manufacturer of the product and should fulfil the requirements of the Directive. If the product is approved under the Directive, it can be labelled with the CE mark. Although most of the recommendations of the good manufacturing practice (GMP) and other standard documents are acceptable, some of them are considered rather excessive in terms of microbiological requirements, especially routine sampling (Atfield, 1991), for example in rooms used for packing instruments and dressings, which will subsequently be sterilized. However, packs should be assembled in a room, which is as clean and dust free as is reasonably practicable. Inadequate cleaning of instruments could be associated with a much greater bioburden on an instrument than exposure to unfiltered air. Appropriately controlled conditions are necessary to meet the European Directive, but these are not defined. However, quality systems to meet the Directive are available (BS EN 46001; BS EN 46002, British Standards Institution, 1976).

Manufacturers are legally responsible for providing instructions on the decontamination of reusable equipment under the Medical Devices Directive 93/42/EEC (European Union, 1995). The instructions should include compatibility with decontamination methods and instructions on assembly and disassembly of the instruments. EN 17664 (British Standards Institution, 2004) describes the information to be provided by the supplier of the reusable medical device.

DESIGN OF DEPARTMENTS AND WORK FLOW

The design features for an SSD are described in HBN 13 (NHS Estates, 2004). The design provides for two distinct flow lines:

- for routine processing of surgical instruments/utensils; and
- for medical equipment.

The typical work flow for surgical instruments and utensils is as follows:

1 sorting, washing, heat disinfection and drying;
2 inspection, setting trays and assembling packs;
3 sterilization;
4 transfer to sterile goods store;
5 distribution to wards and other units.

The work flow should be in one direction only, and all stages of the decontamination process should be documented (Medical Devices Agency, 1993, 1996, 1999, 2006).

Other medical equipment is similarly treated, but may require stripping down to component parts before cleaning, re-assembling and checking after processing.

COLLECTION AND RETURN OF USED EQUIPMENT TO THE STERILE SERVICES DEPARTMENT

Equipment should be effectively contained so that there is no risk to personnel during transport to the SSD. Single-use items should be correctly disposed of by the user, especially sharps (e.g. needles and blades), and not returned with re-processable equipment. Delicate items must be well protected. Body fluids in suction bottles or hollow-ware should preferably be discarded by the user. Used surgical instruments are commonly returned in sets in their original trays or metal boxes, and are checked before processing. The reception area in the SSD should be separate from clean areas and have readily cleanable surfaces.

PROCESSING PROCEDURES FOR USED EQUIPMENT

Sterile services staff (and most other health service staff) have become increasingly concerned about the hazard of acquiring hepatitis B virus and human immunodeficiency virus infection, despite the extremely low risk. However, staff must assume that there is a possibility of infection from any used item that is returned to the SSD. The risk can be reduced by wearing gloves (household), visors and plastic aprons when handling all items, particularly those that are bloodstained, and exercising care when handling sharp instruments. Any existing cuts or damaged skin on the hands should be covered with a waterproof dressing, and the hands should be thoroughly washed after removal of gloves. All staff handling potentially contaminated instruments or equipment should be immunized against hepatitis B.

Known high-risk equipment should be decontaminated as soon as possible after receipt with minimal handling. All returned items that require cleaning should be disinfected by heat after cleaning (see also Chapter 6). Forceps and scissors require opening before washing in a machine to ensure penetration of the joints with cleaning agent and hot water. Some items (e.g. tubes or some items contaminated with secretions which have been subject to prolonged drying) may still require washing by hand. Chemical disinfection may be ineffective before cleaning and will thus give a false sense of security. Autoclaving before cleaning will coagulate protein, making it difficult to remove during subsequent washing. A washer–disinfector commissioned and monitored in accordance with BS2745 (British Standards Institution, 1993) and HTM 2030 (NHS Estates, 1997) is desirable, but cleaning by hand or in an ultrasonic machine should be a safe procedure, if it is carried out by trained staff wearing the correct protective clothing. The choice of methods for dealing with contaminated items must be made by the manager in association with the ICT. Washer–disinfectors are also of considerable value for processing anaesthetic and respiratory equipment, as the items can then be dried and packaged without further treatment.

Routine decontamination procedures should be sufficient for equipment from high-infection risk patients, but it may be advisable for SSD managers to be informed of any unusual hazard.

TESTING OF WASHER–DISINFECTORS AND STERILIZERS

If washer–disinfectors are to be used for the decontamination of high-risk items, agreement should be reached with the ICT on what is an acceptable process. Cleaning efficacy and time/temperature parameters should be checked when commissioning washer–disinfectors and at periodic intervals [BS2745 (British Standards Institution, 1993), BS EN ISO 15883 (British Standards Institution, 2006), HTM 2030 (NHS Estates, 1997), HTM 2010 (Department of Health, 1995); see also Chapter 5]. Routine microbiological testing other than possibly during commissioning should be unnecessary if the process is well controlled and monitored. Sterilizers should be routinely monitored according to HTM 2010 (Department of Health, 1994) and the Medical Devices Agency (1993, 1996, 1999, 2006).

QUALITY SYSTEMS AND AUDIT

Fulfilling the requirements for good manufacturing practice and conducting internal audits by SSD managers, possibly with a member of the ICT, will provide evidence of a quality service. However, external assessment and audit by a certification body is being increasingly required for evidence of conformation with quality standards for the BS EN ISO 9002 (British Standards Institution, 1994) quality systems model; for quality assurance in productions, installations, servicing and EN 46002 (specification for application of EN ISO 9002 to the manufacture of medical devices) and other regulations and requirements to comply with the Medical Devices Directive. External assessment is not required if products are not sold to other establishments.

RETURNING EQUIPMENT FOR SERVICING OR REPAIR

It is a requirement of the Department of Health that certificates are issued stating that equipment returned for servicing or repair is microbiologically safe (MHRA, 2005). However, it is not always possible to ensure that the internal surfaces of some items of equipment have been adequately decontaminated. It may also be necessary to return equipment that has not been decontaminated due to failure in use (e.g. an endoscope with a blocked channel). In these circumstances, a note should be attached to the returned equipment indicating safe methods of handling and suitable decontamination methods.

All single-use components should be removed and discarded as clinical waste. Non-disposable components should be cleaned and preferably autoclaved (if heat tolerant) or disinfected in a washing machine. If this is not possible, immersion in a disinfectant such as 70 per cent ethanol, a solution of a chlorine-releasing agent (1000 ppm available chlorine) or a peroxygen compound is acceptable provided that it is effective against the probable contaminating organisms and compatible with the surface (see Chapters 5 and 6 for a choice of disinfectants, and the advantages and disadvantages of their use).

Following immersion, items should be thoroughly rinsed and dried. If there are difficulties in decontaminating the internal surfaces, all external surfaces should be cleaned before returning an item to the manufacturer. Maintenance staff should be provided with suitable protective clothing, disinfectants and decontamination equipment. They should also be trained in handling and disinfection procedures.

Ambulance service

Avril Weaver

INTRODUCTION

The infection status of the vast majority of patients conveyed by ambulance will be unknown. However, patients known or suspected to be suffering from an infectious disease need to be looked after with sensitivity and compassion, irrespective of the risks that the infection may carry.

All staff should approach this important part of ambulance service work with a good grasp of the principles of infection control as well as a reasonable understanding of the nature of any infections from which patients may be suffering. Over-reaction to infectious disease can cause alarm, feelings of isolation or rejection in the patient. Under-reaction may lead to the risk of infection not only to ambulance staff, but also to other patients and persons.

It is normal practice, where a patient's infection status is known and there are no confidentiality issues, that this information should be available to ambulance staff. However, standard principles for infection control should be used at all times, so it is rarely necessary to know whether patients are carrying an infection and, if they are, the exact diagnosis.

On the occasions that ambulance crews are required to transfer patients with open wounds (e.g. external fixators, etc.), advice should be sought from the hospital's Infection Control Team. This is to ensure that the intended journey plan is compatible with the needs of both the patient, and any other patients who may be travelling at the same time.

In general, very few infectious patients require special procedures or action by ambulance staff, other than closely following the principles of standard precautions (see Chapter 13). Equally, the majority of patients do not require the provision of special travel arrangements, as these are normally only necessary in high-risk (e.g. Category 4) cases.

As a consequence, the need to convey patients with infections routinely as a single patient journey is now negated. Similarly, there is no longer any justification to restrict the travel of these patients to accident and emergency (A&E) ambulances only, as the principles of exercising standard precautions apply equally to staff of the Patient Transport Service.

TRAINING

Basic

While infection control is included as a module of the 'basic training' for technicians and paramedics, provision should also be made at induction for those working in other parts of the service, for example, station and vehicle cleaners (external contactors are responsible for their own employees training), control room operatives, information management and maintenance staff. The detail of this training should be appropriate to the level of risk for each group.

All ambulance service personnel should receive education on the basics of infection control at induction, which includes: effective hand hygiene, personal hygiene, appropriate use of personal protective equipment, handling and disposal of used sharps, linen and waste, management of blood or body-fluid spillage, cleaning and decontamination of equipment, preparation and use of disinfectants with the emphasis on Control of Substances Hazardous to Health regulations (Health and Safety Executive, 1999a) and occupational safety (i.e. immunization schedules and the importance of prompt reporting of accidents/incidents, particularly those following accidental inoculation injuries). Infection control updates should also be included as part of annual mandatory training.

Training for operational staff should also incorporate details on management of communicable diseases. This again can be tailored to the risks involved (i.e. those working on emergency vehicles, patient transport and control room staff).

Chemical, biological, radiation and nuclear

Further extensive training on chemical, biological, radiation and nuclear exposure should be provided for operational staff to ensure they are prepared for the unknown and unexpected, particularly on the issue of deliberate release. Training should cover potential viruses, toxins and weaponized organisms, transmission routes and methods of decontamination, with an emphasis on maintaining normal hygiene precautions at all times.

Resources

All staff should have access to infection control guidelines, such as the *Basic training manual of the Ambulance Service* (Institute of Health and Care

Development, 1999) and the *UK Joint Royal Colleges Liaison Committee clinical guidelines* (Ambulance Service Association, 2004). Training resources are constantly being developed to meet the specific needs of the service (e.g. 'e-learning, self-assessment tools and distance learning) all of which need to be assessed for accessibility and suitability. There should also be suitable access to an occupational health service.

PROCEDURES FOR SPECIFIC COMMUNICABLE DISEASES

Gastrointestinal diseases

When dealing with patents who have diarrhoea (with or without vomiting), staff should adopt standard precautions. These include the wearing of gloves and disposable aprons when staff are performing hands-on care, environment cleaning or decontamination. Other than closely adhering to these precautions, there are no special procedures required for the management and conveyance of these patients. The environment needs to be cleaned and decontaminated with a suitable disinfectant (e.g. chlorine-releasing agent) after such a patient has been transported.

Hepatitis B and C and human immunodeficiency virus

Other than closely adhering to standard precautions, there are no special procedures required for the management and conveyance of these patients. If there is a blood spillage, then this needs to be decontaminated, ideally with a chlorine-releasing agent in granule form.

Tuberculosis

Patients with tuberculosis (TB) should be cared in an environment that protects staff. This will usually require appropriate ventilation and the adoption of standard precautions (see Chapter 13). Even minimal ventilation in an ambulance will provide a very high rate of air changes, thus avoiding the need for the use of masks by ambulance staff in the majority of patients. Ventilation in ambulances can be provided by turning the ventilation fan on (the minimum setting should be adequate) and this should be done when the vehicle is stationary for longer than a few seconds (Interdepartmental Working Group on Tuberculosis, 1998).

Infectious patients (e.g. those with open pulmonary TB, who have not completed 2 weeks' treatment) with an uncontrolled cough should wear a surgical facemask, if available, or cough into disposable tissues. The exception to this is where the patient is infected with multi-drug resistant tuberculosis (see Chapter 12), in which case masks satisfying the requirements of the FFP3 standard should be worn. Any masks, be they surgical or FFP3 must be carefully discarded as clinical waste, followed by careful attention to handwashing procedures. Face masks are for single use only, and should be discarded as clinical waste on completion of the assignment. This also applies to single-use respiratory equipment (e.g. masks, oxygen, suction and intubation tubing, etc.).

If a patient has been prone to episodes of unprotected coughing and sneezing whilst in the ambulance, local cleaning and disinfection is appropriate. This should include wiping over those areas that have been in close proximity to the patient, using a detergent solution or detergent wipes followed by the appropriate disinfectant (see Chapter 6). Particular attention should be given to horizontal surfaces, as these are where droplets from an aerosol origin are likely to settle. All used tissues, cleaning/disinfection materials and disposable items of PPE should be discarded as hazardous waste and placed in a yellow waste bag (see Chapter 7).

Methicillin-resistant *Staphylococcus aureus*/extended spectrum β-lactamase-producing Gram-negative organisms.

Infection caused by these organisms poses no special hazard to ambulance personnel or their relatives. Standard infection precautions should be applied and are sufficient to provide a safe environment.

Infestations – scabies, lice, fleas

The best means of defence to safeguard against infestation is by the use of standard precautions. This dictates that high standards of personal hygiene must be maintained at all times, particularly with regard to handwashing procedures. Disposable gloves should be worn if there is any suspicion of infestation, together with a disposable apron, if necessary.

In general, following transport of a patient with an infestation, no specific cleaning of the vehicle is required, other than close attention to the area immediately occupied by the patient. This will involve utilizing a detergent cleaner on the seat or trolley mattress, as well as the adjacent wall and floor surfaces.

In cases where the patient is visibly infested with fleas, crews may wish to request a return to the station for a shower and uniform change. This would normally follow confirmation of an infestation by hospital staff; as such conditions usually become evident as the patient is undressed.

Category 4 disease (smallpox, viral hemorrhagic fever)

Diseases requiring Category 4 infection control measures are extremely rare in the UK. Most patients who could have a Category 4 disease are likely to present to A&E departments either directly or via their general practitioner. The patient will present with pyrexia (fever) of unknown origin shortly after having returned from abroad, but these early symptoms could indicate any number of far less serious conditions and a positive diagnosis can only be made following extensive tests. It is therefore likely that A&E crews may already have had contact with such patients before their illness is formally diagnosed. The Advisory Committee on Dangerous Pathogens have issued guidance that most pre-diagnosis Category 4 patients can be safely managed by following Standard Principles of Infection Control and the safe disposal of clinical waste. Any resuscitation regimen must include the use of either the bag and mask, or resuscitation pack. Under no circumstances should any form of direct oral resuscitation be carried out. However, should a Category 4 disease be subsequently diagnosed, the attending ambulance crew will be required to undergo surveillance for a period of 21 days from the last possible date of exposure to infection. There need be no restriction on work or movement within the UK, surveillance will entail daily monitoring of body temperature and the reporting of any suspicious symptoms.

Decontamination

There is limited space for equipment on vehicles and, crews often only have access to water and detergent when at station or visiting A&E departments. It is appropriate therefore that all vehicles are equipped with disposable detergent wipes, alcohol wipes and 'spill kits' containing sodium dichloroisocyanourate (NaDCC) granules and tablets to deal with blood spillages and an absorbent compound for other body fluid spillages.

Hands

Handwashing facilities are not always accessible to operational staff and therefore alcohol hand gel should be readily available at all times as personal issue. It must be remembered that alcohol hand gel is not effective on soiled hands and, in such instances, washing with soap and water will be necessary. If access to washing facilities is not available, detergent wipes should be used. All staff should be aware that the wearing of jewellery, nail varnish and acrylic nails impedes effective hand hygiene, and that any lesions should be kept covered.

Equipment

Prior to purchasing any piece of vehicle equipment, it is essential to check that it can be easily cleaned and decontaminated and withstand cleaning chemicals (this should include all carry bags, e.g. paramedic bags). All sterile equipment used by ambulance staff should, where possible, be designated as 'single use' and disposed of in accordance with waste regulations immediately after use.

Other contaminated equipment will require cleaning and/or disinfection to render it safe for re-use. This should be undertaken as soon as is practically possible after use (i.e. before use on the next patient or prior to storage). It is important to follow agreed procedures for cleaning and disinfection, and guidance on the safe use of chemicals involved. Staff using equipment should be familiar with the manufacturer's recommendations for cleaning individual items. Any items that are heavily soiled and unable to be decontaminated effectively should be disposed of in line with Trust policy. Complex items that need to be sent for repair should be decommissioned and will need to be sent for repair accompanied by a 'decontamination certificate'. This certificate which outlines whether the item is safe from an infection control viewpoint and, if not, how it should be decontaminated.

Vehicle

As it is not possible to identify all infected patients, standard precautions should be adopted (see Chapter 13). However, as blood and body fluids are important sources of infection, ambulance crews must be familiar with the techniques used to disinfect areas that have become contaminated with such material. Other than general day-to-day cleaning activities, the only areas that will require disinfection are those where blood or body-fluid contamination has occurred.

Interior of the vehicle

The nature of ambulance work is such that interior surfaces are prone to becoming dirty and dusty during normal everyday use. If not cleaned regularly, dirt can accumulate, which creates an ideal environment for micro-organisms to survive and grow. It is therefore important that all staff contribute to keeping the ambulance clean, and thus help to reduce the risks of cross-infection to themselves, their colleagues and their patients. This can best be accomplished by all participating in frequent and routine cleaning activities.

During each shift, all interior surfaces that become directly contaminated should be cleaned as soon as possible (in between patient use). This process must always include the use of detergent as the primary cleaning agent, followed by the use of an appropriate disinfectant, if the contamination is likely to contain either blood or body fluids. It is also advisable to provide as much ventilation as possible during cleaning activities, so ambulance doors and windows should be opened accordingly.

In addition, regular 'damp dusting' should be undertaken throughout the shift. This simply involves cleaning the area with detergent wipes, paying particularly attention to the horizontal surfaces in the ambulance, as well as all fixtures and fittings that are regularly handled.

The ambulance floor should be mopped clean on a regular basis throughout the shift. As the floor carries a comparatively low risk of cross-infection, this does not require disinfection and cleaning with hot water and a detergent is sufficient. However, if blood or body fluids have been involved, then disinfection with a chlorine-releasing agent (or suitable equivalent) should take place. In addition all ambulance interiors should be adequately cleaned on a weekly basis. In addition all ambulance interiors should be adequately cleaned on a weekly basis. This would be a good time to ensure stock times are rotated and used within use-by dates.

Detachable items should first be removed in order that all surfaces can be accessed. When cleaning and disinfecting the interior, ensure that appropriate items of PPE are worn, and that doors and windows have been opened, if a disinfectant with strong odour is used (e.g. chlorine-releasing agents). Detachable items which have already been removed should be cleaned (and disinfected, if appropriate) prior to being re-positioned in the vehicle. The process of drying is an important element of good infection control, so this should be aided wherever possible by leaving the vehicle in a well-ventilated position.

It is recognized that operational demands may restrict opportunities for the weekly clean to be undertaken as a singular activity at a designated time. This factor is further complicated by local shift patterns and vehicle resourcing issues; therefore, vehicle cleaning arrangements must be devised and agreed at station level.

Ambulance stations

The role of domestic cleaning on station premises is normally undertaken by staff employed for this purpose. Cleaning schedules and specifications should be clearly set out to meet the needs of the station, with particular focus on kitchens, handwashing facilities, toilets and shower facilities. Cleaning staff should be provided with the appropriate PPE, disposable colour-coded cleaning materials (with clear instruction on the decontamination methods for re-usable items) and appropriate storage facilities for the safe containment of cleaning materials.

FURTHER READING (AMBULANCE SERVICE)

Ambulance Service Association (ASA) (2004) *National Guidance and Procedures for Infection, Prevention and Control – Managing Healthcare Associated Infection and Control of Serious Communicable Diseases in Ambulance Services.*

Fisher JD, Brown SN, Cooke M (2006) *UK Ambulance Service Clinical Practice Guidelines.* Joint Royal Colleges Ambulance Service Liaison Committee. www.jrcalc.org.uk

Institute of Health and Care Development (1999) *The Ambulance Service: Basic Training Manual.*

Pathology laboratories

Adam Fraise and Christina Bradley

Reports of outbreaks of laboratory-acquired infection and the introduction of the Health and Safety at Work Act (1974) and Health Services Commission (1988) have been followed by the publication of guidelines from several committees and other publications. As new evidence emerges, these guidelines continue to be modified (Collins and Kennedy, 1999; Health and Safety Executive, 2003).

The Advisory Committee on Dangerous Pathogens (ACDP) has classified organisms into four hazard and containment categories (ACDP, 2004). Category 1 includes agents unlikely to cause human disease, and requires no special precautions. Category 2 includes most organisms isolated in clinical laboratories, and requires good microbiological practice. Category 3 includes organisms of special risk to laboratory workers (e.g. *Salmonella typhi* and *Mycobacterium tuberculosis*), and requires special containment facilities. Category 4 includes organisms that are extremely hazardous to laboratory workers and which may cause serious epidemic disease (e.g. Lassa, Ebola and Marburg viruses), which require particularly stringent containment. It is recognized that Category 3 organisms may be isolated in routine laboratories, and on identification subsequent work on them must be carried out in the appropriate containment category. Modified requirements are adequate for handling samples from patients with hepatitis B virus (HBV) or HIV antibody, but work in a cabinet may be preferred. These viruses are transferred by contact with blood and not by the airborne route.

The recommendations in these codes and guidelines are extensive and demand much from the laboratory worker and also from those who design or direct laboratories. They comprise all the sensible and feasible precautions that need to be taken in diagnostic clinical (and research) laboratories, although no code of practice can prevent infections due to negligence or poor technique of the laboratory worker. Everyone who works in a pathology department must develop habits of safe and careful technique. However, precautions against laboratory-acquired infection should be reasonable and, whenever possible, based on scientific or clinical evidence. Rituals should be discouraged. For example, ventilated rooms cannot be expected to influence the transmission of blood-borne infections such as HBV or HIV, or organisms transferred by the faecal–oral route, such as *Salmonella typhi*.

SPECIAL RISKS OF INFECTION

There are several ways in which the pathology department may be involved in the spread of infection in hospital. Patients are at risk from infection carried from the laboratory by laboratory staff collecting specimens in wards or outpatient departments, and may also be infected by procedures performed by the technician involving transfer of microbes from one patient to another. Laboratory staff are at risk both from patients and from specimens of biological material and cultures examined in the laboratory. This risk to laboratory staff from biological specimens is in practice the most likely to have serious consequences. Many risks are well known and precautions are taken to prevent spread, but infections can also arise from unsuspected sources (e.g. a request form contaminated by faeces and handled by clerical staff, or serum containing HBV examined in the biochemistry department).

There are many routes by which infections are acquired in pathology departments (e.g. infected aerosols or sprays generated from pipetting or pouring liquids in the laboratory may be inhaled by workers, or HBV or HIV may enter through skin abrasions). Tuberculosis and HBV have been particularly important in hospital and laboratory infections in the UK, but HBV has been acquired less in microbiological than in biochemical and haematology laboratories. In recent years, such infections have become less frequent as a result of better training in safe working. There is no evidence that HIV has been transferred to laboratory workers from clinical samples, but despite the very low risk of transmission, HIV infection is such a dangerous infection that particular care is necessary. In general, it is not usually a specimen that is already known to be infective that causes an infection, but one which is not suspected of being dangerous. Some areas (e.g. animal houses, tuberculosis laboratories and hospital mortuaries) are especially hazardous and require special precautions.

Prevention of infection

All samples should be handled with care (e.g. transported in sealed plastic bags and handled with disposable gloves), as the diagnosis may not be known until laboratory tests have been completed. However, many laboratories still label high-risk specimens (containing category 3 pathogens) as 'biohazard' or 'danger of infection', although this should not be necessary. Specimens must be received in an area used exclusively for this purpose. The general office can be used if the reception area is separated from the clerical area. Staff handling specimens should be adequately trained. A hand wash-basin with pedal or elbow taps should be readily available, as well as appropriate materials and disinfectants for cleaning up any spillage, and a container for disposal of spillage.

Laboratory staff, including phlebotomists, visiting the wards should be trained in barrier-nursing techniques, and must follow the instructions for handling infected patients carefully. Advice on protection against bloodborne infections in the workplace is given by ACDP (1995).

TRANSPORT OF SPECIMENS

Attention should be given to the containers used to transport specimens from patient areas to laboratories. The specimen containers should be leakproof, robust and transported in trays or boxes, which will hold the specimens upright. Laboratories generally seal all specimens in plastic bags with a pocket to keep the forms free from contamination. Simple, clear rules need to be formulated for staff who are involved in transporting specimens. Staff involved in the transport of specimens should be trained to cope with spillage. Transport of laboratory specimens should comply with the Transport of Dangerous Goods Regulations (2004) and Postal Regulations (see http://www.opsi.gov.uk/si/si2007/uksi_20071573_en_1).

PROCEDURES WITHIN THE LABORATORY

Details of hazards and their avoidance are given in several publications (e.g. Collins and Kennedy, 1999). When specimens are handled, particular attention should be given to centrifuges and other possible sources of infective aerosols. Infected materials (e.g. slides and pipettes) should be discarded into jars containing a phenolic or chlorine-releasing disinfectant, which is replaced daily (see Chapters 5 and 6). Plastic pipettes should be used whenever possible to reduce the hazards of trauma when handling. The elimination of unnecessary glassware is one of the most important measures for reducing risks of bloodborne infection. Plastic petri dishes involve problems of disposal. If possible, they should be made safe before removal from the laboratory, and this is best achieved by autoclaving in a suitable container or in stainless-steel buckets. The resultant lumps of polyethylene can be handled by the refuse collectors, but should be kept in sealed plastic bags. Difficulties have arisen when plates have been discarded without treatment and subsequently appear on local refuse sites. Incineration, preferably on site, without prior autoclaving is acceptable, provided that the waste is effectively contained during transport. Incineration of plastic plates in bulk may lead to an unacceptable level of smoke pollution. Used glass petri dishes should be autoclaved by trained staff before being handled by domestics. Other glass containers (e.g. bijou bottles containing infective material) should be similarly autoclaved before leaving the laboratory, whether they are going to be reprocessed or disposed of.

Care is needed during selection of the container for autoclaving. Failure to remove air from bags or buckets is likely to cause failure of decontamination. Various designs of containers are available that facilitate removal of air. Sterilizing temperatures are usually recommended, but are rarely required to achieve adequate decontamination, unless the work of the laboratory involves spore-bearing organisms that are hazardous to workers (e.g. *Bacillus anthracis,*

Clostridium tetani or *Clostridium botulinum*). It is important that temperatures in the coolest part of the load are regularly checked with thermocouples.

IMMUNIZATION OF LABORATORY STAFF

Infections against which immunization should be offered to laboratory staff include tuberculosis, poliomyelitis and tetanus. Hepatitis B vaccine should be offered to all laboratory staff who handle clinical specimens, and may be a condition of employment if the member of staff is involved in invasive procedures. Female staff should also be offered rubella vaccination, preferably after testing their immune state. Tuberculin-negative staff, who have been given BCG (bacille Calmette–Guérin) must be excluded from work with material that contains or is likely to contain tubercle bacilli until conversion has taken place (British Thoracic Society, 2000). Other protective measures should be strongly encouraged to all staff on joining the laboratory (see Chapter 11).

TRAINING AND INSTRUCTIONS FOR STAFF

Training of staff in aseptic procedures and in methods of handling infected material is part of the routine education in microbiology departments. In most hospitals, the various branches of pathology recruit their own staff and, as multidisciplinary training is now rare, there is often no opportunity for biochemists or technicians to acquire experience in microbiology departments. In these cases, some basic instruction should be given on methods of spread of infection, aseptic procedures and handling of potentially infected biological or toxic materials. The Code of Practice and other relevant documents should be readily available for consultation. The COSHH regulations (Health Services Commission, 1988) apply to micro-organisms as well as to toxic chemicals, and each laboratory should produce its own Safety Code, which includes the most important rules.

PRECAUTIONS AGAINST LABORATORY INFECTION

The following is an example of such information given to laboratory staff:

'Any specimen entering the laboratory may be infectious, and some will certainly contain the agents that cause HBV, hepatitis C virus (HCV) and HIV infection, typhoid, tuberculosis and other infections. Your own and your family's safety, and that of your colleagues, depend on observing the following instructions.'

General

There must be no smoking, no eating and no drinking in the laboratory. Keep your bench clean and tidy.

Wash your hands thoroughly on leaving the laboratory before taking food or drink or handling personal possessions, after handling specimens, after changing tubing or dialysers or diluters in the auto-analysers, and if you think you have contaminated them, thoroughly wash with soap and water. If contamination with bacterial cultures has occurred, and in 'high-risk' laboratories, use an antiseptic handwashing method. Thorough application of 70 per cent alcohol after washing is particularly effective.

Handwashing

This is your most important safeguard. Wear gloves when dealing with high-risk specimens or spillage. Wash hands after removing gloves (see Chapter 6).

Cuts and abrasions

Wash well in running water. Cover with waterproof protective dressing. If you splash your eye with serum or a culture, wash it thoroughly with saline or tap water. Report to the laboratory manager or their deputy at once, and enter the incident in the accident book (needlestick injuries must be entered and immediately reported).

Spilt specimens – treatment of contaminated area, floor or other surfaces

Swab with a chlorine-releasing agent containing 10 000 ppm available chlorine when cleaning up blood or organic materials that possibly contain viruses; 1000 ppm is adequate for small amounts of spillage or routine cleaning. Rinse well, particularly if a metal surface is involved. Thoroughly covering the spillage with a chlorine-releasing or peroxygen powder or granules before removal with paper towels is also effective. Do not use a chlorine-releasing powder or granules for large amounts of spillage, as excessive amounts of chlorine may be released. Wear gloves when handling contaminated materials or disinfectants.

Pipettes

Avoid mouth suction. Single-use pipettes may be preferable. Use automatic pipettes, rubber bulbs or teats. Discard all reusable pipettes into a chlorine-releasing solution – 0.25 per cent (2500 ppm available chlorine) – to cover them completely. It is preferable to use a jar with a screw lid.

Other equipment

Plastic disposables should be incinerated. Slides should be autoclaved in the discard jars in which they have been placed. Syringes and needles should be discarded into an approved container (see Chapter 7).

Centrifuging

Use only closed centrifuges with sealed buckets, which should be opened only within a protective exhaust cabinet if dangerous pathogens are involved or a breakage is suspected. Clean the centrifuge bowl with a detergent solution, dry and disinfect with 70 per cent alcohol. Wear disposable gloves. If a breakage occurs, autoclave the bucket and its contents. Disinfect the bowl as described above.

White coats

A plentiful supply of white coats is necessary. Coats must be changed immediately if they become contaminated, all coats should be treated as infected linen in the laundry, and coats known to be contaminated with particularly hazardous pathogens should be autoclaved in the laboratory autoclave. Fully protective coats should be worn when handling Category 3 pathogens.

Do not wear your laboratory coat to visit the wards. Do not wear *any* white coat to visit the coffee room or toilet.

CONTAINMENT LEVEL 3 LABORATORIES

The room will contain a cabinet with exhaust ventilation that is filtered before discharge, usually to the outside (ACDP, 2001). The cabinet and system should be disinfected with formalin both before maintenance and after a spillage, and air flows should be regularly checked. The room itself should be sealable in the event of a spillage and possible fumigation (Health and Safety Executive, 2006). Gloves should be worn for all manipulations, and staff must be adequately trained in order to avoid a false sense of security when using a cabinet. Careful work on an open bench may often be safer, particularly if one is working with viruses such as HBV or HIV, which do not spread in the air. It is therefore recommended that for the clinical examination of samples containing HBV or HIV the work may be carried out at a defined workstation, which allows sufficient seclusion to avoid inoculation accidents.

A fully protective gown or plastic apron and a visor should be worn, as well as disposable gloves, for more dangerous manipulations. Staff must be adequately trained in the use of aseptic measures in addition to provision of this protective clothing, otherwise a false sense of security may lead to simple errors, which would not arise if gloves were not being worn.

Fungi

Cultures of fungi that cause communicable systemic infection (e.g. *Histoplasma*) should be processed in a ventilated cabinet, as recommended for tubercle bacilli.

POST-MORTEM ROOM AND MORTUARY

The dead body, whether previously infected or not, may be a source of infection, and mortuary and post-mortem staff are at risk. As in the ward, bacteria may spread by air or by contact, but there are special hazards when a post-mortem examination is being performed. Contaminated aerosols or splashes may be released through squeezing sponges; cutting tissues, such as the lung, or incising abscesses, and the sawing of bones may also release small contaminated chips into the air. Cutting or pricking a finger with a contaminated instrument or ragged bone edge is one of the commonest modes of infection. Although most organisms in the dead body are unlikely to infect healthy individuals with intact skin, there are some specific hazards.

Tubercle bacilli may be spread in large numbers in aerosols. Salmonella, shigella and other intestinal pathogens may be transmitted from the intestinal tract. Following a break in the skin of the operator, large numbers of *Staphylococcus aureus* or *Streptococcus pyogenes* may be introduced, and unless treatment with appropriate antibiotics is given promptly, these may cause a severe local infection and sometimes septicaemia. HBV, HCV or HIV introduced by a cut or needle-prick are a major potential hazard. The conjunctiva may be infected by splashes or aerosols, and a severe local infection may follow. Bloodborne viruses may also enter the body by this route (see Chapter 9).

The mortuary should be designed to provide dirty, clean and transition areas. The dirty area would include the post-mortem room, dirty utility room and refrigerated body store. The clean area would include reception and waiting areas, viewing rooms, stores, offices and post-mortem observation area.

(See also Health Services Advisory Committee, 2003.)

Prevention of infection

The risks of infection are not high if adequate precautions are taken. Cleanliness of the mortuary, refrigerator and post-mortem room, as well as good personal hygiene of members of staff, are essential. The post-mortem room should be mechanically ventilated and designed so that cleaning can be readily achieved. Fly-proofing arrangements in the mortuary and post-mortem room should be efficient. A shower, with soap and towels supplied, should be available for the post-mortem room staff. When performing post-mortem examinations, the pathologist and mortuary technicians should completely change their outer clothing, and a disposable plastic apron, disposable gloves and rubber boots should be worn. Clean white trousers, vests and jackets should be supplied daily, if possible, or at least several times a week or if they become contaminated. Visitors to the post-mortem room who are not going to be in close contact with the body should wear a gown and overshoes. A wash-basin with disposable paper towels, soap and an antiseptic handwashing preparation (povidone–iodine or chlorhexidine detergent, or 70 per cent ethanol) should be available in the post-mortem room.

Staff should wash their hands thoroughly after handling any contaminated surface or material, irrespective of whether gloves are worn, and always on leaving the post-mortem room. If the hands are likely to have become contaminated, they should also be washed before handling case-notes or any other clean items.

If the skin or eye is splashed, it should be thoroughly washed. An eyewash bottle containing sterile saline should be available. Any cut or finger-prick should be immediately reported to the pathologist, after thorough washing under running water. All pre-existing cuts or open lesions on the hands should be covered with a waterproof dressing. Open injuries, other than minor ones, should be treated in the casualty department.

Instruments should be routinely cleaned before disinfection, as the presence of organic matter may protect the organisms from the disinfectant. A small washer–disinfector is preferred, as washing by hand would be avoided. Chemical disinfectants may be used and should have a wide range of antimicrobial efficacy and be compatible with the instruments. After treatment with a disinfectant, all instruments should be rinsed and dried. For the disinfection and cleaning of instruments and the room used at autopsies of patients with infections caused by the agents of the transmissible spongiform encephalopathies, see below. The room and other equipment should be thoroughly cleaned after use with a chlorine-releasing agent (1000 ppm available chlorine or an alternative equally effective agent). If chlorine-releasing agents are used on metal surfaces, they should be rinsed immediately in order to avoid corrosion.

Linen should be sent in a sealed bag and treated as 'infected' by the laundry. Dressings, waste materials and body tissues should be sealed in plastic bags and treated as clinical waste.

Special precautions should be taken with certain infections. In post-mortem examinations of patients with untreated pulmonary tuberculosis, filter-type masks should be worn by operators. Post-mortems on patients with known or suspected HBV, HCV or HIV infection should be avoided unless absolutely essential (for general precautions, see Chapter 13). Special care is necessary to avoid cuts and needle-pricks.

Agents such as prions that cause transmissible spongiform encephalopathy (e.g. Creutzfeldt–Jakob disease) are relatively resistant to heat and are also resistant to most chemical disinfectants, especially aldehydes (ACDP, 2003). The environment should be disinfected with a strong chlorine-releasing solution (containing 0.25 per cent available chlorine), and blood should be mopped up with a solution containing 1 per cent (10 000 ppm) available chlorine or following the application of a chlorine-releasing powder. If the skin is contaminated, wash thoroughly with soap and water. Instruments should be autoclaved at 134°C for 18 min (e.g. six 3-min cycles) after thorough washing (see also

Chapter 6). Immersion in 2 M sodium hydroxide is a possible alternative if autoclaving is not possible (see p. **122**).

Formaldehyde used for the preservation of tissues is an effective antimicrobial agent. Thorough penetration should be ensured before handling, particularly if lesions are caused by potentially dangerous infections (e.g. tuberculosis, typhoid or hepatitis). It is ineffective against prions.

It is most important that the mortuary staff and undertakers should be informed about the bodies of patients who have died or were suffering from a communicable disease. These should be enclosed in a plastic bag, and it would be useful to attach a warning label to them in the ward. Training of mortuary staff in prevention of infection is also necessary. Immunization should be offered as for laboratory staff.

Dental practice

Andrew J Smith

BACKGROUND

There are several million episodes of dental treatment undertaken each year in the UK. The challenging aspect for infection control in dental practice lies in the diverse nature of the surgical procedures undertaken, the complexity and expense of items of equipment, the relatively high throughput of patients and the low numbers of staff employed in many practices, which necessitates many staff undertaking several different roles. Facing these challenges, it is surprising then that more incidents of cross-infection are not reported. There may, however, be several reasons for the under reporting of cross-infection in dental practice:

- lack of active surveillance data;
- lack of microbiological analysis of oral infections;
- asymptomatic infection/colonization.

There have been reports of transmission of infectious agents in dental practice such as hepatitis B (Hadler *et al.*, 1981; Reingold *et al.*, 1982; Shaw *et al.*, 1986), herpes simplex (Lewis, 2004), *Mycobacterium tuberculosis* (Smith *et al.*, 1982; Cleveland *et al.*, 1995), MRSA (Martin and Hardy, 1991) and respiratory tract viruses (Davies *et al.*, 1994). It would seem imprudent therefore to ignore the fundamental principles of good clinical practice and infection control merely on the limited data on outbreaks of infection in dental practice.

BASIC PRINCIPLES

The basic principles of infection control in dental practice can be explained by referring to the chain of infection, there are six links in the chain.

1. *The infectious agent*, which has the ability to cause disease. The infectious agent may be one of several different types of micro-organism such as viruses (e.g. hepatitis B), bacteria (e.g. *Staphylococcus aureus*) or fungi (yeast; e.g. *Candida albicans*). The infectious agent may form part of our normal resident flora (e.g. *Streptococcus anginosus*) or it may be overtly pathogenic (e.g. *Mycobacterium tuberculosis*). The likelihood of infection being caused will depend on the disease-causing ability of the micro-organism – its virulence potential. Virulence factors are substances produced from micro-organisms that increase the likelihood of infection (e.g. bacterial toxins). The health of the host (see the sixth chain link) will also affect the ability of the micro-organism to cause disease.

2. *The reservoir* refers to where the source of the microbe can be found (e.g. patients, staff or the surgery environment). The reservoir of infection may be endogenous (from within/on the patient) or exogenous (external source). An endogenous reservoir means that the source of the infection arises from our own bacterial flora – these micro-organisms usually do no harm but following a surgical operation gain access to the inside of our bodies; this may occur following dental surgery in the oral cavity.

An external reservoir of infection can comprise many different sources. It can be useful to divide these into active and passive reservoirs of infection. Active reservoirs are those where the number of micro-organisms can increase over time, for example, people incubating colds or ultrasonic baths containing dirty cleaning solutions. Passive reservoirs are those where the number of micro-organisms does not increase over time; these include environment areas such as work surfaces and door handles.

3. *The portal of exit* (means of escape) from the reservoir of infection. A common reservoir of infection is people; micro-organisms may escape from people in the form of excretions (stools, vomiting), secretions (body fluids – saliva), droplets (coughing, talking) and skin (skin cells). Other means of exit may be through poorly designed and operated decontamination equipment, for example, using ultrasonic baths without a lid.

4. *Mode of transmission* describes how the microbes are moved or transported from one site to another. The mode of transmission can be via a number of routes. This can include direct spread (e.g. the hands of dental staff), indirect spread (e.g. contaminated surgical instruments) or airborne spread (patients coughing or water-cooled high-speed dental instruments).

5. *Portal of entry* into the host. The portal of entry can be via a number of different routes, this could include surgical treatment, a needlestick injury or through inhalation (influenza), mucous membranes (herpes simplex) or ingestion (*Helicobacter pylori*).

6. *The susceptible host*; this part of the chain describes the ability of the body to defend itself against infection and is termed immunity. This comprises non-specific or innate immunity, and includes the normal mechanical and physiological properties of the body, such as intact skin and mucous membranes. Specific immunity is acquired (naturally or artificially) during a patient's lifetime. It depends on the action of antibodies and the body's lymphocytes (white blood cells), for example staff who are not immunized against hepatitis B virus are extremely likely to become infected with hepatitis B if exposed to the virus.

APPLIED INFECTION CONTROL IN DENTAL PRACTICE

An awareness of the chain of infection allows us to apply these principles to the prevention of infection in dental practice. The application of infection control measures can be summarized into the infection control cycle (Figure 15.1).

THE DENTAL PATIENT

Although it is important that a comprehensive medical history is taken at the patient's initial visit and regularly updated, it is vital that the same infection control procedures are used for all patients, since those with asymptomatic disease or in the latent stages of infection will be unaware of their condition.

This means that patients with HIV infection (or any other bloodborne pathogen) can be safely treated in any dental practice and no form of discrimination is justified on the grounds of infection control. For patients with a history of or at-risk from Creutzfeldt–Jakob disease (CJD) in any form, there are concerns over the possibilities of transmission via contaminated instruments. Current UK guidance recommends no special precautions be taken for instrument re-processing; however, it would be prudent to liaise with infection control colleagues and recent guidelines as advice is updated frequently in this area.

STANDARD (UNIVERSAL) PRECAUTIONS

More recently, the term 'standard precautions' has replaced the term that most practitioners have been familiar with as 'universal precautions' (British Dental Association [BDA], 2003; Centers for Disease Control and Prevention [CDC], 2003; Molinari, 2003; Pratt *et al.*, 2007). In principle, there is no fundamental change in philosophy for dental practice (Box 15.2). The fundamental principle is that all blood and body fluids, such as saliva that may contain blood, should be treated as infectious, since many patients with bloodborne viruses may either be unaware of their infectivity, asymptomatic or fail to disclose the full nature of their medical history. It is perhaps worth highlighting that standard precautions do extend some of the boundaries that some have associated

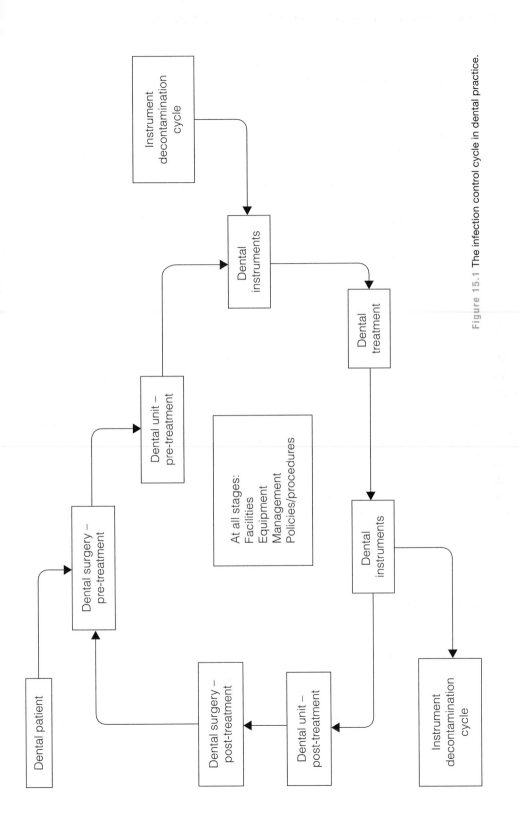

Figure 15.1 The infection control cycle in dental practice.

Box 15.2 Standard precautions in dental practice to minimize cross-infection

- Hand hygiene
- Personal protective equipment
- Prevention of occupational exposure (includes immunization of dental staff against communicable diseases, safe handling of sharps and management of sharps injuries)
- Management of blood and body fluid spillage (includes use of rubber dam and high-volume aspiration to reduce aerosolization and splatter of oral secretions)
- Decontamination of equipment (includes cleaning and sterilization of dental instruments and disinfection of dental impressions)
- Cleanliness of the environment
- Safe handling of linen
- Safe disposal of waste

---

with universal precautions, and now standard precautions apply to contact with all body fluids (regardless of blood content) and mucous membranes. The same infection control precautions are therefore required for all dental patients.

DENTAL SURGERY PREPARATION

The dental surgery is the area in which dental treatment occurs. The dental treatment area should be dedicated to providing treatment and not be used for reprocessing used instruments or preparing and eating food and beverages (BDA, 2003; CDC, 2003). Items of equipment and various paraphernalia should be restricted to that which is strictly necessary for the treatment of an individual patient. This will leave unit tops and surfaces readily cleanable. The surgery should have a dedicated sink for handwashing. Dental prosthetic material (i.e. when returned from dental laboratories) must be disinfected and an appropriate transfer record completed to record this process prior to fitting into a patient (BDA, 2003; CDC, 2003).

DENTAL UNIT PREPARATION

The dental unit comprises the dental chair, spittoon and bracket table, this equipment may also be self-contained with suction apparatus and integral compressed air and water to supply the dental handpieces. It is incumbent on dental unit manufacturers that the dental units are designed to allow cleaning of the various services and permit 'no-touch' operation of the functions of the unit. For poorly designed units, it may be appropriate to cover difficult to clean areas with removable coverings to minimize contamination and allow ease of cleaning.

As a result of the large surface area to volume ratio of the water supply to the dental handpieces in the dental unit, the water supplying dental handpieces and the air/water syringe is frequently contaminated with environmental micro-organisms and occasionally isolates of human origin (Walker *et al.*, 2000; Smith *et al.*, 2002). The problem of contaminated water lines in dental units has arisen as a result of poor engineering and inadequate material construction of dental units. Long-term resolution of the microbial contamination of dental unit water line will only be resolved when these shortcomings are addressed. In the interim, since dental units are classed as medical devices (Medical Devices Directive 93/42/EEC), the manufacturers of dental units are required under the Medical Devices Directive to provide validated instructions on disinfection of the dental unit water lines (BS EN ISO 17664, 2004). It is incumbent on dental practitioners to review these instructions prior to purchase and assess their long-term practicality, monitoring and revenue costs. Some work has been undertaken to assess the efficacy of disinfectants in controlling the biofilms (Walker *et al.*, 2003); however, care must be undertaken in their selection and compatibility with the materials of the dental unit must be checked with manufacturers prior to use (Pankhurst, 2003).

DENTAL INSTRUMENTS

Dental treatment by its very nature uses a wide range of instruments that range in invasiveness from non-critical to critical devices (Spaulding, 1968). It seems illogical in busy dental surgeries to attempt to segregate dental instruments on their degree of invasiveness and all instruments should be steam sterilized, with critical devices such as extraction forceps and scalers supplied as sterile at point of use. Such a system would require the use of vacuum sterilizers to process wrapped instruments. The use of bench-top steam sterilizers should be integrated into the decontamination cycle (Figure 15.2) with particular emphasis on the cleaning stage.

DENTAL TREATMENT

Having prepared the dental surgery environment for treatment of the patient and assembled the appropriate wrapped instruments, the next stage in the infection control cycle is treatment of the patient. The key to infection prevention at this point is effective hand hygiene and control of aerosol generation (McColl *et al.*, 1994; Bennett *et al.*, 2000). Direct contact of hands with surfaces or fomites is an important mode of transmission of bacteria, such as MRSA, or viruses, such as respiratory tract viruses or herpes viruses (Pratt *et al.*, 2007). By the simple act of handwashing the majority of the more

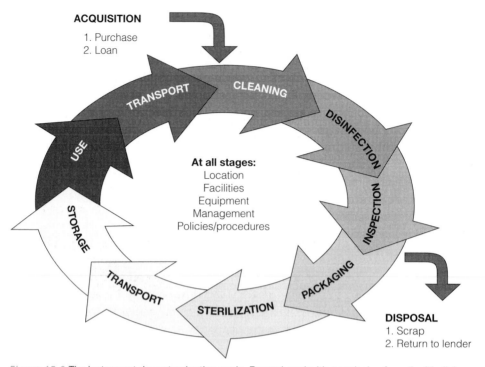

ACQUISITION
1. Purchase
2. Loan

TRANSPORT

CLEANING

DISINFECTION

USE

At all stages:
Location
Facilities
Equipment
Management
Policies/procedures

INSPECTION

STORAGE

TRANSPORT

STERILIZATION

PACKAGING

DISPOSAL
1. Scrap
2. Return to lender

Figure 15.2 The instrument decontamination cycle. Reproduced with permission from the Medicines and Healthcare products Regulatory Agency, *MAC Manual Part 2*: Figure 1, p. 12. © 2005 Crown Copyright.

pathogenic transient micro-organisms can be removed from the skin. The introduction and efficacy of alcohol hand gels and solutions has done much to improve the compliance of hand hygiene for use on clean hands. Hands should be washed with soap and water that are visibly soiled (Pratt *et al.*, 2007). Gloves should be routinely used as highlighted in standard precautions, and since gloves can be frequently perforated or torn these must be changed after each treatment episode including simple examinations (Murray *et al.*, 2001).

In addition to protective gloves other items of personal protective equipment that should be worn include protective eyewear such as goggles or visors, surgical facemasks and uniforms (tunics). Dental practice is by its nature prone to the generation of aerosol and splatter, which can frequently contaminate work wear and the environment. Work wear should be changed daily and uniforms visibly contaminated with blood or body fluids should be changed following treatment of that patient. Consideration should be given to the use of disposable plastic aprons to minimize the contamination of work wear (CDC, 2003; Pratt *et al.*, 2007). In order to minimize the generation of aerosols and splatter of oral secretions, the use of rubber dams in conjunction with high volume aspiration will reduce the risk of transmission from respiratory secretions and microbial aerosols from contaminated dental unit water lines.

Care should be taken in the handling of dental instruments with sharp working ends to avoid sharps injuries. Needles should be re-sheathed only using an appropriate safety device and each practice should have a documented and rehearsed policy for dealing with sharps injuries (Gore *et al.*, 1994; Smith *et al.*, 2001).

For surgical procedures such as surgical removal of wisdom teeth, periodontal surgery or dental implant placement, it would be prudent to adopt aseptic protocols in accordance with good surgical practice (CDC, 2003).

MANAGEMENT OF DENTAL INSTRUMENTS FOLLOWING USE

Following dental treatment, the patient will leave the dental surgery, and the process of clean up and preparation for the next patient begins. Re-usable dental instruments should be returned to the dedicated instrument re-processing area for the decontamination process. The instruments will then enter the decontamination cycle (Figure 15.2). Single-use instruments and sharps must be segregated from instruments that are to be re-processed. It is the dental surgeon's responsibility to make sharps safe for further handling or disposal. Burs must not be left in dental handpieces and must be disposed of in appropriate sharps containers. The sharps box must be compliant with appropriate national or international standards (e.g. BSI, 1990). Instruments for re-processing should be replaced in their trays and transported in an appropriate container to the instrument reprocessing area. Ideally this should be located outside the dental treatment area (BDA, 2003; CDC, 2003).

There are a number of methods used to clean instruments, ranging from manual washing to ultra-sonication and automated washer–disinfectors. This should be followed by steam sterilization in a bench-top steam sterilizer (preferably a vacuum sterilizer that will re-process devices that are wrapped and have lumens). Expert advice must be sought if other methods of instrument sterilization are to be used (BDA, 2003; CDC, 2003).

MANAGEMENT OF THE DENTAL UNIT FOLLOWING TREATMENT

Following dental treatment, waste generated must be disposed of following the appropriate waste stream. Care must be taken by the dental team when clearing trays of used instruments. It is the responsibility of the dental surgeon to dispose of any non-reusable sharps generated during the intervention safely (e.g. local anaesthetic and suture needles into sharps boxes). Clinical waste must be segregated from domestic waste and disposed of in appropriate colour-coded bags. Clinical waste bags are usually coloured yellow but may vary locally. Amalgam and extracted teeth containing amalgam must be disposed of separately, usually in red-topped containers from which amalgam is extracted prior to disposal. Extracted teeth not containing amalgam should be disposed of in a sharps container (small containers that can be disposed of frequently eliminate the generation of odours). Local anaesthetic cartridges part/fully discharged must be disposed of into the appropriate waste stream according to local policy. All clinical and special waste should be collected by a registered agent and appropriate consignment notes kept for a minimum of 3 years.

Impression material used during restorative or prosthetic treatment will require disinfection prior to dispatch to the dental laboratory (BDA, 2003; CDC, 2003; Pankhurst, 2006). This is a legal requirement in some countries. There are several proprietary disinfectants available for this purpose, although it is important to check that the disinfectant has been tested for its efficacy in disinfecting impression material. The manufacturer's instructions for the disinfectant must be followed, and suitable management policies and procedures are in place to control its use, including appropriate control of substances hazardous to health (COSHH) documentation (Health and Safety Executive, 2002). Instruments must not be disinfected in these solutions and glutaraldehyde solutions must be avoided. Accessories used during treatment that are difficult to clean, such as aspirators, must be disposed of after single use. Pathological or microbiological specimens are designated UN 3373 and must only be transported and labelled in accordance with United Nations and postal regulations.

MANAGEMENT OF THE DENTAL SURGERY FOLLOWING TREATMENT

Following cleaning of the dental unit, the dental chair, bracket table and cabinetry in the immediate facility of the patient must be wiped down with a detergent-impregnated cloth to clean the clinical area. At the end of a clinical session, the same areas should be wiped down with a suitable disinfectant compatible with the materials of the dental chair and cabinetry.

RECOMMENDATIONS APPLICABLE AT ALL STAGES

Location

The ideal location for a dental practice is in purpose-built surroundings that have been specifically designed and built for this purpose with due diligence accounting for types of dental interventions and patient throughput (CDC, 2003). However, the vast majority of dental practices in the UK are located in converted residential properties, which will physically restrict good infection control practice. Therefore, steps should be taken to segregate instrument reprocessing from the treatment area wherever feasibly possible and provide a linear work flow from dirty to clean.

Health Facilities Scotland (2008) recommend that the interior of the surgery should be designed to avoid dust traps and permit ease of cleaning. The junctions between walls, floors and ceilings should be coved where possible. Walls, floors and other surfaces should be of a smooth water-resistant finish and able to withstand frequent cleaning. Non-slip materials should be used where spillage of liquids may occur, and carpets must not be used in the treatment or instrument decontamination areas. Fittings should have smooth cleanable surfaces free from sharp corners, which may act as dirt traps. Within the surgery and instrument decontamination areas all horizontal surfaces must be smooth, intact, easy to clean, able to withstand frequent cleaning, resistant to mechanical damage and not shed particulate matter. Joints between fittings should be smooth, cleanable, resistant to mechanical damage and non-shedding. Where surfaces meet walls, edges must be coved.

Whilst there appears to be no definitive guideline on ventilation for dental surgeries, the functions of such a system are the extraction of odours and aerosols, dilution and control of airborne pathogenic material, removal of heat generated by equipment and reduction of moisture levels generated by equipment. For areas re-processing dental instruments, an extract ventilation system should be used to ensure that the room is maintained at negative pressure while in use to prevent egress of contaminated air. A dual motor/fan extract unit could be used, equipped with automatic changeover, and providing an extraction rate of not less than 10 air changes per hour. Where practical, the discharge vent from washer–disinfectors should be vented outside the building. Supply and extract ventilation (providing an extract rate of not less than 10 air changes per hour) can be used for treatment areas. The complexity of the ventilation system will depend on local circumstances and may range from simple wall-mounted fans to a ducted distribution system. The air supplied by air compressors to dental handpieces must be of sufficient quality and undergo periodic testing and maintenance.

Management

It would be beneficial both to the operation of infection control and the management of a dental practice if the principles of a quality management system were developed for dental surgeries. Such a system could not be as extensive as that used for sterile service departments but would still require documented policies, procedures and records for all the key elements of the infection control cycle. Stepwise procedures should be written for each stage of the infection control and instrument decontamination cycle. These procedures may then be used as in-practice training documents and as part of audit tools. Part of the quality system records should include non-batch-related records such as testing and maintenance records of equipment and batch-related records (e.g. sterilizer cycle and sterile product release records). Records must be maintained, securely stored and readily accessible. As part of the management of infection control, it is also essential that staff have access to occupational health services and are fully vaccinated according to recommended national guidelines.

Policies and procedures

Each practice must have a written infection control policy outlining the roles and responsibilities of key personnel, surgery and dental unit set-up protocols, instrument decontamination protocols, waste disposal, disinfection policy and management of sharps injuries (BDA, 2003; CDC, 2003; Pankhurst, 2006). Possession of advice sheets (e.g. BDA A12; BDA, 2003) by itself is insufficient.

Policies and procedures should be audited periodically to ensure staff compliance, relevance to activities and compliance with regulatory requirements and guidance. A documented review of policies and procedures should be undertaken on at least an annual basis.

Medicolegal requirements

It is essential that in assembling all the practical elements for effective infection control that appropriate guidelines and standards are followed to ensure compliance with relevant legislation. Key legislative instruments are summarized in Box 15.3.

Box 15.3 Examples of relevant legislation that may impact on infection control in dental practice

- Health and Safety at Work Act 1974
- Management of Health and Safety at Work Regulations 1999
- Workplace (Health, Safety and Welfare) Regulations 1992
- Provision and Use of Work Equipment Regulations 1999
- Electricity at Work Regulations 1989
- Health and Safety (First Aid) Regulations 1981
- Control of Substances Hazardous to Health Regulations (COSHH) 2002
- Manual Handling Operation Regulations 1992
- Reporting of Injuries, Diseases and Dangerous Occurrences Regulations (RIDDOR) 1985
- Pressure Systems Safety Regulations 2002

Equipment

Dental surgeries contain a wide variety of equipment and medical devices. In general terms, the key parameters relating to each piece of equipment are the equipment specification, required services, validation requirements, routine testing, maintenance and operation. These documents should form part of the practices quality management system.

CONCLUSIONS

One of the more frequent criticisms of infection control standards by members of the dental team is the paucity of evidence to demonstrate a real detrimental effect on patient well-being following dental surgery. However, there is evidence to demonstrate the transmission of a wide range of pathogens in the dental surgery and application of standard infection control principles such as hand hygiene, control of aerosolization and instrument decontamination is well established in the scientific literature. One of the challenges in obtaining the evidence base for cross-infection in dental practice has been the lack of surveillance data, which in turn is challenging to collect owing to confounding variables, not least being the operation within a heavily contaminated surgical field. Nevertheless, it is prudent to observe the lessons from other surgical specialities, *in-vitro* work and application of basic principles of infection control, since these apply equally to dental surgeries as they do to other surgical specialities.

The debate over standards of instrument re-processing continues especially with the threat of transmission of iatrogenic CJD, which has raised the bar in terms of instrument re-processing standards. One of the benefits of the raising of standards is also to reduce the risks from iatrogenic transmission of other pathogens. The move to the use of dental instruments sterile at the point of use will align the dental profession alongside other surgical professions. This will not be without its challenges and the dental profession requires considerably more technical and financial support to aid in the design, installation, validation and periodic testing of decontamination equipment in order to meet these standards.

USEFUL WEBSITES

British Dental Association: http://www.bda.org
Environment Agency: http://www.environmental-agency.gov.uk
Health Protection Agency: http://www.hpa.org.uk
Health Protection Scotland: http://www.hps.scot.nhs.uk
Health and Safety Executive: http://www.hse.gov.uk/cdg/pdf/infect-subs.pdf
Medicines and Healthcare Products Regulatory Agency: http://www.mhra.gov.uk

Chiropody

Rebecca Evans

This section aims to provide the chiropodist/podiatrist with a practical overview of how to apply the principles of infection, prevention and control to daily practices whether in hospital or community, and should be used in conjunction with other associated professional and national guidelines.

The prevention and control of healthcare-acquired infections should be paramount to all clinical practice. Healthcare-associated infections not only place an increased financial burden on healthcare organizations, but also have an associated morbidity and mortality (Plowman *et al.*, 1999; National Audit Office, 2000; Department of Health, 2003). While it is recognized that not all HCAIs are preventable, the application and adherence to policies, procedures and guidelines will facilitate a reduction in the level of HCAI. To ensure compliance to practice, infection prevention and control should form a core element of all education and training programmes, and should be an integral part of clinical practice and care pathways.

Chiropodists/podiatrists offer a diverse service, involving the assessment, diagnosis and treatment of abnormalities/diseases of the lower limbs, which involves the application of minor to complex invasive techniques/procedures, with patients often having associated risk factors (e.g. rheumatoid arthritis, peripheral vascular disease, peripheral nerve damage, diabetes).

Appropriate reduction of the risk of cross-infection is largely dependent on the susceptibility of the patient, the procedures undertaken and environment in which the patient/client is seen. Owing to the diversity and complexity of procedures, risk assessments should form an integral part of the management and care and should include:

- suitability of the location at which practices are being undertaken (e.g. hospital, community general practitioner's surgery, clinics, patient's home);
- environment – can procedures be undertaken safely (e.g. clean, fit for purpose);
- equipment used and decontamination methods required;
- facilities available to decontaminate equipment;
- complexity of procedures being undertaken;
- clinical condition of the patient/client and any associated risk factors (e.g. diabetes);
- contamination risk (e.g. transmission of micro-organisms; solutions; dressings; environment; equipment);
- use and availability of personal protective equipment;
- ability to transport equipment and waste safely.

There should be clearly defined operational procedures in place based on local and national policy which identify the risk and action taken to minimize the risk of patients acquiring a HCAI.

MODE OF TRANSMISSION

The mode of transmission of micro-organisms will influence the methods required to minimize cross infection. Micro-organisms are primarily transmitted by four routes: airborne; contact; blood/bodily fluids and enteric Practices required to reduce transmission will be dependent upon the mode of spread. Table 15.1 (p. 395) outlines the primary modes of transmission. Prior to undertaking any procedures, risk assessments should identify other associated factors that may increase or alter the mode of transmission, for example, fungal infections of nails are primarily spread by contact but, if nail drills are used, the mode of transmission is also airborne, requiring staff to wear facemasks to reduce aerosol contamination (Gatley, 1991; Davies et al., 1983).

LOCATION/ENVIRONMENT

The optimum environment is one which allows treatments to be undertaken with the minimum of risk of infection to the patient and staff member. Whether in hospital or community, it is essential that the principles of asepsis are maintained. Determining the suitability of the environment/location will largely depend upon the functionality of the department; complexity of procedures; associated patient risk factors and the ability of the environment to allow the practitioner to undertake defined procedures or treatments with minimum risk.

When new builds or upgrades are planned, it is essential that operational policies clearly identify the complexity and diversity of procedures being undertaken; decontamination processes; equipment/facilities required and adequate storage, to ensure the design complements the functionality of service requirements.

PREVENTING/REDUCING THE RISK OF CROSS-INFECTION

Outlined below are key principles for the prevention and control of infection that can be applied to practices whether in hospital, clinics or the community. These guidelines should be used in conjunction with local infection control guidelines.

Identification of patients

Early identification of susceptible patients and patients with known or suspected communicable infections facilitates better management of patient case loads and reduces the risk of cross-infection. Ideally, this should be incorporated as part of the referral process whether via hospitals or general practitioners. Identification of patients can either be electronically through 'patient administration systems' or manually. To maintain patient confidentiality, it is more practical to identify risk by mode of transmissions as outlined above as opposed to diagnosis (e.g. hepatitis B and C, and HIV).

Scheduling of patients

Should be based on clinical need and risk of infectivity with the lowest risk of infectivity reviewed first (e.g. immunocompromised/immunosuppressed) and patients with infected wounds/lesions and communicable infections reviewed last. Where this cannot be achieved owing to clinical need, risk assessments should identify the justification, associated risk and action taken to minimize the risk.

In hospitals and nursing or residential homes, practitioners should check with the person in charge to ascertain if there are other associated risk factors (e.g. outbreaks of diarrhoea and/or vomiting). If so, consideration should be given to re-scheduling appointments.

Hand hygiene

- Compliance with good hand decontamination is the single most effective action that can be taken to prevent the spread of infection. Hand decontamination should be carried out:
  - between all patient contact;
  - following any task where contact with body fluids has taken place;
  - prior to performing an aseptic technique;
  - following contact with any contaminated or potentially contaminated equipment.
- Wrist watches and stoned rings should not be worn in clinical areas or when undertaking clinical procedures.
- Alcohol hand rubs/gels are recommended for use on physically clean hands and should be available at key locations within departments and within the community.

Use of personal protective equipment

Personal protective equipment should be used to protect both the practitioner and patient from any potential risk of cross infection.

Personal protective equipment should be readily available within each department for use as appropriate. Staff should be trained and understand the correct use and application of PPE. Where chemical or hazardous substances are used, compliance with legislation is essential (Health and Safety Executive, 1974, 1992, 1999a, b).

The type of PPE worn should be based on a risk assessment of:

- the proposed risk of transmission of any potential organisms;
- the patient's status (e.g. infectivity and susceptibility to infection);
- the procedure being undertaken;
- the type of equipment used.

Types of personal protective equipment

See Box 15.1, **p. 399**. In addition, masks should be worn by practitioners when using or cleaning nail drills to reduce the risk of contamination from dust particles.

Care of blood and bodily fluids

- Care should be taken when handling all blood and bodily fluids.
- Gloves should be worn when in contact with blood or bodily fluids
- The use of solidifying agents should be considered to contain liquids.
- Goggles/face visors should be used if there is a risk splashing may occur.

Safe management of sharps and clinical/hazardous waste

- All sharps, clinical/hazardous waste should be handled in accordance with Waste Regulations (NHS Estates, 1995; Department of Health, 1997; Department of Health, 2006).
- Sharps should be disposed of at the point of use (where practical), into an approved container which must comply to national standards (e.g. UK – BS7320).
- There should be systems in place for the storage, collection, transportation and disposal of waste.

Safe handling of linen

- Clean and dirty linen should be segregated in a designated area.
- Any infected linen should be handled according to local infection control policy.

Equipment

- When purchasing equipment, consideration should be given to the use of disposable, single-use items where practical. Where single-use items are used, it is essential that equipment is disposed of and transported in accordance with waste regulations.
- Items of equipment not designated as single use but have direct contact with the patient must be able to be decontaminated between use. Equipment can be divided into high-, intermediate- and low-risk categories depending on the purpose of its use (see Table 15.2, **p. 401**). Examples with high risk are cutting equipment and theatre instruments; nail clippers are intermediate risk and wash bowls low risk.

- It is essential that risk assessments are undertaken to determine the suitability of equipment to be decontaminated. Cleaning, disinfection and sterilization are all processes that remove or destroy micro-organisms. The method and ability to decontaminate equipment will depend on the facilities available, the decontamination process required, the complexity of equipment (e.g. lumens, size, sharps), the integrity of the equipment to withstand the decontamination process (e.g. chemical or steam disinfection) and the infection risk associated with the equipment/medical device.

- Prior to purchasing any equipment, it is the responsibility of the user to ensure that the equipment can be decontaminated adequately. Within any department, there should be a programme for cleaning and maintaining all items of equipment based on the local and national policy.

- Where practical, equipment designated as re-usable should be decontaminated in a sterile services department to ensure adequate decontamination and compliance to national guidelines. Where local decontamination is employed, it is essential consideration is given to dedicated decontamination facilities and the effectiveness of the decontamination processes being used. Where bench-top sterilizers/autoclaves are used, only instruments fit for purpose should be processed. Organic matter should be removed prior to inserting any instruments in an autoclave. This is ideally achieved by use of an ultrasonic washer. If ultrasonic washers are not available, suitability for manual cleaning needs to be assessed. Care must be taken to reduce an inoculation accident when handling any instruments/sharps.

- If local sterilizers are used, there should be a maintenance programme in place and a monitoring system to ensure each load achieves the correct temperature. Instruments with lumens should only be processed in a vacuumed autoclave, which should comply with national guidelines (Medical Devices Agency, 1998, 2001).

- As part of any cleaning programme where solutions or disinfectants are used, consideration should be given to the following, that:
  - surfaces can withstand cleaning with detergent and water and disinfectants (e.g. chlorine-releasing agents, 70 per cent alcohol);
  - no patients or staff are put at risk where disinfectants are used;
  - the appropriate PPE is available for use;
  - products used comply with national policy, Control of Substances Hazardous to Health Regulations (Health and Safety Executive, 1999a) and health and safety legislation.

Details of the specific equipment used in chiropody/podiatry and the methods for its decontamination are given in Table 15.4.

Table 15.4 Specific equipment used in chiropody/podiatry

Examples of types of equipment	Method of decontamination	Comments
Couches/chairs	General use – detergent and water[a]	Disposable roll should be used between patients
Dressing trolleys/work surfaces	Detergent and water[a]	Dressing trolleys/work surfaces
Instruments (e.g. nail files, scissors, scalpel handles, nippers)	Single use	Care should be taken to prevent an inoculation accident
	If reusable – autoclave organic matter should be removed prior to autoclaving	
	The use of an ultrasonic washer is preferred[b]	
Nail drills	Follow manufacturer's guidelines	Masks should be worn when cleaning equipment
Scalpel blades	Single use only	Dispose of in an approved sharps container
Suction tubing	Disposable	Dispose of as clinical waste
Treatment units	Follow manufacturer's guidelines	Should be part of a cleaning schedule

[a]Cleaning should be followed by a chlorine-releasing agent (1000 ppm) or an alcohol-impregnated wipe if used on a patient with a known or suspected infection.
[b]Where instruments require manual cleaning, a risk assessment should be undertaken to ensure that the equipment can be decontaminated effectively and safely.

REFERENCES

Advisory Committee on Dangerous Pathogens (1995) *Protection against blood-borne infections in the workplace: HIV and hepatitis.* London: HMSO.

Advisory Committee on Dangerous Pathogens (2001) *The management, design and operation of microbiological containment laboratories.* London: HMSO.

Advisory Committee on Dangerous Pathogens (2003) *Transmissible spongiform encephalopathy agents: safe working and prevention of infection.* Available online at: http://www.advisorybodies.doh.uk/acdp/tseguidance (last accessed January 2007).

Advisory Committee on Dangerous Pathogens (2004) *Approved list of biological agents.* London: HMSO.

Allwood M, Stanley A and Wright P (eds) (2002) *The cytotoxics handbook*, 4th edn. Oxford: Radcliff Medical Press Ltd.

Anon. (1977) *Guide to good manufacturing practice.* London: HMSO.

Anon. (2005) *The supply of unlicensed relevant medicinal products for individual patients* (MHRA Guidance Note No. 14, revised May 2005). London: MHRA.

Atfield RD (1991) Hospital hygiene – a continuing assessment: a microbiological view of sterile services production. *Journal of Hospital Infection* 18(Suppl A), 524.

Beaney A (ed.) (2006) *Quality assurance of aseptic preparation services*, 4th edn. London: Pharmaceutical Press.

Bennett AM, Fulford MR, Walker JT, Bradshaw DJ, Martin MV and Marsh PD (2000) Microbial aerosols in general dental practice. *British Dental Journal* 189, 664.

Breckenridge A (1976) *Report of the working party on the addition of drugs to intravenous infusion fluids*, HC(76)9 (Breckenridge report). London: Department of Health and Social Security.

British Dental Association (2003) Advice Sheet A12: *Infection control in dentistry*. London: British Dental Association.

British Standards Institution (1976) *Environmental cleanliness in enclosed spaces. BS 5295: Parts 1, 2 5c 3*. London: British Standards Institution.

British Standards Institution (1990) *BS7320. Specification for sharps containers*. London: British Standards Institution.

British Standards Institution (1993) *BS2745. Washer disinfectors Parts 1–3*. London: British Standards Institution.

British Standards Institution (1994) *Quality systems: model for quality assurance in production, installation and servicing*. BS EN ISO 9002. London: British Standards Institution.

British Standards Institution (2004) BS EN ISO 17664:2004 *Sterilization of medical devices. Information to be provided by the manufacturer for the processing of resterilizable medical devices*. London. British Standards Institution.

British Standards Institution (2006) EN ISO 15883:2006 *Washer disinfectors (Parts 1–4)*. Milton Keynes: British Standards Institution.

British Thoracic Society (2000) Control and prevention of tuberculosis in the United Kingdom. *Thorax* **55**, 887.

Centers for Disease Control and Prevention (2003) Guidelines for infection control in dental health care settings. *MMWR* **52**, rr-17.

Cleveland JL, Kent J, Gooch BF, Valway SE, Marianos DW, Butler WR and Onorato IM (1995) Multidrug-resistant *Mycobacterium tuberculosis* in an HIV dental clinic. *Infection Control and Hospital Epidemiology* **16**, 7.

Collins CH and Kennedy IDA (1999) *Laboratory-acquired infections. History, incidence, causes and prevention*, 4th edn. Oxford: Butterworth Heinemann.

Cystic Fibrosis Trust (2002) *Clinical guidelines for the physiotherapy management of cystic fibrosis*. Bromley, Kent: Cystic Fibrosis Trust.

Cystic Fibrosis Trust (2004) *The* Burkholderia cepacia *complex: suggestions for prevention and infection control*, 2nd edn. Bromley, Kent: Cystic Fibrosis Trust.

Davies K, Herbert A-M, Westmoreland D and Bagg J (1994) Seroepidemiological study of respiratory virus infections among dental surgeons. *British Dental Journal* **176**, 262.

Davies RR, Ganderton MA and Savage MA (1983) Human nail dust and precipitating antibodies to *Trichophyton rubrum* in chiropodists. *Clinical Allergy* **13**, 309.

Department of Health (1994) HTM 2010: *Sterilizers*. London: Department of Health.

Department of Health (2003) *Winning ways: working together to reduce healthcare associated infection in England*. Report by the Chief Medical Officer. London: Department of Health.

Department of Health (2006) Health Technical Memorandum 07-01: *Safe management of healthcare waste*. Peer review consultation draft 7 July 2006. London: Department of Health.

Department of the Environment (1997) Health Technical Memorandum (HTM2065): *Healthcare waste management – segregation of waste*.. London: Department of Health.

European Union (1995) 93/42/EEC *Council Directive, Medical Devices Directive*. Brussels: European Union.

Farwell J (1995) *Aseptic dispensing for NHS patients* [Farwell report]. London: Department of Health.

Gatley M (1991) Human nail dust: hazard to chiropodists or merely nuisance?. *Journal Society of Occupational Medicine* **41**, 121.

Gore SM, Felix DH, Bird AG and Wray D (1994) Occupational risk and precautions related to HIV infection among dentists in the Lothian region of Scotland. *Journal of Infection* **28**, 209.

Hadler SC, Sorley DL, Acree KH *et al.* (1981) An outbreak of hepatitis B in a dental practice. *Annals of Internal Medicine* **95**, 133.

Health and Safety Executive (1974) *The Health and Safety at Work Act.* London: HMSO.

Health and Safety Executive (1992) *Personal protective equipment* (EC Directive). Regulation. Sudbury: HSE Books.

Health and Safety Executive (1999a) *Control of substances hazardous to health regulations.* Approved Code of Practice. Sudbury: HSE Books.

Health and Safety Executive (1999b) *Management of health and safety at work.* Approved Code of Practice L21 HMSC. Sudbury: HSE Books.

Health and Safety Executive (2002) *The control of substances hazardous to health regulations,* 4th edn. Sudbury: HSE Books.

Health and Safety Executive (2003) *Safe working and the prevention of infection in clinical laboratories and similar facilities.* London: HMSO.

Health and Safety Executive (2006) *Sealability of microbiological containment level 3 and 4 facilities.* Available online at: http://www.hse.gov.uk/biosafety/gmo/guidance/sealability (last accessed January 2007).

Health and Safety Executive and Health Protection Agency (2006) *Management of spa pools: controlling the risk of infection.* London: Health Protection Agency.

Health Facilities Scotland (2008) *Scottish Health Planning Note 13 Part 2 – Decontamination Facilities: Local Decontamination.* Available online at: http://www.hfs.scot.nhs.uk/online-services/publications/propertly/scottish-health-planning-notes/ (last accessed February 2009).

Health Services Commission (1988) *Control of substances hazardous to health: approved code of practice.* London: HMSO.

Infection Control Nurses Association (2001) *Guidelines for preventing intravascular catheter-related infection.* Bathgate: Fitwise Publications.

Infection Control Nurses Association (2004) *Audit tools for monitoring infection control standards 2004.* Bathgate: Infection Control Nurses Association.

Institute of Decontamination Science (2007a) *Quality standards and recommended practices.* Available online at: http://www.idsc-uk.co.uk.

Institute of Decontamination Science (2007b) *Sterile services teaching and training manual.* Available online at: http://www.idsc-uk.co.uk.

Institute of Sterile Services Management (1989) *Guide to good manufacturing practice for national health sterile services departments.* London: Institute of Sterile Services Management.

The Interdepartmental Working Group on Tuberculosis (1998) *The prevention and control of tuberculosis in the United Kingdom: UK guidance on the prevention and control of transmission of 1. HIV-related tuberculosis, 2. drug-resistant, including multiple drug resistant tuberculosis.* London: Department of Health.

Lewis MAO (2004) Herpes simplex virus: an occupational hazard in dentistry. *International Dental Journal* **54**, 103.

Martin MV and Hardy P (1991) Two cases of oral infection by methicillin resistant *Staphylococcus aureus. British Dental Journal* **170**, 63.

McColl E, Bagg J and Winning S (1994) The detection of blood on dental surgery surfaces and equipment following dental hygiene treatment. *British Dental Journal* **176**, 65.

Medical Devices Agency (1993, 1996, 1999, 2006) *Sterilization, disinfection and cleaning of medical equipment.* London: HMSO.

Medical Devices Agency (1998) MDA DB 9804: *The validation and periodic testing of benchtop vacuum steam sterilizers.* London: Medical Devices Agency.

Medical Devices Agency (2001) MDA DB 2002(06): *Benchtop steam sterilizers – guidance on purchase, operation and maintenance.* London: Medical Devices Agency.

Medicines and Healthcare products Regulatory Agency (2003) Device Bulletin 2003(06): *Community equipment loan stores – guidance on decontamination.* London: Medicines and Healthcare Products Regulatory Agency.

Medicines and Healthcare products Regulatory Agency (2005) *Management of medical devices prior to repair, service or investigation DB 2003(05).* London: Medicines and Healthcare Products Regulatory Agency.

Medicines and Healthcare products Regulatory Agency (2006) *Single use medical devices: implications and consequences of reuse.* DB 2006(04). London: MHRA.

Midcalf BW, Phillips J, Neiger and T. Coes (eds) (2004) *Pharmaceutical isolators: a guide to their application, design and control.* London: Pharmaceutical Press.

Molinari JA (2003) Infection control: its evolution to the current standard precautions. *Journal of the American Dental Association* **134**, 569.

Murray CA, Burke FJT and McHugh S (2001) An assessment of the incidence of punctures in latex and non-latex dental examination gloves in routine clinical practice. *British Dental Journal* **390**, 377.

National Audit Office (2000) *The management and control of hospital acquired infection in acute NHS trusts in England.* London: National Audit Office.

National Institute for Clinical Excellence (2003) *Infection control: prevention of healthcare associated infection in primary and community care.* London: National Institute for Clinical Excellence.

NHS Estates (1995) *Safe disposal of clinical waste. Health service guidance notes whole hospital policy guidance.* London: HMSO.

NHS Estates (1997) HTM 2030: *Washer disinfectors.* London: NHS Estates.

NHS Estates (2004) HBN 13: *Sterile services department.* London: NHS Estates.

Pa L, Ng YS and Tay BK (2004) Impact of a viral respiratory epidemic on the practice of medicine and rehabilitation: severe acute respiratory syndrome. *Archives of Physical Medicine* **85**, 1365.

Pankhurst CL (2003) Risk assessment of dental unit water line contamination. *Primary Dental Care* **10**, 5.

Pankhurst CL (2006) *Control of infection guidelines for general dental practice*, 2nd revised edn (Jan 2006). London: Southwark Primary Care Trust.

Pike JH and McLean D (2002) Ethical concerns in isolating patients with methicillin resistant *Staphylococcus aureus* on the rehabilitation ward: a case report. *Archives of Physical Medicine* **83**, 1028.

Plowman R, Graves N, Griffin MA *et al.* (1999) *The socio-economic burden of hospital acquired infection.* London: Public Health Laboratory Service.

Pratt RJ, Pellow C, Loveday HP *et al.* (2001) Standard principles for preventing hospital-acquired infections. *Journal of Hospital Infection* **47**, s21.

Pratt RJ, Pellowe CM, Wilson JA *et al.* (2007) epic2: National evidence-based guidelines for preventing healthcare-associated infections in NHS hospitals in England. *Journal of Hospital Infection* **65**(Suppl), S1.

Public Health Laboratory Service (1999) *Hygiene for hydrotherapy pools.* London: Public Health Laboratory Service.

Reingold AL, Kane MA, Murphy BL, Checko P, Francis DP and Maynard JE (1982) Transmission of hepatitis B by an oral surgeon. *Journal of Infectious Diseases* **145**, 262.

Rimland D (1985) Nosocomial infections with methicillin and tobramycin resistant *Staphylococcus aureus* – implications of physiotherapy in hospital-wide dissemination. *American Journal of the Medical Sciences* **290**, 91.

Royal College of Nursing (2005) *Standards for infusion therapy.* London: Royal College of Nursing.

Schabrun S, Chipchase L and Rickard H (2006) Are therapeutic ultrasound units a potential vector for nosocomial infection? *Physiotherapy Research International* **11**, 61.

Sclech WF, Simonson N, Sumarah R and Martin RS (1986) Nosocomial outbreak of *Pseudomonas aeruginosa* folliculitis associated with a physiotherapy pool. *CMAJ* **134**, 909.

Sharp J (2000) *Quality in the manufacture of medicines and other healthcare products.* London: Pharmaceutical Press.

Shaw FE Jr, Barrett CL, Hamm R *et al.* (1986) Lethal outbreak of hepatitis B in a dental practice. *JAMA* **255**, 3260.

Smith AJ, Kennedy D, Cameron S and Bagg J (2001) Management of needlestick injuries in general dental practice. *British Dental Journal* **190**, 645.

Smith AJ, McCormick L, Stansfield R, McMillan A and Hood J (2002) Microbiological quality of water from units in general dental practice. *British Dental Journal* **193**, 645.

Smith WH, Davies D, Mason KD and Onions JP (1982) Intraoral and pulmonary tuberculosis following dental treatment. *Lancet* **1**, 842.

Spaulding EH (1968) Chemical disinfection of medical and surgical materials. In: Block SS (ed.) *Disinfection, sterilization and preservation,* 4th edn. Philadelphia: Lea & Febiger.

Spaulding EH (1972) Chemical disinfection and antisepsis in the hospital. *Journal of Hospital Research* **9**, 5.

Underwood E (1999) Good manufacturing practice. In Russell AD, Hugo WB and Ayliffe GAJ (eds) *Principles and practice of disinfection, preservation and sterilization,* 3rd edn. Oxford: Blackwell Science, 374.

Walker JT, Bradshaw DJ, Bennett AM, Fulford MR, Martin MV and Marsh PD (2000) Microbial biofilm formation and contamination of dental-unit water systems in General Dental Practice. *Applied and Environmental Microbiology* **66**, 3363.

Walker JT, Bradshaw DJ, Fulford MR and Marsh PD (2003) Microbiological evaluation of a range of disinfectant products to control mixed-species biofilm contamination in a laboratory model of a dental unit water system. *Applied and Environmental Microbiology* **69**, 3327.

16 INFECTION PREVENTION AND CONTROL IN THE COMMUNITY

Iain Blair

INTRODUCTION

The community is defined as all settings that are outside major hospitals. Care settings in the community are those that provide healthcare, social care and other welfare services. These include Primary Care Trusts (PCTs), community hospitals, care homes, hostels, day-care and home-care services, schools, colleges, nurseries and prisons. Other community settings are workplaces, leisure centres, hotels, restaurants, shops, places of entertainment, communal areas, transport, and homes and gardens.

Infectious diseases result from an interaction between an infectious agent, a susceptible host and the environment. Most infectious diseases have the capacity to spread within community settings where people, some of whom may be particularly susceptible, share eating and living accommodation.

In recent years the prevention and control of infection has become an important consideration in all community settings, but particularly in care settings where the risks and consequences of infection are greatest. There are several reasons for this (Box 16.1).

To address the challenges posed by infection in community settings community infection control services have developed. These services comprise surveillance, investigation and risk assessment followed by advice, support and leadership on standard precautions, development and implementation of policies and guidelines, training, audit, advice on immunization, decontamination, management of outbreaks and use of antimicrobials.

ADMINISTRATIVE ARRANGEMENTS FOR THE PREVENTION AND CONTROL OF INFECTION IN THE COMMUNITY

Prevention and control of infection in the community depends on joint working between many different agencies and individuals (Box 16.2).

Primary Care Trusts

In England there are 152 PCTs serving populations which vary in size between 0.2 and 1 million. PCTs take responsibility for all aspects of the health of their

Box 16.1 Reasons for the increasing importance of community infection control

- Increase in the number of services providing health and social care in the community
- Increase in the scope and complexity of healthcare interventions provided in the community
- Declining length of stay in acute hospitals, more day surgery and ambulatory care
- Patients cared for in the community are increasingly very dependent; they undergo invasive procedures and have risk factors for infection
- The ratio of trained to untrained staff in the community is lower than in hospitals
- More children are placed in day care, often at an early age
- Demand from service providers for advice and guidance on the prevention and control of infection has increased
- There is an increasing public and media interest in healthcare-associated infections
- There is growing awareness amongst patients, their relatives and care givers of the importance of a clean and safe environment.

Box 16.2 Agencies, individuals and organizations involved in community infection control

HEALTH PROTECTION AGENCY (HPA)

- Local Health Protection Unit staff
- Regional HPA laboratory
- National centres

HOSPITALS

- Director for Infection Prevention and Control
- Infection Control Doctor
- Medical microbiologist
- Infection Control Nurse
- Infectious disease specialist
- Tuberculosis (TB) specialist, TB nurse advisers
- Genitourinary medicine (GUM) specialist, GUM health adviser

LOCAL AUTHORITY DEPARTMENTS (ENVIRONMENTAL HEALTH, EDUCATION, SOCIAL SERVICES)

- Environmental Health Officers
- Trading Standards Officers
- Teachers, social workers, home carers
- Residential home managers, health and safety managers

Box 16.2 – *contd*

PRIMARY HEALTH CARE SERVICES

- General practitioners
- Practice nurses
- Community pharmacists
- General dental practitioners
- Opticians

PRIVATE CARE HOMES

- Managers
- Nursing staff
- Carers

OCCUPATIONAL HEALTH DEPARTMENTS

- Occupational health doctors and nurses

DAY NURSERIES

- Managers
- Nursery nurses

NHS DIRECT 24-HOUR PHONE LINE STAFFED BY NURSES AND OTHERS PROVIDING HEALTHCARE ADVICE TO THE PUBLIC

- Managers
- Nurses
- Call handlers

MENTAL HEALTH TRUSTS: SPECIALIST MENTAL HEALTH SERVICES, INPATIENT AND OUTPATIENT

- Clinical staff
- Social care staff
- Carers

AMBULANCE TRUSTS: EMERGENCY ACCESS TO HEALTHCARE

- Immediate care doctors
- Paramedics
- Other ambulance staff

GENERAL PUBLIC

- Citizens, consumers, newspapers, radio, television

population, including providing and commissioning health services. They are responsible for health protection and health emergency planning but receive, assistance from the Health Protection Agency to do this. PCTs are also responsible for a range of preventative and public health services including immunization. Some PCTs provide genitourinary medicine (GUM) services and tuberculosis services while in other areas they commission these services from hospital trusts.

Primary Care Trusts provide infection control services in their community facilities (which may be extensive) and in general practice, and usually employ one or more Community Infection Control Nurses (CICNs) to do this. PCTs have a Director Of Public Health and, like hospitals, have a Director of Infection Prevention and Control (DIPC) and an Infection Control Committee (ICC). They may also have an Infection Control Doctor (ICD).

The NHS devotes considerable time and resources to controlling healthcare-associated infections (HCAIs). In the past, acute hospitals have been the focus for much of this effort but now action is being taken across the whole health economy. PCTs have an important part to play in the prevention and control of HCAIs both as providers and commissioners of care and as local leaders of the NHS (Department of Health, 2008a). PCTs are increasingly subject to the same requirements as acute hospitals (Department of Health, 2007, 2008b) and are being held accountable for levels of HCAI in the healthcare premises within their areas.

Health Protection Agency

Health protection describes activities aimed at protecting public health from infectious diseases and environmental hazards such as chemical contamination and radiation. Historically, in the UK, the National Health Service (NHS) was the main provider of health protection services. However, in 2003, following the publication of a strategy document *Getting ahead of the curve* (Department of Health, 2002), the Health Protection Agency (HPA) was established by the merger of NHS resources with the Public Health Laboratory Service (PHLS). Further changes took place in 2005 when the Agency merged with the National Radiological Protection Board (NRPB). The HPA has three national centres of expertise covering emergency preparedness, infections, and chemical, radiological and environmental threats to health. There is also a local services division comprising nine regional offices, eight regional microbiology laboratories and 28 local Health Protection Units (HPUs) each serving a population of between 1 and 2 million. At a local level, HPUs provide advice, support and leadership to the NHS and other stakeholders. HPUs are staffed by Consultants in Communicable Disease Control (CCDCs), consultants in health protection, health protection nurses and support staff, and work directly with PCTs, hospital trusts and local authorities on surveillance, investigation and management of incidents and outbreaks, and the delivery of national action plans.

Health Protection Units

Health Protection Units have local responsibility for health protection and community infection prevention and control. Although they are not responsible for providing an infection control service directly to PCT facilities or private care homes, they will ensure that appropriate arrangements are in place. HPU staff maintain professional links with other infection control staff, and attend local infection control committees and outbreak control groups. They will also assist in the investigation and management of outbreaks of infection in the community and in hospitals. Key tasks for the HPU include advocacy and support for infection control within the NHS and wider community, including practical assistance where appropriate, ensuring that surveillance data and information are shared by those who need to know, and ensuring compliance with statutory requirements and relevant guidelines. The HPU develops relationships with local stakeholders to consult on HPU-wide strategies and policies and encourage collaboration.

Care homes

Care homes include nursing homes and residential homes. They may be owned and managed by the NHS, social services or the private sector. The owner of a home is responsible under health and safety legislation for maintaining an environment that is safe for residents, visitors and staff, and this includes having suitable arrangements for the control of infection. There should be a written infection control policy and an annual infection control report. The registered manager of the home should have 24-hour access to infection control advice from a suitably qualified person. The person in charge of the home should ensure that infection control policies and procedures are available, in use and are understood by all members of staff.

General practitioners

General practitioners (GPs) provide care for patients with infection, including diagnosis and treatment. They should be prepared to advise on hygiene and other infection control measures including immunization. The GP should consider the implications of infection for other people. GPs should report cases of infection to and seek advice from the local HPU.

Hospitals

National Health Service hospitals have service agreements with their local PCTs. The agreements specify the services that are to be provided and the standards that are to be achieved. These include satisfactory infection control arrangements, access to patients and clinical records for HPU staff, and ensuring that a comprehensive range of diagnostic tests are offered by the microbiology laboratory. Private hospitals are expected to achieve similar standards.

Local government authorities

Local government in England and Wales is based on elected councils, which are accountable to the residents that they serve. Councils consist of elected members and salaried officers. Officers acting on behalf of a council must ensure that the powers they exercise have been lawfully delegated to them by the elected members. Often the council exercises its power through a specific officer, the proper officer, which for some public health legislation is the CCDC or another HPU staff member. Councils arrange themselves in a series of functional departments. These departments include environmental health, education, social services, housing and leisure

Environmental Health Departments and Environmental Health Officers

The responsibilities of Environmental Health Departments include food safety, air quality, noise, waste, health and safety, water quality, port health controls at air and sea ports, refuse collection and pest control. Environmental Health Officers (EHOs) investigate outbreaks of foodborne and waterborne infections, advise on and enforce food safety legislation, inspect food premises, investigate complaints and provide food hygiene training. EHOs liaise with a wide range of other professionals including HPU staff, GPs, teachers, microbiologists and veterinary surgeons.

Commission for Social Care Inspection

The Commission for Social Care Inspection (CSCI) is the independent body responsible for the inspection and regulation of public and private social care services in England. CSCI registers services and carries out local inspections against nationally agreed standards.

The Healthcare Commission

The Healthcare Commission promotes improvement in the quality of the NHS and independent healthcare by reviewing, assessing and rating performance. There are explicit care standards that include standards for infection control. In April 2009 the Healthcare Commission will merge with CSCI to form a new health and adult social care regulator, the Care Quality Commission.

Occupational Health Services

Occupational Health Services advise managers and employees about the effect of work on health and of health on work. They devise risk management programmes to ensure that the hazards that staff face during their work are minimized.

Health and Safety Commission and Executive.

The Health and Safety Commission (HSC) and Health and Safety Executive (HSE) are statutory bodies whose aims are to protect those at work and those who may be affected by any work-related activity. In particular, the HSE is the enforcement agency for the Health and Safety at Work etc Act 1974, the Control of Substances Hazardous to Health (COSHH) Regulations 1994 and the Management of Health and Safety at Work (MHSW) Regulations 1994. The COSHH regulations require employers to assess the risk of infection for their employees and members of the public. The MHSW regulations require an assessment of risks to health, provision of health surveillance, if appropriate, and information for employees. The Reporting of Incidents, Diseases and Dangerous Occurrences Regulations 1985 (RIDDOR) require employers to report acute illness requiring medical treatment where there is reason to believe that this resulted from an exposure to a pathogen or infected material.

Other agencies with a role in infectious disease control

These are listed in Box 16.3.

SURVEILLANCE

The effective management of infectious disease depends on good surveillance. This is true whether infection occurs in hospital or the community. Surveillance has been defined as the continuing scrutiny of all aspects of the occurrence and spread of a disease through the systematic collection, collation and analysis of data, and the prompt dissemination of the resulting information to those who need to know so that action can result.

The advantages of surveillance are that:

- it allows individual cases of infection to be identified so that action can be taken to prevent spread;
- it measures the incidence of infection, changes in which may signal an outbreak;
- it tracks changes in risk factors for infection, which may need new interventions;

Box 16.3 Other agencies with a role in infectious disease control

DEPARTMENT FOR THE ENVIRONMENT, FOOD AND RURAL AFFAIRS (DEFRA)

Defra is a UK Government department that promotes sustainable development and a better environment and safeguards public health in relation to foodborne disease and zoonoses.

DRINKING WATER INSPECTORATE (DWI)

The DWI regulates the safety of public water supplies and the performance of water companies.

ANIMAL HEALTH (FORMERLY THE STATE VETERINARY SERVICE)

Animal Health is an executive agency sponsored by Defra that is responsible for animal health and managing outbreaks of notifiable animal diseases such as avian influenza, which may have an impact on public health.

VETERINARY LABORATORIES AGENCY (VLA)

The VLA is a regional network of 16 veterinary laboratories that provides animal disease surveillance, diagnostic services and veterinary scientific research.

ENVIRONMENT AGENCY (EA)

The EA concerns itself with the effect of the environment on health, including waste disposal.

FOOD STANDARDS AGENCY (FSA)

The FSA protects the public from risks connected to the consumption of food, safeguards the interests of consumers, provides the government response to outbreaks of foodborne disease, operates the food hazard warning system and develops policies for microbial, chemical and other hazards associated with food. The FSA has set targets for the reduction of foodborne disease.

- it allows existing control measures to be evaluated;
- it allows the emergence of new infections to be detected and described.

A good surveillance system consists of the following steps:

- case-definition based on clinical and/or microbiological criteria;
- identification of cases through reports from clinicians and laboratories;
- collection of a dataset (Box 16.4) for each case by telephone, visit or letter, using suitable data collection forms, and entry on a database.

Box 16.4 Dataset for case investigation

FOR ALL INFECTIONS

- Name
- Date of birth
- Sex
- Address
- Ethnic group
- Place of work
- Occupation
- Name of general practitioner
- Recent travel
- Immunization history
- Date of illness
- Clinical description of illness

FOR FOODBORNE INFECTIONS

- Food histories
- Food preferences

FOR INFECTIONS WITH AN ENVIRONMENTAL SOURCE

- Places visited
- Journeys made

FOR INFECTIONS THAT ARE SPREAD FROM PERSON TO PERSON

- Names and addresses of contacts

Surveillance data should be used in the following way:

- to ensure that the cases satisfy the case-definition;
- to produce summary statistics including frequency counts and rates (if suitable denominators are available);
- to describe epidemiology in terms of person, place and time;
- to track trends and detect clusters or outbreaks;
- to share local data and merge data to produce regional and national datasets;
- to analyse data and share resulting information so that action can be taken.

Reporting can take place in a variety of ways. Increasingly data are available online, but may also be found in local and national newsletters and journals. Feedback to local data providers is important. It demonstrates the usefulness of the data and creates reliance on them. This in turn will lead to improvement in case ascertainment and data quality. Local data may be sent to GPs, hospital clinicians, microbiologists and EHOs.

Data sources

A number of data sources are available for the surveillance of infectious diseases. Cases of infection that are sub-clinical or do not lead to a medical consultation can only be detected by population surveys. Cases that are seen by a doctor or nurse may be reported via a primary care reporting scheme or statutory notification system, and cases that are investigated by laboratory tests may be detected by a laboratory reporting system.

Statutory notifications of infectious disease

The current list of notifiable infectious diseases in England and Wales is shown in Box 16.5. Any clinician suspecting these diagnoses is required to notify the proper officer of the local authority, who is usually the CCDC. The data are collated by the HPA and published on their website (http://www.hpa.org.uk).

Box 16.5 Statutorily notifiable infectious diseases in England and Wales

Very rare infections	Rare infections	Common infections
Anthrax	Leptospirosis	Food poisoning
Leprosy	Yellow fever	Viral hepatitis
Typhus	Cholera	Whooping cough
Relapsing fever	Diphtheria	Tuberculosis
Plague	Poliomyelitis	Malaria
Smallpox	Typhoid fever	Meningitis
Viral haemorrhagic fever	Paratyphoid fever	Meningococcal septicaemia
	Rabies	Ophthalmia neonatorum
	Tetanus	Measles
	Encephalitis	Mumps
		Dysentery (amoebic and bacillary)
		Rubella
		Scarlet fever

Laboratory reporting system

The HPA's laboratories, NHS hospital laboratories and private laboratories should be able to offer a full diagnostic service for all common pathogenic micro-organisms. If a laboratory is unable to carry out the work, then specimens are forwarded to a suitable reference laboratory. Medical microbiologists ensure that results of clinical significance are notified to the requesting clinician. Micro-organisms of public health significance are also notified to the local HPU in accordance with previously agreed arrangements. Typical arrangements for reporting to the HPU are shown in Box 16.6. The method of reporting will vary depending on the urgency with which public health action is required. Increasingly, electronic reporting is in use.

In England, laboratory reports are also sent to the HPA. These data are collated and analysed, and are published regularly in the online Health Protection Report available each week on the HPA website (http://www.hpa.org.uk/hpr/).

Although the data are usually of high quality, they are limited to infections for which there is a suitable laboratory test; infections that are easy to diagnose clinically tend to be poorly covered. Trends are difficult to interpret, since the data are sensitive to changes in testing or reporting by laboratories. In addition, because data are based on place of treatment rather than place of residence, denominators are not usually available and because negatives are not reported, neither the number of specimens tested nor the population at risk is known with certainty.

Surveillance of healthcare-associated infection

In England surveillance of some healthcare-associated infection (HCAI) is mandatory:

- MRSA bacteraemia;
- glycopeptide-resistant enterococcal bacteraemia;
- *Clostridium difficile*-associated disease;
- orthopaedic surgical site infection.

Data from these schemes can be found at: http://www.hpa.org.uk/infections/topics_az/hai/mandatory_report_2006.htm.

Although it is assumed that these infections are healthcare associated, they are increasingly reported from the community albeit usually in patients who have recently been in hospital or had contact with other healthcare settings. The true incidence of HCAI in patients in primary and community care settings in the UK is not known with certainty. Some other infections may be either hospital or community acquired. These include *Streptococcus pneumoniae*, *Acinetobacter* species, extended-spectrum beta-lactamase-producing *Escherichia coli*, *Candida* spp and norovirus.

Other sources of surveillance data

Primary care

Around 40 per cent of the UK population consult their GP each year because of infection and 80 per cent of antibiotics are used in primary care. Primary care surveillance data from the Royal College of General Practitioners Weekly Returns Service, the QResearch bulletin and NHS Direct can be found at: http://www.hpa.org.uk/infections/topics_az/primary_care_surveillance/menu.htm.

Box 16.6 Reporting of laboratory isolations to the Health Protection Unit

INFECTIONS TO BE REPORTED THE SAME DAY ELECTRONICALLY, BY TELEPHONE OR FAX

Common	Uncommon
Campylobacter	Malaria
Salmonella	Hepatitis E
Other forms of food poisoning	Amoebic dysentery
Shigella	Yersinia
Hepatitis A	*Vibrio parahaemolyticus*
Tuberculosis	*Clostridium perfringens*
Cryptosporidium	*Listeria*
Escherichia coli 0157	Rubella
Giardia	
Mumps	
Norovirus	
Chronic hepatitis B and C	

INFECTIONS OF PUBLIC HEALTH SIGNIFICANCE AND/OR UNUSUAL INFECTIONS TO BE REPORTED IMMEDIATELY BY TELEPHONE

Regularly identified	Rare
Meningococcal infection	Parvovirus
Other forms of meningitis	Leptospirosis
Legionella	Lyme disease
Typhoid and paratyphoid	*Coxiella burnetii*
Invasive group A streptococcal infection	

Occasional	Very rare
Measles	Viral haemorrhagic fever including Lassa fever and Marburg disease
Influenza viruses	Leprosy
Haemophilus influenza type B	Yellow fever
Tetanus	Anthrax
Cholera	Typhus
Clostridium botulinum	Plague
Acute hepatitis B	Poliomyelitis (acute)
Chickenpox	Rabies
Diphtheria	Relapsing fever
Chlamydia psittaci	
Pertussis	

Hospital data

Data are available from hospital information systems on infectious diseases that result in admission to hospital. This is a useful source of data on more severe diseases likely to result in admission to hospital, although data are often not sufficiently timely for some routine surveillance functions.

Sexually transmitted diseases

Surveillance data on human immunodeficiency virus (HIV) infection and other sexually transmitted infection can be accessed at: http://www.hpa.org.uk/webw/HPAweb&Page&HPAwebAutoListName/Page/1191942172144?p=1191942172144.

Death certification and registration

Mortality data on communicable disease are of limited use since communicable diseases rarely cause death directly. Exceptions are deaths due to influenza, acquired immunodeficiency syndrome (AIDS), tuberculosis and HCAI. However, not all deaths due to infection are coded as such, and data may not be sufficiently timely for all surveillance functions. Recently there has been interest in the mortality caused by HCAI (Office for National Statistics, 2008)

International surveillance

International surveillance data can be found on the website of the World Health Organization (http://www.who.int/en/). Surveillance is undertaken by individual European countries and summary data are available through Eurosurveillance (http://www.eurosurveillance.org).

Enhanced surveillance

In England, the HPA has established enhanced surveillance systems for infections and hazards of particular public health importance. Systems have been established for meningococcal disease, tuberculosis, HCAI, antimicrobial resistance, travel-associated *Legionella* infection, zoonoses, influenza, infections in prisons, outbreaks of infectious intestinal disease and waterborne infections and water quality. Output from these systems can be found on the HPA website.

Occupationally acquired infection

Active surveillance of selected occupationally acquired infections is carried out by the Surveillance of Infectious Diseases at Work (SIDAW) Project at the Centre for Occupational Health at the University of Manchester (http://www.coeh.man.ac.uk/thor/sidaw.htm).

CONTROL MEASURES FOR COMMUNITY INFECTION

The control of an infection in the community requires a detailed knowledge of its epidemiology, clinical features, reservoir, mode of transmission, incubation period and communicable period. Detailed summaries for selected infections are available (Hawker *et al.*, 2005). To prevent and control infection measures can be taken to control the source of infection and the route of transmission, and susceptible people can be offered protection with antibiotics or immunization. These measures are directed at the person or case, his or her contacts, the environment and the wider community (Box 16.7).

Box 16.7 Control measures for community infection

PERSON

The case is contacted and details are recorded on a case report form.

Further diagnostic samples may be requested.

An assessment is made of the risk that the case may spread infection. Guidelines are available to assist with this risk assessment. Most of these can be found on various websites, such as the HPA website. With gastrointestinal infections, the case may be assigned to one of four risk groups: food-handler, health or social care worker, child aged less than 5 years or older, child or adult with low standards of personal hygiene (Working Group of the former PHLS Advisory Committee on Gastrointestinal Infections, 2004). Factors such as type of employment, availability of sanitary facilities and standards of personal hygiene should be taken into account.

The risk assessment will help to determine the control measures that are needed.

- The case may be isolated until no longer infectious. Usually isolation at home will be sufficient. It may be necessary to exclude infectious cases from school or work.
- The case may be kept under surveillance, examined clinically or subjected to laboratory investigations.
- The case may be treated to reduce the communicable period.
- The case, his or her family and household contacts, and medical and nursing attendants may be advised to adopt certain precautions to reduce the risk of transmission. These may be standard precautions, droplet precautions or contact precautions. Occasionally admission to hospital may be necessary to ensure these precautions are in place. The case may be advised to restrict contact with young children and others who may be particularly susceptible to infection. He or she may be advised not to prepare food for other household members.
- Advice should be reinforced with written material such as leaflets or a video may be available. Leaflets are available from various websites including the HPA website and the websites of individual HPUs. Legal powers are available but these are rarely used.

Box 16.7 – *contd*

CONTACT

Contacts of a case of infectious disease may be at risk of acquiring infection themselves or they may risk spreading infection to others. It is important to have a definition of a contact and conduct a risk assessment.

For example, a contact of a case of gastrointestinal infection is someone who has been exposed to the vomit or faeces of a case. With typhoid, this definition would be extended to those exposed to the same source as the case, such as those who were on the same visit abroad. A contact of a case of meningococcal infection is someone who has spent a night under the same roof as the case in the 7 days before onset or has had mouth-kissing contact (see later).

Contacts may be subjected to clinical or laboratory examination (e.g. contacts of a case of diphtheria or typhoid). They may be offered advice, placed under surveillance or offered prophylaxis with antibiotics or immunization. In some circumstances, contacts may be excluded from school or work. Legal powers are available.

ENVIRONMENT

In some circumstances, it may be appropriate to investigate the environment of a case of infection. This may involve inspection and laboratory investigation of home or work. Examples are foodborne infections, gastrointestinal infections and legionnaires' disease. There are legal powers to control the environment including powers to seize, destroy and prohibit the use of certain objects. This may be necessary in the event of infection caused by a contaminated foodstuff. It may be appropriate to advise on cleaning and disinfection.

COMMUNITY

The occurrence of cases of infection will have an effect on the wider community. For example, a case of legionnaires' disease or tuberculosis may generate considerable anxiety in the workforce. Meningitis and hepatitis B will have a similar effect in schools on staff, pupils and parents. Scabies in day-care centres and head lice in schools are other examples.

It is helpful to keep all sections of the community informed about cases of infection. This can be done by letter or public meeting. In some circumstances, it may be appropriate to set up a telephone advice line. In addition, it can be helpful to inform local newspapers, radio, television and politicians.

All sections of the community have information needs with respect to the prevention and control of infectious disease. Advice is available from a range of health professionals. This can be reinforced by leaflets, videos, websites and through the media.

In community settings, such as schools, nursing homes, residential homes and primary care, it is helpful to make available written guidelines on infection control in the form of a manual or handbook. These materials can subsequently form the basis for training and audit in infection control.

HPA, Health Protection Agency; HPU, Health Protection Unit; PHLS, Public Health Laboratory Service.

Public health law

The Public Health (Control of Disease) Act 1984 and the Public Health (Infectious Diseases) Regulations 1988 give local authorities wide-ranging powers to control communicable disease. Some powers, such as those that deal with the notification of diseases, are purely administrative. However, there are powers to control things, premises and people. Many of these powers have their origin in the social conditions of the nineteenth and early twentieth centuries. Public health law reform is long overdue. The Health and Social Care Bill 2007-08 currently before Parliament will introduce new, more flexible provisions to control health threats from infectious diseases and contamination by chemicals and radiation.

PREVENTION OF INFECTIOUS DISEASE

Measures to prevent infection can be directed at the host or the environment (Box 16.8).

Box 16.8 Measures to prevent infectious disease

HOST

Risk behaviour may be changed by health education campaigns. These may be national or local, and may be aimed at the general population or targeted at those who are particularly at risk. Infections that have been the subject of national health education campaigns include human immunodeficiency virus (HIV) infection, sexually transmitted diseases (STDs), salmonella, *Listeria* and verocytotoxin- producing *E. coli* (VTEC) infection. Health services offer diagnosis, screening, treatment, prophylaxis and immunization. Examples are routine and selective immunization, services for tuberculosis screening and treatment for newly arrived immigrants and services for STDs.

ENVIRONMENT

Local authority environmental health departments have responsibilities and legal powers to ensure that supplies of food and water are wholesome, and will not harm health and that there are adequate arrangements for the disposal of sewage, waste collection and disposal and pest control.

Over 99% of the population in the UK receives mains water supplies. These supplies are provided by private water companies in England and Wales. The quality of these supplies is very high and all are safe to drink. Regulations require that water supplies must not contain any element, organism or substance at a concentration which would be detrimental to public health. There are legally enforceable standards for 55 different parameters. Water companies are legally obliged to test samples of the water they supply

---

Box 16.8 – *contd*

and report the results to the Drinking Water Inspectorate, which, since privatization, has monitored quality on behalf of the government.

The Food Safety Act 1990 provides a framework for a range of food hygiene regulations that govern the activity of food businesses and implement European Community (EC) directives. The enforcement of food law is usually the responsibility of local authorities. There are statutory codes of practice which provide guidance.

The 1990 Act contains new definitions of contaminated food and provides for a registration system for food businesses. There is also a requirement for hygiene training for food-handlers. The Act gives Environmental Health Officers (EHOs) powers to inspect any stage of food production, manufacturing and distribution and to take samples for testing. EHOs can issue warnings, improvement notices or initiate prosecutions. Regular routine inspection of food businesses is used to achieve agreed standards. Giving advice forms a large part of this activity. The system for the inspection of food premises is based on an assessment of risk with high-risk businesses being inspected more frequently than lower risk premises. These inspections are an EC requirement and the results of inspections are published regularly. The Food Safety Act 1990 Code of Practice No. 6 requires that incidents of illness and contamination of food products should be reported by the local authority to the appropriate central government department.

The Food Safety (General Food Hygiene) Regulations 1995 apply to all types of food businesses from a hotdog van to a five-star restaurant. They do not apply to food cooked at home for private consumption. They require food businesses to identify all steps which are critical to food safety and ensure adequate safety controls are in place, maintained and reviewed. This is the formal system known has hazard analysis and critical control points (HACCP). EHOs advise businesses on how to approach HACCP. However, ultimately, it is the responsibility of the food business to ensure compliance. In some cases, enforcement officers may need to take action to avoid any risk to the consumer. Guidance notes and explanatory booklets are available.

The 1995 Regulations changed the arrangements governing food-handlers fitness to work (Department of Health, 1995). The aim of the changes is to prevent the introduction of infection into the food-business workplace by advising staff of their obligation to report to management any infectious or potentially infectious conditions, and to leave the workplace immediately if they should have such a condition. The conditions are diarrhoea and vomiting, gastrointestinal infections, enteric fever and infected lesions of skin, eyes, ears and mouth. Before returning to work following illness owing to gastrointestinal infection, there should be no vomiting for 48 hours, a normal bowel habit for 48 hours and good hygienic practices, particularly handwashing.

Some EC food hygiene directives require medical certification of employees in selected food businesses. The view in the UK is that there is no evidence that medical certification prevents the spread of infection from infected food-handlers since it only provides information about a prospective employee's health status at one point in time.

Other regulations include the Food Safety (Temperature Control) Regulations 1995, which detail the temperatures at which particular types of food should be stored before consumption. There are also a range of product specific regulations covering fresh meat, wild game, minced meat and shellfish aimed at dairies, meat processors or wholesale fish markets.

The government and local authorities carry out publicity campaigns on food safety and food hygiene aimed at food businesses and the general public.

The Meat Hygiene Service is an executive agency of the Food Standards Agency, and has responsibility for hygiene and animal welfare inspection and enforcement in slaughter houses and meat-cutting plants.

There is a comprehensive food surveillance programme with over 140 000 analyses carried out each year for a wide range of food contaminants. The annual EC coordinated food control programmes require member states to carry out inspection and sampling of specified categories of food items (e.g. refrigerated salads for *Listeria*).

Measures for the prevention and control of infection in specific community settings

Box 16.9 provides a checklist for the community infection prevention and control measures that should be in place in a range of community settings. These settings include community hospitals, care homes, GP and primary care clinics, dental clinics, home-care services, schools, nurseries and prisons. Other settings include tattooists and body-piercing premises, swimming pools and gyms. Not all these measures will be relevant for every setting.

Box 16.9 Checklist for community infection prevention and control (CIPC) measures

- Clear management accountability for CIPC.
- CIPC is part of clinical governance and quality framework.
- Named person with operational responsibility for CIPC.
- Programme of policy review and updating, training and audit.
- Arrangements for seeking advice on risk assessment and application of appropriate control measures.
- Arrangements for surveillance, recording and reporting of cases of infection and outbreaks and incidents. Outbreaks and incidents should be reported to the Health Protection Unit (HPU), which will advise what action is required. Care homes also have an obligation under the Care Homes Regulations to report to Commission for Social Care Inspection. Symptoms in two or more residents that may indicate a possible outbreak are cough and/or fever (e.g. influenza), diarrhoea and/or vomiting (e.g. *Clostridium difficile*/norovirus/food poisoning) and itchy skin lesion or rash (e.g. scabies).

Box 16.9 – *contd*

- Handbook or procedure manual detailing
  - Standard precautions
    - hand hygiene
    - use of personal protective equipment (gloves, aprons, masks, eye protection)
  - Aseptic technique for clinical procedures to prevent contamination of wounds and other susceptible body sites (including minimizing exposure of the susceptible site, using a 'no-touch' approach if appropriate, hand decontamination, using sterile or non-sterile gloves as appropriate, use of disposable plastic aprons, ensuring all equipment and materials are sterile, not re-using single-use items)
  - Safe handling and disposal of sharps
  - Management of waste
  - Managing spillages of blood, vomit and diarrhoea
  - Collection and transport of specimens
  - Decontaminating equipment and the environment including cleaning, disinfection and sterilization
  - Maintaining a clean and safe clinical environment including vaccine storage
  - Laundry and linen management
  - Placing patients with infections in appropriate accommodation including isolation
  - Circumstances where droplet, airborne or contact precautions are required
- Arrangements for meeting the occupational health needs of staff
  - Prevention of occupational exposure to bloodborne viruses (BBV) including prevention of sharps injuries
  - Management of occupational exposure to BBVs and post-exposure prophylaxis
  - Management of exposure to rash illnesses
  - Health of pregnant staff
  - Pre-employment assessment (tuberculosis; human immunodeficiency virus, HIV)
  - Immunization of staff (influenza; varicella; combined vaccine for measles, mumps and rubella; hepatitis B)
- Antibiotic formulary or equivalent to ensure appropriate use of antimicrobials
- Information for patients, relatives, visitors and staff
- Access to reference books or posters detailing the epidemiology and control measures for common infections of public health significance
- Guidance on specific procedures and practices such as that published by the Health Protection Agency, the Department of Health, the National Institute for Health and Clinical Excellence and professional bodies such as the Royal College of Nursing (this guidance covers management of urinary catheters, enteral feeding, peripheral and central vascular devices, and respiratory support equipment)
- Arrangements for responding to outbreaks of infection including reporting, closure of wards, departments and premises to new admissions, restrictions on visitors, staff absenteeism and business continuity planning

Infection control guidelines for specific community settings

In response to the need to develop robust community infection prevention and control arrangements, a range of manuals, handbooks and guidelines have been developed covering selected community settings. These are summarized in Box 16.10.

Box 16.10 Infection control guidelines for specific community settings*

CARE HOMES

- Best practice guidance on the control of infection in care homes, and the clarification of roles and responsibilities are detailed in the recent publication from the Department of Health. This is available online at: http://www.dh.gov.uk/en/Publicationsandstatistics/ Publications/PublicationsPolicyAndGuidance/DH_4136381
- 'Essential steps to safe, clean care' provides a framework for community organizations to apply best practice to prevent and manage infections. Available online at: http://www.clean-safe-care.nhs.uk/public/default.aspx?level=2&load=Tools& NodeID=125

GENERAL PRACTITIONER AND PRIMARY CARE CLINICS

- Guidance is available from the Infection Control Nurses Association (Rayfield *et al.*, 2003)

DENTAL CLINICS

- Guidance is available from the British Dental Association online at: http://www.udp.org.uk/resources/bda-cross-infection.pdf#search=%22infection%20 control%20in%20dentistry%22

SCHOOLS AND NURSERIES

- Guidance is available from the Health Protection Agency (HPA) online at: http://www.hpa.org.uk/webw/HPAweb&HPAwebStandard/HPAweb_C/1203496946639? p=1158945066455
- Several Health Protection Units (HPUs) have produced detailed guidance, which is published online and can be found by searching within the HPA website
- Similarly leaflets and factsheets for most infections affecting school-age children can be found by searching online

PRISONS

- Prisons should have a comprehensive written policy on communicable disease control, including an outbreak control plan. Guidance is available from Offender Health (a partnership between the Ministry of Justice and the Department of Health). Available online at: http://www.dh.gov.uk/en/Healthcare/Offenderhealth/index.htm
- Guidance is also available on the HPA Prison Infection Prevention Team website:

Box 16.10 – *contd*

http://www.hpa.org.uk/webw/HPAweb&Page&HPAwebAutoListName/Page/11919421264
63?p=1191942126463

- In addition, several HPUs have produced guidelines that can be found by searching within the HPA website

TATTOOISTS AND BODY-PIERCING PREMISES

- Under the Local Government (Miscellaneous Provisions) Act 1982, no person may carry out procedures that involve skin penetration (electrolysis, acupuncture, tattooing, ear-piercing) unless they are registered with their local environmental health department. Medical practitioners are exempt. Many local authorities publish guidelines. An example can be found at:
  http://www.salford.gov.uk/piercinginfectioncontroladvice.pdf#search=%22infection%20control%20guidelines%20for%20tattooists%22
- The Health and Safety Executive has produced guidance related to body piercing, tattooing and scarification. See: http://www.hse.gov.uk/LAU/LACS/76-2app.htm
- In addition, trade organizations publish guidelines for their members. An example is Habia, which serves the hair, beauty, nails and spa industries; see: http://www.habia.org

SWIMMING POOLS

- The risks of *Legionella* infection in spa pools are covered in: http://www.hpa.org.uk/web/HPAweb&HPAwebStandard/HPAweb_C/1200471665170
- The Pool Water Treatment Advisory Group is an independent, industry group that publishes standards for swimming pool water treatment and quality. See: http://www.pwtag.org/home.html
- The Federation of Tour Operators has published guidelines for hotel swimming pool operators. See: http://www.fto.co.uk/assets/documents/fto_cryptosporidum%20Global%20V2.pdf

UNDERTAKERS AND FUNERAL HOMES

- Guidance on infection control for funeral workers (Bakhshi, 2001) and the infection risk from human cadavers can be found at: http://www.hpa.org.uk/cdph/issues/CDPHVol4/no4/funeral%20workers.pdf#search=%22deceased%22 and http://hse.gov.uk/pubns/web01.pdf#search=%22funeral%22

---

* All internet links were valid at September 2008.

Measures for the prevention and control of specific infections of community relevance

A number of specific infections are of particular importance in community settings. These are listed in Box 16.11 together with references to best practice guidelines for their prevention and control in community settings.

Box 16.11 Control measure for specific infections

BLOODBORNE VIRUSES

- Guidelines on managing all aspects of hepatitis B, hepatitis C and human immunodeficiency virus (HIV) infection, including occupational health aspects , are available on the Health Protection Agency (HPA) and Department of Health websites at: http://www.hpa.org.uk/infections/topics_az/bbv/bbmenu.htm and http://www.dh.gov.uk/PolicyAndGuidance/HealthAndSocialCareTopics/BloodSafety/BloodborneViruses/fs/en
- Some individual Health Protection Units (HPUs) have produced helpful guidelines for responding to needlestick injuries in the community. These can be located by searching within the HPA website.

MENINGOCOCCAL INFECTION

- Guidelines for the public health management of meningococcal infection are available online at: http://www.hpa.org.uk/webw/HPAweb&HPAwebStandard/HPAweb_C/1195733852962?p=1201094595231

TUBERCULOSIS

- Guidelines on the clinical management of tuberculosis and measures for its prevention and control in a range of settings are available online from the National Institute for Health and Clinical Excellence at: http://www.nice.org.uk/page.aspx?o=CG033 quickrefguide

GASTROINTESTINAL INFECTION

- Guidelines on the control of gastrointestinal infections (Working Group of the former PHLS Advisory Committee on Gastrointestinal Infections, 2004) can be accessed online at: http://www.hpa.org.uk/cdph/issues/CDPHvol7/No4/guidelines2_4_04.pdf

METHICILLIN-RESISTANT *STAPHYLOCOCCUS AUREUS* (MRSA)

- Historically MRSA has been acquired as a result of hospital treatment or other healthcare interventions. Guidelines are available for managing healthcare-associated MRSA (Coia *et al.*, 2006). MRSA infections presenting in the community are becoming more frequent. Most of these are healthcare associated, occurring in patients who have had direct or indirect contact with hospitals.
- Community healthcare staff should be able to suspect, diagnose and treat MRSA infection in the community and take appropriate measures to prevent transmission. Good lines of communication are required when patients with MRSA are transferred between community and hospital and vice versa. Increasingly, community staff are being asked to help with pre-admission screening and decolonization and post-discharge management of MRSA infection. They may also be asked to assist with the investigation of cases of MRSA bacteraemia including root cause analysis.
- New strains of community-associated MRSA are emerging that are genetically distinct

Box 16.11 – *contd*

from hospital strains and which cause infection in community patients with no apparent link to healthcare settings. Guidelines for managing community-associated MRSA are now available (Nathwani et al., 2008).

- Some strains of *Staphylococcus aureus* produce the Panton–Valentine leucocidin (PVL) toxin. Specific guidelines on the management of PVL-producing strains is available online at: http://www.hpa.org.uk/webw/HPAweb&HPAwebStandard/HPAweb_C/1195733827175
- Guidance on MRSA for nursing staff is available online at: http://www.rcn.org.uk/resources/mrsa/downloads/Wipe_it_out-MRSA-guidance_for_nursing_staff.pdf
- Information leaflets are available for hospital patients (see http://www.hpa.org.uk/webw/HPAweb&HPAwebStandard/HPAweb_C/1203496949853?p=1153846674382) and for patients in the community (see http://www.hillingdon.nhs.uk/uploads/MRSA_Advice.pdf).
- The 'Clean, Safe Care' website is a good resource for healthcare staff (see http://www.clean-safe-care.nhs.uk/public/default.aspx?level=1&load=HomeNews).

CLOSTRIDIUM DIFFICILE-ASSOCIATED DISEASE (CDAD)

- CDAD is increasingly presenting in community settings. Community healthcare staff should be prepared to suspect, diagnose and treat CDAD and implement appropriate measures for prevention and control.
- Guidelines on prevention and control and an information leaflets for health professionals are available online at: http://www.hpa.org.uk/webw/HPAweb&Page&HPAwebAutoList Name/Page/1179745281238?p=1179745281238 and the 'Clean, Safe Care' website (see earlier).
- Many hospitals and patient groups have produced patient information leaflets. An example is: http://www.nnuh.nhs.uk/viewdoc.asp?ID=653&t=Leaflet

SCABIES AND HEAD LICE

- Guidelines on the control of scabies in community settings is available from most HPUs and can be found online by searching within the HPA website.
- Updated evidence-based guidelines on head lice management are available online from the UK Public Health Medicine Environmental Group (see http://www.phmeg.org.uk).

NOROVIRUS

- Guidelines on the management of norovirus outbreaks in hospitals and on cruise ships can be accessed online at: http://www.hpa.org.uk/webw/HPAweb&HPAwebStandard/HPAweb_C/1195733840182?p=1191942172932
- Guidelines on managing norovirus outbreaks in tourist and leisure industry settings is available online at: http://www.hps.scot.nhs.uk/search/guidedetail.aspx?id=18578

SEASONAL INFLUENZA

- Guidelines on seasonal influenza immunization for staff and patients, and the use of antivirals for treatment and prophylaxis can be accessed via the HPA website at:

http://www.hpa.org.uk/web/HPAweb&Page&HPAwebAutoListName/Page/
1191942171468

AVIAN INFLUENZA

- Guidance relating to the management of all aspects of the human health consequences of avian influenza can be accessed online at: http://www.hpa.org.uk/webw/ HPAweb&Page&HPAwebAutoListName/Page/1160495617087?p=1160495617087

PANDEMIC INFLUENZA

- Guidance on planning for pandemic influenza in primary care and community settings is available online at: http://www.dh.gov.uk/en/Publicationsandstatistics/Publications/ PublicationsPolicyAndGuidance/DH_080757
- Guidelines on infection control for pandemic influenza in healthcare and community settings is available online at: http://www.dh.gov.uk/en/Publichealth/Flu/PandemicFlu/ DH_085433

MANAGING INFECTIOUS DISEASE INCIDENTS AND OUTBREAKS

An infectious disease outbreak may be defined in one of the following ways:

- two or more persons with the same disease or symptoms or the same organism isolated from a diagnostic sample; or
- a greater than expected rate of infection compared with the usual background rate.

The control of an outbreak of infectious disease depends on early detection followed by a rapid structured investigation to uncover the source of infection and the route of transmission. This is followed by the application of appropriate control measures to prevent further cases. Outbreaks of infectious disease are usually investigated and managed by an informal team of HPU staff, medical microbiologist and EHO. In large complex outbreaks, an *outbreak control team* may meet to oversee the management of the episode. Each HPU will have a written outbreak control plan.

Detection

An outbreak will be recognized by case reports, complaints or as a result of routine surveillance.

Systematic investigation

A systematic approach to the investigation of an outbreak comprises the following stages:

- establishing that a problem exists;
- confirming the diagnosis;
- immediate control measures;
- case finding;
- collection of data;
- descriptive epidemiology;
- generating a hypothesis;
- testing the hypothesis.

Several of these stages will often occur simultaneously. Once an outbreak has been successfully controlled, a written report should be prepared and circulated, and any recommendations implemented.

Establishing that a problem exists

A report of an outbreak of infection may be mistaken. It may result from increased clinical or laboratory detection of cases, changes in the size of the population at risk or false-positive laboratory tests.

Confirming the diagnosis

Cases can be diagnosed either clinically or by laboratory investigations. At an early stage, it is important to produce and adhere to a clear case definition. This is particularly important with previously unrecognized diseases in which proper definitions are needed before epidemiological studies can proceed.

Immediate control measures

Control measures involve either controlling the source of infection, interrupting transmission or protecting those at risk.

Case finding

In an episode of infection, the cases that are first noticed may only be a small proportion of the total population affected and may not be representative of that population. Efforts must be made to search for additional cases. This allows the extent of the incident to be quantified and provides a more accurate picture of the range of illness that people have experienced. It also allows individual cases to be treated and control measures to be taken, and provides subjects for further descriptive and analytical epidemiology.

There are several ways of searching for additional cases:

- statutory notifications of infectious disease;
- requests for laboratory tests and reports of positive results;
- people attending their GPs, or the local accident and emergency department;
- hospital inpatients and outpatients;
- reports from the occupational health departments of large local businesses;

- reports from schools of absenteeism and illness;
- household enquiries;
- appeals through television, radio and local newspapers;
- screening tests applied to communities and population sub-groups.

Collection of data

A set of data is collected from each of the cases. This includes name, age, sex, address, occupation, name of GP, recent travel, immunization history, the date of illness and a clinical description of the illness.

Data should also be collected about exposure to possible sources of the infection. In the case of a foodborne infection, this would include a recent food history. In the case of infection spread by person-to-person contact, the case would be questioned about contact with other affected persons. In the case of an infection spread by the airborne route, cases would be questioned about places they had visited.

It is preferable to collect these data by administering a detailed semi-structured questionnaire in a face-to-face interview. This allows the interviewer to ask probing questions that may sometimes uncover previously unsuspected associations between cases. Telephone interviews or self-completion questionnaires are less helpful at this stage of an investigation.

Descriptive epidemiology

Cases are described by the three epidemiological parameters of time, place and person. Describing cases by person includes clinical features, age, sex, occupation, social class, ethnic group, food history, travel and leisure activity. Describing cases by place includes home address and work address. Mapping cases can be very helpful. Describing cases by time involves plotting the epidemic curve, a frequency distribution of date or time of onset. This may allow the incubation period to be estimated, which, with the clinical features, may give some clues as to the causative organism. The incubation period should be related to events that may have occurred in the environment of the cases and which may indicate possible sources of infection.

Generating a hypothesis

A detailed epidemiological description of typical cases may well provide the investigators with a hypothesis regarding the source of infection or the route of transmission. A description of atypical cases may also be helpful.

Testing the hypothesis

Finding that consumption of a particular food, visiting a particular place or being involved in a certain activity is occurring frequently among cases is only a first step. These risk factors may also be common among those who have not been ill. To confirm an association between a risk factor and disease, further microbiological or environmental investigations may be required, or an analytical epidemiological study may be required. This can be either a cohort study or a case–control study.

Case–control study

A case–control study compares exposure in people who are ill (the cases) with exposure in people who are not ill (the controls). Case–control studies are most useful when the affected population cannot be accurately defined. Controls can be selected from a GP's practice list, from the health authority patient register, from the laboratory that reported the case, from people nominated by the case or from neighbours selected at random from nearby houses.

Cohort study

The cohort study is a type of natural experiment in which a proportion of a population is exposed to a factor, while the remainder is not. The incidence or attack rate of infection amongst exposed persons is compared with the rate amongst unexposed persons. For example, following a food-poisoning outbreak at a social gathering thought to be due to consumption of contaminated chocolate mousse, the cohort (all those who attended) is divided into those who ate the mousse (the exposed) and those who did not (the unexposed).

Collecting the data

A set of data is collected from both cases and control, or from the exposed and unexposed persons within the cohort. To avoid any bias, the data must be collected from each subject in exactly the same way; this is usually done by questionnaire. Unlike the hypothesis-generating questionnaire, the questionnaire for an analytical study is often shorter, more structured and uses mostly closed questions. It may be administered at interview, by telephone or it may be a self-completion postal questionnaire. Questionnaires should be piloted before use. If several interviewers are used, they should be adequately briefed and provided with instructions to ensure the questionnaire is administered in a consistent way.

Analysis

In both cohort and case-control studies, initial analysis is by a 2×2 table. In cohort studies, the ratio of incidence in exposed to incidence in unexposed is calculated. This is the relative risk. In case-control studies, the odds of exposure in the cases are compared with the odds of exposure in the controls. This is the odds ratio, which approximates the relative risk.

Confidence intervals for these estimates can be calculated and tests of statistical significance applied. Computer programmes, such as Epi Info™ (http://www.cdc.gov/epiinfo/), are freely available that will perform these calculations.

REFERENCES

Bakhshi SS (2001) Code of practice for funeral workers: managing infection risk and body bagging. *Communicable Disease and Public Health* **4,** 283. Available online at: http://www.hpa.org.uk/web/HPAwebFile/HPAweb_C/1200660055420 (last accessed September 2008).

Coia JE, Duckworth GJ, Edwards DI *et al.* (2006) Guidelines for the control and prevention of meticillin-resistant *Staphylococcus aureus* (MRSA) in healthcare facilities. *Journal of Hospital Infection* 66(Suppl 1), 1.

Department of Health (1995) *Food handlers' fitness to work; guidance for businesses, enforcement officers and health professionals.* London: Department of Health.

Department of Health (2002) *Getting ahead of the curve: a strategy for combating infectious diseases (including other aspects of health protection).* London: Department of Health. Available online at: www.dh.gov.uk/assetRoot/04/06/08/75/04060875.pdf (last accessed September 2008).

Department of Health (2007) *Essential steps to safe, clean care: reducing healthcare associated infections.* London: Department of Health. Available online at: http://www.dh.gov.uk/PolicyAndGuidance/HealthAndSocialCareTopics/Healthcare AcquiredInfection/HealthcareAcquiredGeneralInformation/SavingLivesDelivery Programme/fs/en (last accessed September 2008).

Department of Health (2008a) *Clean, safe care: reducing infections and saving lives.* London: Department of Health. Available online at: http://www.dh.gov.uk/en/ Publicationsandstatistics/Publications/PublicationsPolicyAndGuidance/DH_081650 (last accessed September 2008).

Department of Health (2008b) *The Health Act 2006: code of practice for the prevention and control of healthcare associated infections.* London: Department of Health. Available online at: http://www.dh.gov.uk/en/Publicationsandstatistics/Publications/ PublicationsPolicyAndGuidance/DH_081927 (last accessed September 2008).

Hawker J, Begg N, Blair I, Reintjes R and Weinberget J (eds) (2005) *Communicable disease control handbook,* 2nd edn. Oxford: Blackwell Publishing.

Nathwani D, Morgan M, Masterton RG *et al.* on behalf of the British Society for Antimicrobial Chemotherapy Working Party on community-onset MRSA Infections (2008) Guidelines for UK practice for the diagnosis and management of methicillin-resistant *Staphylococcus aureus* (MRSA) infections presenting in the community. *Journal of Antimicrobial Chemotherapy* **61,** 976.

Office for National Statistics (2008) Report: Deaths involving MRSA and *Clostridium difficile* by communal establishment: England and Wales, 2001–06. *Health Statistics Quarterly* **38,** 74. Available online at: http://www.statistics.gov.uk/downloads/ theme_health/HSQ38_MRSA_CDiff.pdf (last accessed September 2008).

Rayfield J, Lawson J and Howard J (2003) *Infection control guidance for general practice.* Bathgate: Infection Control Nurses Association.

Working Group of the former PHLS Advisory Committee on Gastrointestinal Infections (2004) Preventing person-to-person spread following gastrointestinal infections: guidelines for public health physicians and environmental health officers. *Communicable Disease and Public Health* **7,** 362. Available online at: http://www.hpa.org.uk/ cdph/issues/CDPHvol7/No4/guidelines2_4_04.pdf (last accessed September 2008).

INDEX

Indexer: Dr Laurence Errington
Note: *italics* indicate figures and **bold** indicates tables.